Linda Greenwall, Cathy Jameson

Success Strategies for the Aesthetic Dental Practice

Linda Greenwall, Cathy Jameson

Success Strategies for the Aesthetic Dental Practice

QUINTESSENCE PUBLISHING

London, Berlin, Chicago, Tokyo, Barcelona, Beijing, Istanbul, Milan, Moscow, New Delhi, Paris, Prague, São Paulo, Seoul, Singapore and Warsaw

British Library Cataloguing in Publication Data
Greenwall, Linda.
Success strategies for the aesthetic dental practice.
1. Dentistry--Aesthetic aspects.
I. Title II. Jameson, Cathy.
617.6-dc23

ISBN-13: 978-1-85097-221-1

QUINTESSENCE PUBLISHING

Quintessence Publishing Co. Ltd,
Grafton Road, New Malden, Surrey KT3 3AB,
United Kingdom
www.quintpub.co.uk

Cover illustration: © Jan Schuler - Fotolia.com
Editing: Quintessence Publishing Co. Ltd, London
Layout and Production: Quintessenz Verlags-GmbH, Berlin, Germany
Printed and bound in Germany

Foreword

Ronald E Goldstein, DDS

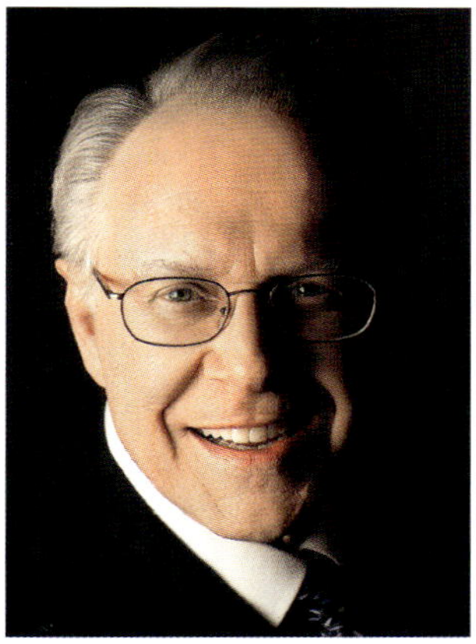

Aesthetic dentistry has become so important in the last several decades that a book which condenses all of the techniques for the business side of aesthetic dentistry is certainly needed. Written by two of the leading authorities on this important aspect of dentistry, both Drs Linda Greenwall and Cathy Jameson have accumulated a tremendous amount of knowledge to condense the important information into easy to read chapters. I have worked with both authors and admire and respect their contributions to dentistry. Perhaps the real reason this book will resonate with the dental reader is that it combines the skills of an excellent dentist with the equal skills of one of dentistry's best practice administrators and coaches.

The book begins where it should, focusing on the individual dentist defining his or her goals for the dental practice. Without vision at the outset it is virtually impossible to make the most out of the next steps in the process of creating the ideal environment for maximum success. Next, it logically proceeds to building the team and here the authors get quite specific, especially in the interview process. This is an area that most dentists are hardly skilled to master, but after reading this chapter they certainly will be. Frankly, this chapter alone is well worth the price of the book.

I found it quite interesting that the next area of discussion is marketing … after all, you need to attract the type of patients you are building your practice for, and so internal and external marketing are covered very well. Both treatment planning and case presentation are well thought out. Most every dentist will take away tips in these areas regardless of how well the processes are handled now. Certainly one of the most important chapters deals with communication skills for the entire dental team. No matter how well your practice communicates now, you will be able to see improvement in your daily contacts with patients and the public.

The concept of using a treatment coordinator was first established by Dr Carl Reider. I published how important I thought it was in the second edition of *Esthetics in Dentistry*, and I am so pleased the authors devote an entire chapter to the role of this person. This leads to the next chapter which deals with the financial aspect of aesthetic dentistry, followed up by what every practice needs to improve on: scheduling. I am delighted to see that a chapter is devoted to the hygienist's role in promoting aesthetic dentistry since this is certainly a prime area that too many dental practices take for granted.

The last chapters are also well placed and deal with the use of technology in building the aesthetic dental practice. Over 25 years ago, Dr Jack Preston and I staged the very first comprehensive show devoted to new technology and how it could enhance our dental practices. Today it is a necessity if dentists want to practice state of the art aesthetics. The ability to have our patients' restorations last as long as possible is directly related to the technical equipment and abilities wrapped up in both diagnosis and treatment. No doubt the future will be even more dependent on sophisticated technology as a major part of every dental practice.

One of the best ideas the authors use throughout the book are action steps at the end of each chapter. These summary tips make it easier to apply the information rather than just reading and forgetting, and to take action where action is needed.

The sum total of the benefit of understanding and using the principles expounded in Success Strategies in Aesthetic Dentistry is that if you want to expand the cosmetic side of your dental practice, then this book is essential reading.

Preface

Linda Greenwall, BDS (Rand), MGDS RCS (Eng), MSc (London), MRD RCS (Eng), FFGDP

Many dentists focus primarily on doing the best clinical dentistry that they can. They concentrate on all the clinical skills that they have been taught at dental school, which leads to a dedication to clinical excellence. This pathway can be frustrating when they do not get to do the dentistry they love as they do not have enough patients saying yes to treatment, or the cases to perform the beautiful aesthetic dentistry that they know they can provide for their patients. Getting patients to say yes takes time. There are certain techniques and systems that should be in place in order to make this happen, including excellent practice management systems and an excellent dental team. Dentists do not like to manage the administrative and management side of the dental practice as they would rather be doing the dentistry at the chairside. They often leave the management aspect of the dental practice to happen haphazardly. This leads to frustration and stress, which is already very high within a dental practice.

As a newly qualified Prosthodontist and Specialist in Restorative Dentistry in 1993, I opened my new dental practice in London the day after completing the specialist examinations. I had very few patients at the beginning, as I started the dental practice from scratch. The end of that same week I had my second child. I took off 8 days from work and returned with the baby in a basket. I thought the dental practice would develop at a slow pace as the baby grew and developed. About 6 months after starting the dental practice, a local journalist came to interview me to coincide with the official launch of the new practice. The article appeared in the local newspaper. The day the article was published, the telephone starting ringing off the hook. We must have had 500 new patients call to schedule an appointment in one day. It was very exciting! However, the excitement soon died down when I realized that these new patients all needed to be seen, assessed, and treatment planned, and we needed to schedule them for treatment. I had no practice systems and thought that we would make it up as we went along, as other dentists do. These great new patients who lived in the local vicinity were used to the best service in restaurants and hotels, and I was not sure that we could live up to their expectations.

I came across a book written by Dr Cathy Jameson called *Great Communication Equals Great Production* (PennWell Books, 1995). It immediately grabbed my attention as it reflected my attitude as to how I would like to look after my patients and manage my dental practice. After delivering my first baby I felt frustrated that I was not part of the decision making process and wanted to be involved in the decisions about my treatment and the way the baby was to be delivered. I felt that if I was the patient, I would like the care giver to discuss the treatment options first and to discuss the process and treatment prior to commencing clinical treatment. Cathy's book reflected what I wanted to put into practice but I did not know how to do it. I contacted Cathy about her book and she offered to travel to London to teach me the systems to run my practice and so develop an excellent dental practice focusing on aesthetic dentistry. My team and I continue to train with Cathy every year since then.

We wanted to write this book together as there are many beautiful clinical textbooks devoted to doing the best clinical dentistry but very few textbooks that focus on the practice management side, which needs to be in place for the clinical side to be excellent. There are few books on how to develop the best dental practice that is patient focused, taking into consideration their hopes and aspirations in order to provide the dental aesthetics that the patients want. The book is meant to be a practical guide to help dentists develop systems in their dental practice that work well and that help the practice to grow and elevate to the next level each year.

As dentists are very busy wearing many different hats or fulfilling different roles in the practice, systems that follow checklists have been developed to assist the dentist and their team to organize themselves practically. Checklists help to reduce stress and to be better prepared for each stage along the patient's journey. Checklists help the dental team to prepare organizationally and clinically and reduce errors and problems. Dr Atul Gawande (2009) wrote a book called The Checklist Manifesto and demonstrated that those professionals who use checklists have fewer errors and complications in all that they do. Checklists for aesthetic dentistry and management aspects have been specially compiled in this book in each chapter. At the end of each chapter there are action points, checklists, and further reading with references. Using these will help focus the dental practice to become well organized in a step-by-step manner.

This book does not deal with the complex compliance issues that are legal requirements in the dental practice within particular states or countries. It deals with the essential aspects that are relevant for all dental practices to develop, regardless of state or country. Many dental practices focus on providing aesthetic dentistry either solely or exclusively, and this book has been formulated especially for those practices. However, all dentists provide aesthetic dentistry whether it is on one tooth, a posterior quadrant, or the whole mouth. Many dentists would like to do more aesthetic dentistry but do not know how to attract those patients who want this treatment. There are also patients within the dental practice who request aesthetic dentistry, whether it is for a major milestone in their lives, to feel better about themselves in general, or to improve their self confidence and their smiles. This book will help dentists to create the organizational structure to make these aesthetic cases happen. A well-organized dental practice reduces stress levels, which helps keep the dentist and their team happy. This happiness reflects on the whole practice and the whole team. Patients notice this and realize that this is a happy dental practice to visit, becoming loyal patients and raving fans.

We hope that you find the book useful and look forward to hearing from you.

References

1. Gawande A. The Checklist Manifesto: How to get things right. New York: Picador, 2009.
2. Jameson C. Great Communication Equals Great Production. Tulsa, OK: PennWell Books, 1995.

Further resources are available at www.jamesonmanagement.com and www.lindagreenwall.co.uk.

Acknowledgements

"

Gratitude to God for his blessings, insight and wisdom.

Do not say I will study when I have the time, for you may never have the time.
Pirkei Avot 2:4

The more study, the more wisdom. *Pirkei Avot 2:8*

"

Linda Greenwall Writing, compiling, and collating this book has taken dedicated time, late nights, and time stolen from many other things. I thank my husband Dr Henry Cohen for his love and encouragement, and sons Andrew, Joseph, Edward, and Rayno for their love, support, and understanding of my absence from them while writing this book.

My mother, Shirley, a feisty lady with high energy and a positive attitude, has always given clear directions on the path to follow and enjoyed the journey even with the bumps along the way. Thank you!

My father, the late Dr Ryno Greenwall, was my inspiration to become a dentist. I enjoyed being part of the family dental practice, practicing together with my father and grandfather, the late Dr Edward Greenwall, in Cape Town, South Africa. I needed the wise counsel and advice, benefitting from your combined 97 years of experience in dental practice and practical tips on treating patients. I miss that now.

To my teachers, mentors, and dental colleagues, I appreciate your input and clear guidance.

To my dental family, my practice team, hygienists, dental therapists, and Diane Rochford for all of your help and assistance. Thank you for all your support, hard work, and fun along the way.

To the dentists who refer their patients to the practice to provide aesthetic dentistry, thank you for your trust and respect.

To my patients, who have given me the honor and privilege of being part of their lives, thank you.

To Sarah Jewell and Rachel Grosvenor who have helped immensely in compiling this manuscript, inserting photos and preparing newsletters, and with many of our projects that we undertake in the practice. Thank you!

To Dr Ron Goldstein, thank you for sharing your wisdom with me and for your foreword.

To Dr Mike Wise, Dr Mervyn Druian, Dr Cherilyn Sheets, Drs Kim and Basil Mizrachi, Dr Gerry Curatola, Drs Larry and Bob Rifkin, thank you for your contributions and sharing your success strategies.

To Dr Oded Bahat and his assistant Reina Ramirez for your help with our implant treatment planning, implant surgery, and CT scan checklists, and constant reality checks!

To Cathy, thank you for your teaching of the Jameson systems, dedication, and being tough talking when things needed to be done, a guiding coach and great friend. Without you I would not have been able to build and grow my aesthetic dental practice in London. Thank you.

Cathy Jameson

Where do I begin to acknowledge the many people who have influenced this body of work – and, indeed, my lifetime? There have been so many people who have supported me on my path. I am grateful to each one of you.

First of all, I acknowledge the love and grace of God Almighty for His strength, guidance, and careful "watch."

My husband, my favorite dentist, and my cowboy hero, Dr John Jameson. Thanks for letting me "test" all my theories of practice management in your practice, which became the launching pad for Jameson Management, Inc. Who could have ever guessed 'the rest of the story'? You are the best.

My wonderful family who don't always understand why I work such long, tedious hours, but always seems to be glad when they see me pop my head up for air! Our son, Dr Brett Jameson, his wife, Amy, and kids, Lauren and Cody. Our daughter, Carrie Jameson Webber, Director of Marketing for Jameson and her husband, Jess Webber, President and CEO of Jameson, and their sons Benjamin and Keller. Thanks to my father, Derry Ebert, where I learned my work ethic and to my mother-in-law, Dorothy Strong Jameson (MiMi) who is always there – for anything.

Thanks to my Jameson Management, Inc. family, which is the best team EVER! Thanks for your willingness to learn from me and for taking such good care of our clients. Your devotion and dedication to our "method" and to the integrity with which we interact with each client has been a major part of the longevity and legacy of Jameson.

A special expression of gratitude to Amy Logan Parrish for her total and complete dedication to me and to the entire Jameson team. You always 'step up to the plate' to help on any project, including this book. You are a blessing to me and to every person with whom you interact. You are amazing.

Rachel Leslie, thank you for sharing your brilliant graphic design and photographic know-how. Your creativity is priceless. To John Jameson, Misty Clark, Dru Halverson and Nancy Dukes, thanks for your contributions to this book.

A special note of gratitude to Alan Cohen, my personal coach. Alan, how do I express my appreciation for your honest and caring support, as well as your personal insights into 'writing from the heart'?

Thank you to Dr Jean Gordon, my faculty mentor from Walden University, where I completed a doctorate in management in June of 2010. Dr Gordon, you epitomize the very best in education. Your unwavering guidance and straightforward instruction made this tedious journey meaningful and successful.

And a special note of heartfelt love and gratitude to my friend, colleague, and mentor, Jeff Gelona.

Thanks to all of the clients throughout time who have given us the privilege of coaching you and your team. You honor us with your trust. Our success is based on your success. A special note of gratitude to the Jameson clients, team members, and friends who have participated in this book: Drs John Jameson, Ken Hamlett, Charles Puntillo, Mark Hyman, Jill Wade, Galip Gurel, Larry Rosenthal, and Bete Johnson from Care Credit.

To all of the people who have come to my lectures and seminars throughout time, thank you. My intention is always to shares ideas and insights that will make a positive difference in your practice and life. May the learning be about "life management," as well as practice management.

To Quintessence, thank you for the trust you have shown by publishing this book, which is a lifetime accumulation of experience, learning, and study. To have you as the publisher of this book is a dream come true. You honor me, and it is my sincere hope that this book will honor you and your readers.

And, finally, a special note of love and thanks to my client, colleague, and friend, Dr Linda Greenwall, one of the most entrepreneurial women I have ever known. You are a visionary, a fine businesswoman, a wonderful wife, daughter, sister, and mother. You are a leader extraordinaire. You never stop learning. Your passion for continuous improvement is steadfast. I honor, respect, and absolutely love you! This book has been a long-term goal of ours, and its time has come. What a privilege to have written it with you. Here's to our lifetime of friendship.

Authors and Contributors

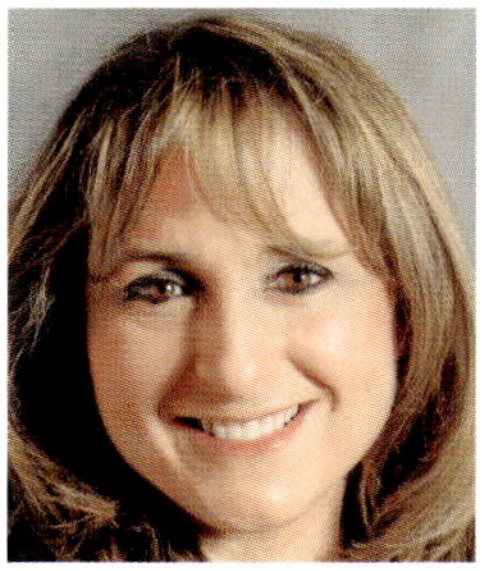

Linda Greenwall, BDS (Rand), MGDS RCS (Eng), MSc (London), MRD RCS (Eng), FFGDP, Private Practice, Hampstead, London; Specialist in Restorative Dentistry; Specialist in Prosthodontics; Editor-in-Chief of Aesthetic Dentistry Today

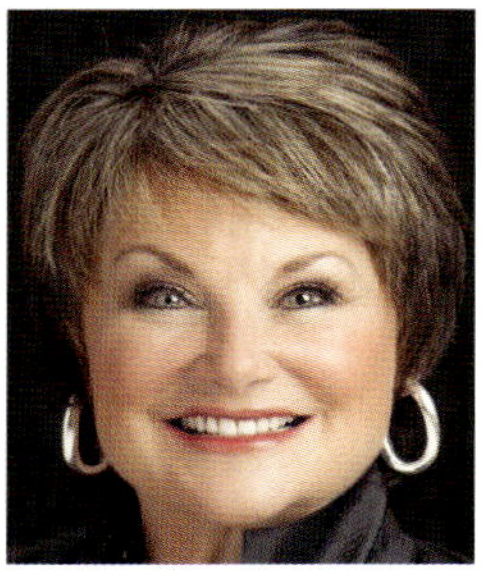

Cathy Jameson, PhD, MA, BS, Founder and CVO of Jameson Management, Inc., Adjunct Faculty Member Oklahoma University College of Dentistry, Member of the Oklahoma State University Board of Trustees

Featured contributors

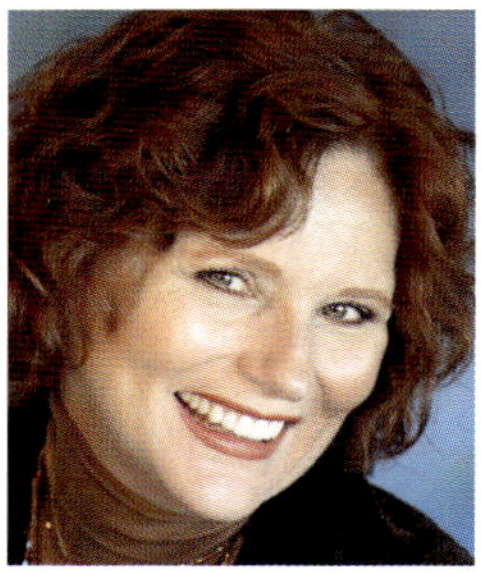

Cindy Butler, Business Administrator, Dr Charles Puntillo's practice

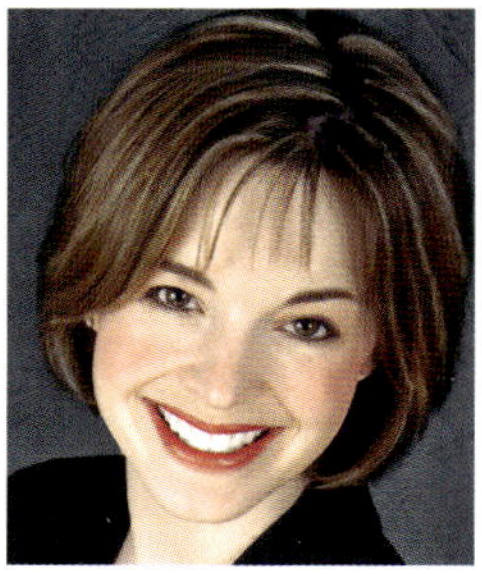

Misty Absher Clark, VP of Creative Services, Jameson Management, Inc

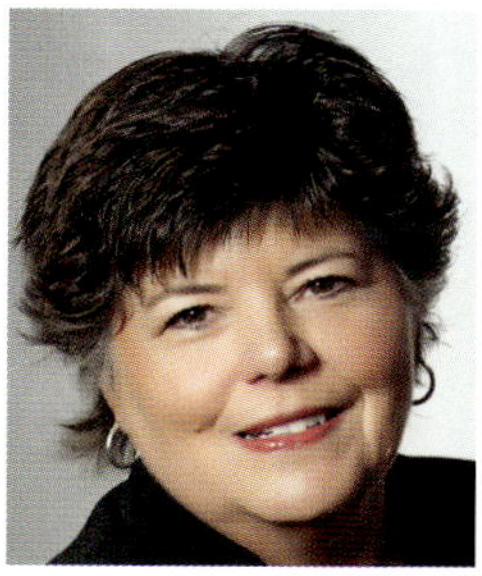

Nancy Dukes, BA, RDH, CBM, Director of Clinical Consulting, Jameson Management, Inc

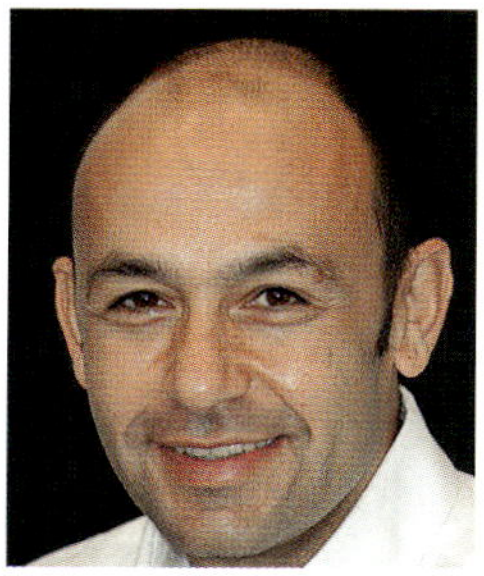

Galip Gürel, DDS, Dentis Dental Clinic, Istanbul, Turkey; Founder and Honorary President of Turkish Academy of Esthetic Dentistry

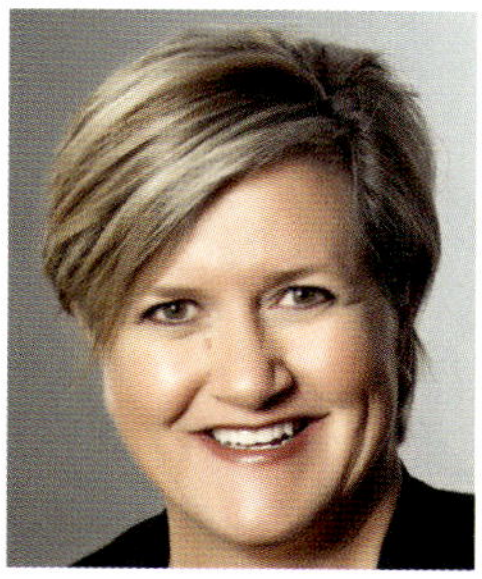

Dru Halverson, BS, RDH, Director of Quality Assurance, Jameson Management, Inc

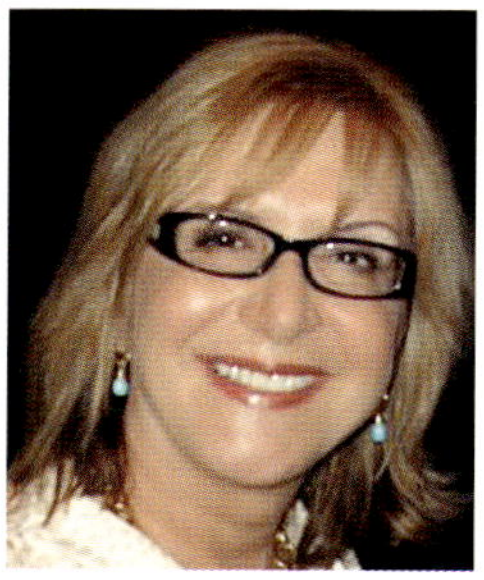

Debra Hamlett, Business Administrator, Kenneth Hamlett, DDS, Dallas, Texas

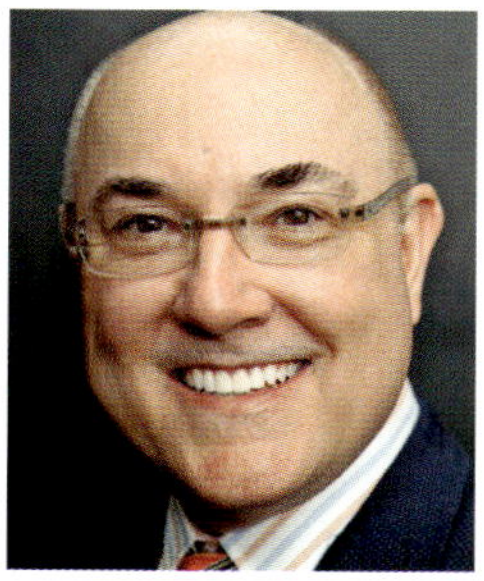

Ken Hamlett, DDS, Clinician at Kenneth Hamlett, DDS, Dallas, Texas; Senior Clinical Instructor at the Rosenthal Institute

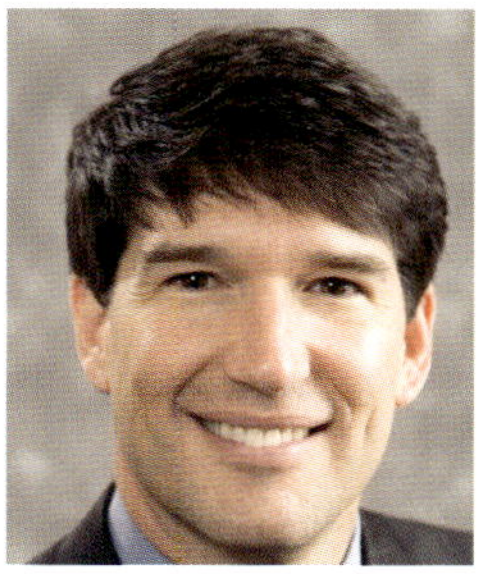

Mark Hyman, DDS, MAGD, Clinician at Mark Hyman, DDS, Greensboro, North Carolina

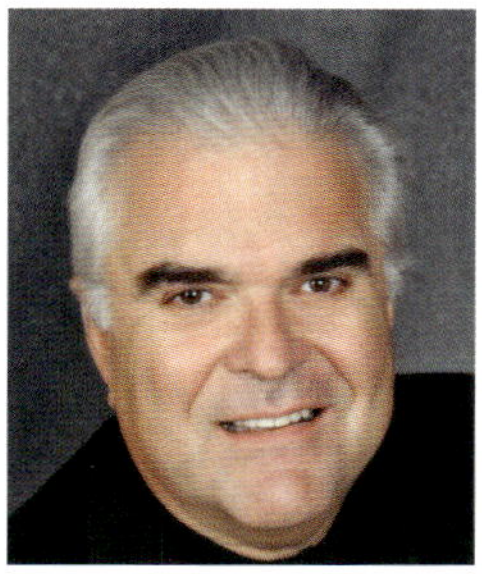

John Jameson, DDS, Chairman of the Board, Jameson Management, Inc

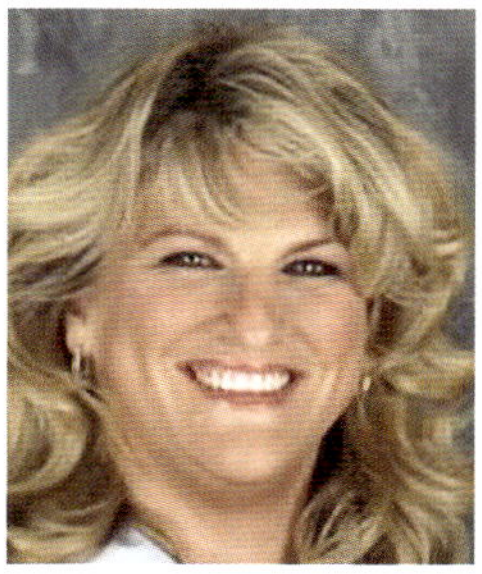

Bete Johnson, Director of Business Development, Care Credit

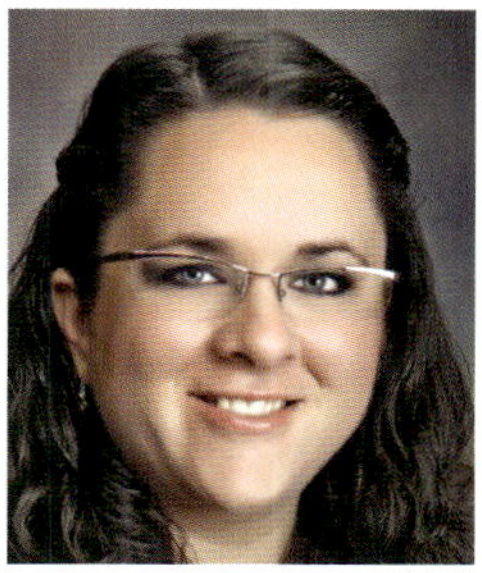

Shana Munson, Treatment Coordinator and Marketing Director, Dr Tuyen Nguyen Soft Dental, Rush City, Minnesota

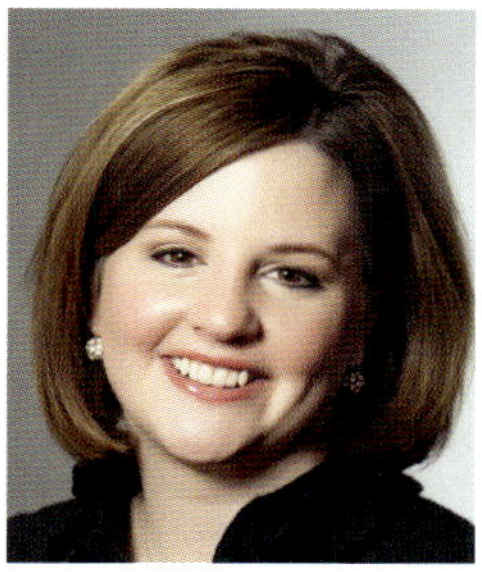

Amy Logan Parrish, VP of Development, Jameson Management, Inc

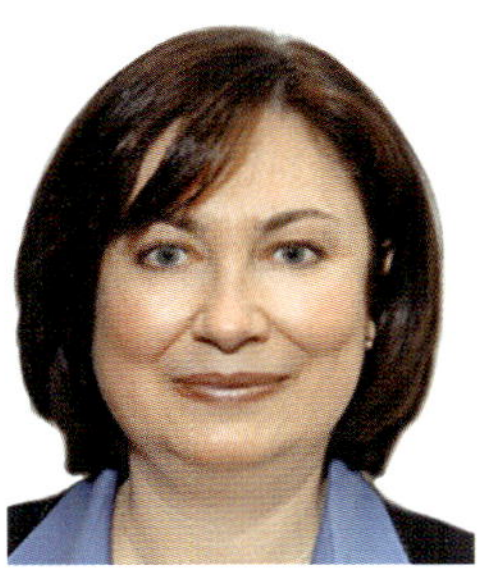

Jacqueline Pastore, Practice Administrator, Rosenthal/Apa Group New York, New York

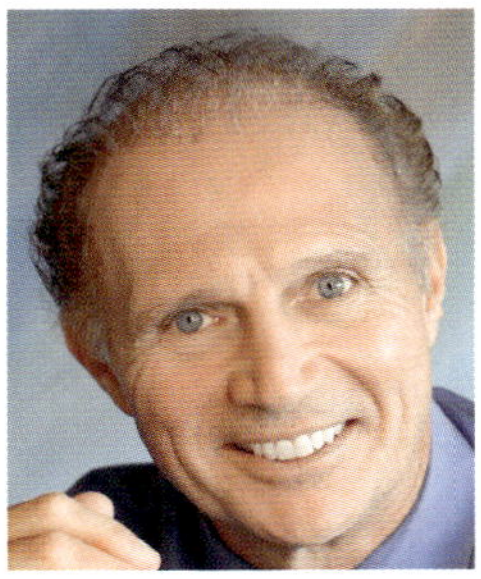

Charles Puntillo, DDS, Clinician at Charles Puntillo, DDS, Burlington, Wisconsin

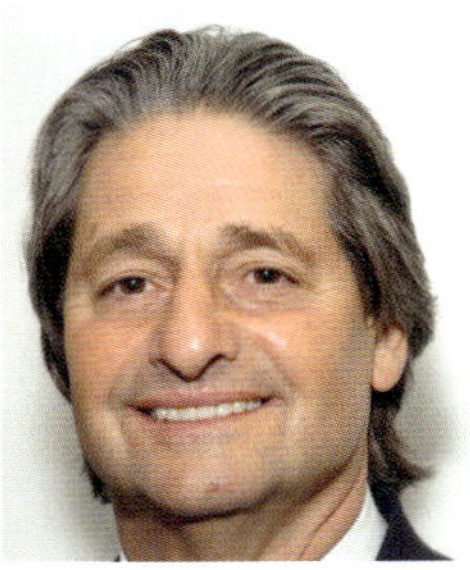

Larry Rosenthal, DDS, PC, Clinician at Rosenthal/Apa Group New York, New York; Founder and Clinical Director of Rosenthal Institute, Aesthetic Advantage and Aesthetic Advantage Continuum

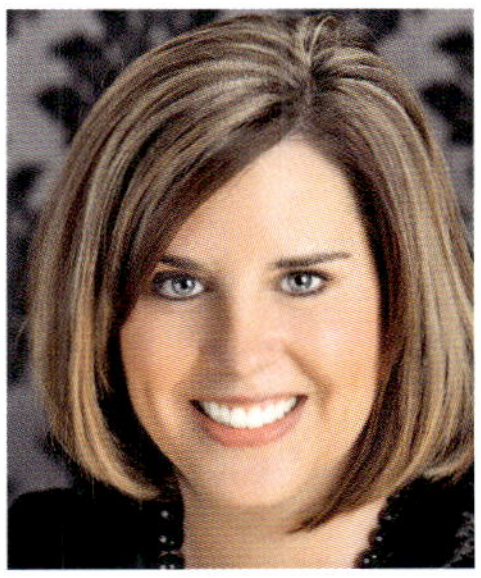

Jill Wade, DDS, MAGD, Clinician at Stonebriar Smile Design, Frisco, Texas

Other contributors

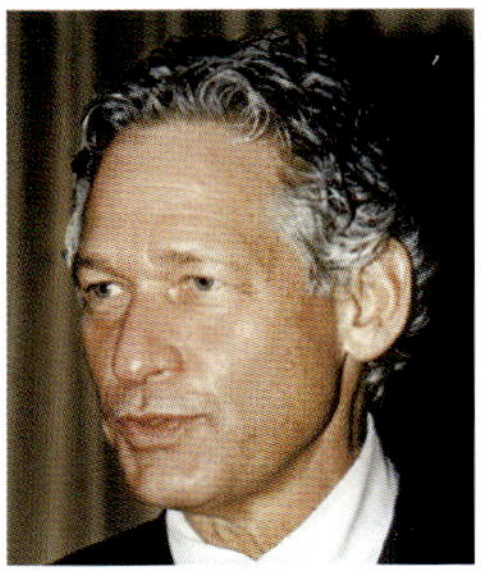

Oded Bahat, DDS, Implant Surgeon and Periodontist, Beverley Hills, California

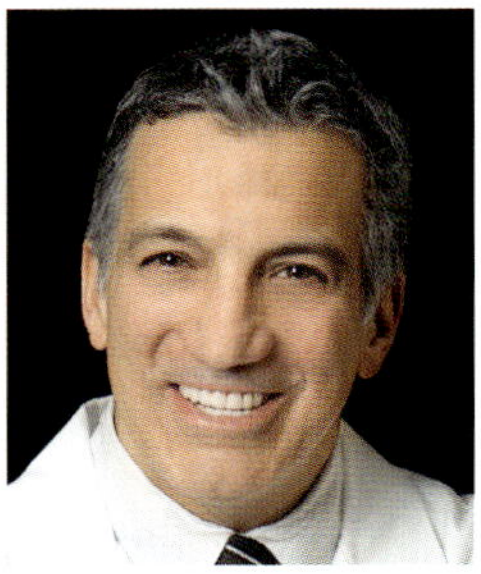

Gerry Curatola, DDS, Aesthetic Dentist, New York, New York

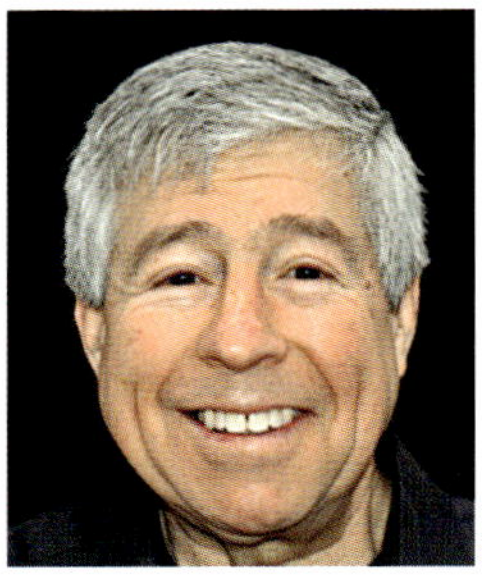

Mervyn Druian, BDS (Rand), DGDP RCS, Cosmetic Dentist, London

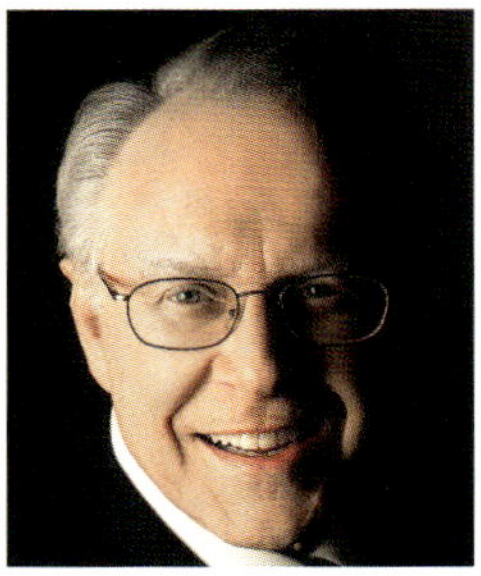

Ron Goldstein, DDS, Clinical Professor, School of Dentistry, Medical College of Georgia, Augusta, Georgia

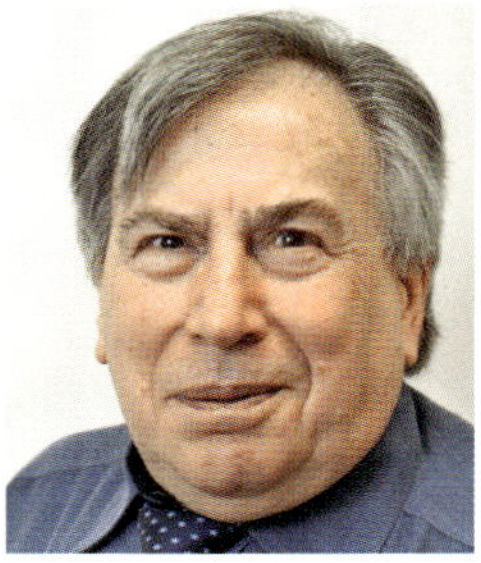

David Klaff, BDS, Prosthodontist and Aesthetic Dentist, London

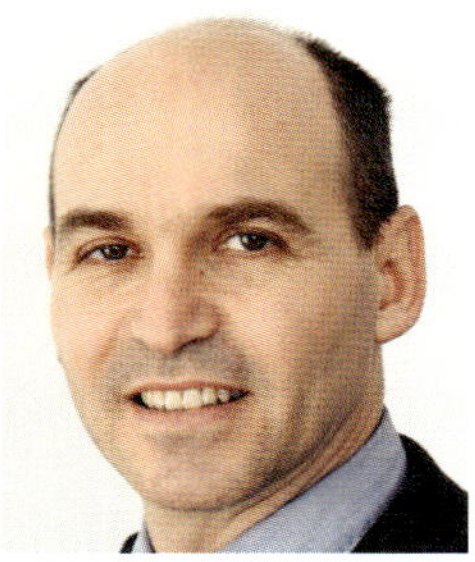

Basil Mizrahi, BDS, MSc (Rand), Prosthodontist, London

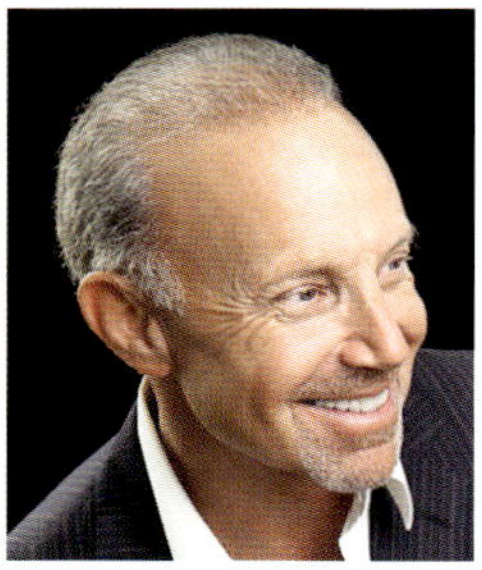

Larry Rifkin, DDS, Cosmetic Dentist and Prosthodontist, Beverley Hills, California

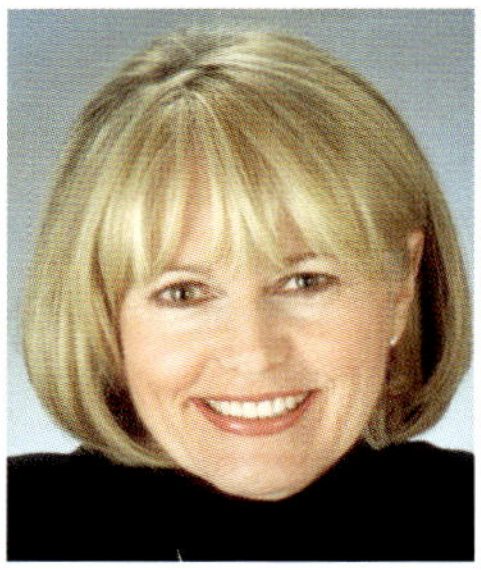

Cherilyn Sheets, DDS, Prosthodontist, Newport Beach, California

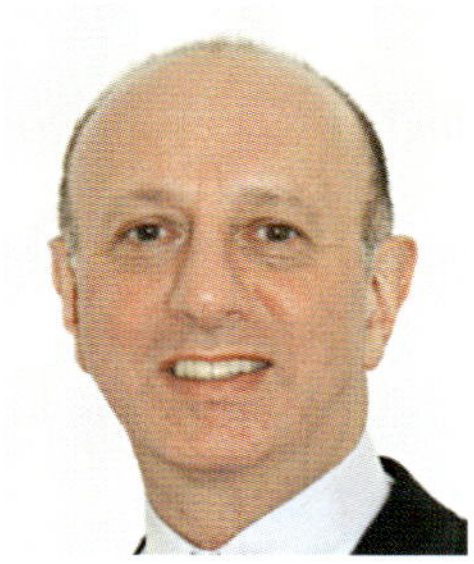

Michael Wise, BDS, MScD, LD SRCS, FDS RCS, Specialist in Restorative Dentistry and Oral Surgery, London

Contents

1 Introduction

Cathy Jameson and Linda Greenwall

Why this book?

Why a book on building the aesthetic aspect of your dental practice? There are two major reasons. First, the general public has an interest in wanting to look good and to improve the appearance of their smile. This interest has inspired dentists who are committed to responding to the growing needs of their patients. Second, providing this type of treatment, where appearance and lives are changed for the better, contributes to dentists' desire to undertake meaningful work and make a difference in the lives of their patients.

In order to respond to the wishes and demands of existing and potential patient populations, dentists need to learn how to build and manage this aspect of their practice. While aesthetic dental care has been a part of dentistry for many decades, very few dental practices are doing as much aesthetic dentistry as they desire. The purpose of this book is to provide dentists with the guidelines and strategies to make that happen.

Generational differences and opportunities

People from all generations are realizing that they can feel good about themselves by improving their unsightly teeth. Baby boomers are currently the largest segment of the population. This enormous segment is beginning to reach middle age and has a continued interest in being at their best throughout life. People of all ages want a beautiful smile, enhanced confidence, and comfort with their appearance. Below are two letters from such patients.

- *"I thought that I would drop you a line to say a big thank you! My teeth are beautiful and I appreciate them every day. I actually smile now and the best thing is people just think they are my own. I absolutely love them and can't tell you how much they have made a difference to me. The three-hour journeys to your office, the timings and the costs are insignificant when I look at what I have now … thank you to you and your fantastic team."*

- *"I thought I was too old to have a smile makeover. But I hated my teeth. I felt ugly, so I just never smiled. Then, my dentist showed me what I could look like with a new smile. I couldn't wait. He helped me find a way to finance the dentistry and I went ahead. Boy, am I glad. I am happier with my smile and with myself than I have ever been. I only wish I had known about this earlier!!"*

By providing this kind of dental care, dentists are rewarded both personally and financially. Like the patients quoted above, there are so many people whose lives can be changed for the better if they just know what is available to them. Most people have no idea of what treatments are available to improve the appearance of their smile. Here is an opportunity and a challenge to the practicing dentist: let people know who you are, what you do, and what kinds of services you offer. This book is designed for those readers who want to do more aesthetic dentistry and want to know how the best dentists have done it. That is what can be found within the pages of this book.

As a practicing dentist and prosthodontist who specializes in restorative dentistry in London, Dr Linda Greenwall focuses on comprehensive dentistry for her patients. Dr Greenwall has worked diligently for many years to establish herself as a dentist who provides aesthetic care and one whom people seek for advice and treatment. She knew the kind of dentistry she wanted to provide and made a commitment to make that happen. Dr Greenwall has published many articles and written the award-winning book *Bleaching Techniques in Restorative Dentistry* (Greenwall, 2001), the *Business of Bleaching* e-learning program (Greenwall, 2007), and contributed to *Tooth Whitening in Esthetic Dentistry* (Kwon et al., 2009). She is editor-in-chief of the journal *Aesthetic Dentistry Today* (FMC Publications) and lectures internationally on the subject of tooth whitening and aesthetic dentistry. A renowned author, lecturer, and practitioner, Dr Greenwall brings practical advice to this book and shares her own experiences. She realized early in her career that the success of her dental practice is dependent upon excellent systems of management. She wanted to accomplish ultimate success, and needed and wanted a coach by her side. That coach and mentor is Dr Cathy Jameson and her team of experienced consultants. She has been a client of Jameson Management since 1994 and has been recognized as the "Best New Practice" and "Best New Business" in the United Kingdom based on the management of her dental practice.

Cathy Jameson, PhD, is the founder and Chief Visionary Officer of Jameson Management, Inc., an international dental management and consulting organization. Dr Jameson's academic qualifications in education, psychology, and management, combined with her years of hands-on experience in the practice of her dentist husband, Dr John Jameson, have given her the background necessary to develop effective personnel and business systems of management that create and support successful dental practices. She and her team of consultants/advisors have worked with dental practices in every state in the US. Cathy says that "the success of Jameson Management, Inc. is in direct proportion to the success of our clients." She has lectured in 29 countries throughout the world and brings practical experience to her teaching through books, articles, lectures, seminars, and in-office management coaching. Her books, *Great Communication Equals Great Production* (editions 1 and 2) and *Collect What You Produce* (editions 1 and 2) provide "tried and true" teaching for dental practices. JF Jelenko published her book, *Cosmetic Dentistry Workbook*, which has been foundational for those who wish to incorporate aesthetics into their practices. The present book takes that goal to new heights.

Along with Drs Greenwall and Jameson, the reader will hear from some of the best aesthetic dentists around the world. Each chapter is interspersed with interviews of these successful dentists and members of their organizations. Outstanding members of their teams give you their insights along with the thoughts and reflections of the dentists.

Throughout the book, there are photographs and support data from Dr Greenwall in London, Dr Ken Hamlett in Dallas, TX, Dr Mark Hyman of Greensboro, NC, and Dr Charles Puntillo of Burlington, WI, as well as others. All of these dental practices are clients of Jameson Management, Inc.

The photographs demonstrate certain aspects of each chapter. Each dentist and dental practice is required to comply with their country or state legislation on all aspects of the admininstration, management and compliance of their dental practice.

The authors want you to see both the similarities and the acceptable differences in dental practices from different states and different countries. They do not want you to think that what they are teaching will not work in your dental practice and in your country. As has been noted, the authors have traveled and taught throughout the world. These systems will and do work in all countries. Read and study with an open mind and adapt the principles taught within this book to your own situation.

Below follows a summary of what you can expect in each chapter.

Chapter 2: The Foundation: Mission, Vision, Goals

The first step to developing a successful aesthetic practice is to determine what that looks like to you, the dentist. The development of your vision follows the clarification of your purpose and is brought to reality through careful strategic planning or goal setting. In Chapter 2, the reader will be provided with the guidelines necessary to do all three imperative protocols: establish the mission/purpose, clarify the vision, and perform strategic planning or goal setting.

Chapter 3: The Critical Factors of the Business of Dentistry

Each of the dentist's management systems will have goals established. These are the "Critical Factors." Defining these critical factors allows the dentist, as the leader of the team members, to track, monitor, and assess whether or not the systems are working. If they are working, celebration will be in order. The dentist will see and feel the benefits. If the systems are not working, the dentist will want to know this immediately, determine why they are not working, and make alterations to rectify the situation. The only way to know this critical information is to monitor the progress of those systems. Set goals, determine how those goals are going to be accomplished, and monitor whether the goals are being reached. As an astute leader, the dentist accepts the challenge of rapidly changing aspects that are not working and inhibiting revenue growth. Chapter 3 gives the reader the essential management strategies that are fundamental to a successful business.

Chapter 4: The Most Critical Factor: the Team

In the comprehensive and complex world of dentistry today, especially in those dental practices that wish to add an aesthetic dimension, having a dynamic and productive team is essential. Determining the "ideal" dental practice involves getting the right people on the dentist's team and leading them in a way that makes it possible to accomplish that "ideal." To that end, dentists should surround themselves with people whose company they enjoy and who are on the same path as their vision. Team members are more productive when given the ability to shine in that work situation. Goals can be set and worked toward that are mutually generated and supported. A healthy work environment is created where people can thrive and where constructive communication is a part of the culture. This will benefit the dentist, the team, and the dentist's patients.

Chapter 5: Internal Marketing

An internal marketing program introduces aesthetic options to existing patients. Some of the patients within the dental practice have never had smile makeover options discussed with them and do not even know that the practice provides such services. This chapter will teach the dentist how to open doors for aesthetic discussions with existing patients and how to market to the established client base.

Marketing is an integral part of the growth of the aesthetic portion of the dentist's practice. Each member of the team needs to understand their role in the building of this particular aspect of the dental practice. Job descriptions for each team member need to be generated so that everyone knows what his/her responsibilities are to be. Then, appropriate training must take place so that there is comfort and confidence in undertaking each task.

Chapter 6: External Marketing

Through external promotion, you, the dentist, will be educating your community about the benefits of aesthetic dentistry and the opportunities available in dentistry today. The general public does not know, for the most part, about new opportunities in aesthetic dentistry. Through a well-developed external marketing plan, you will inform your community/potential patients who you are, where you are, and what services you provide in your dental practice. You will introduce yourself to your community and help people understand why coming to your dental practice is a good idea. In addition, you can introduce aesthetic options to potential new patients. Many people may wish to improve their smiles but do not know what is available in dentistry. The introduction of smile options to potential new patients is a critical element for developing an excellent aesthetic dental practice.

For certain countries this chapter poses futuristic ideas. For other countries, these external promotional protocols are a possibility for dentists now.

Chapter 7: Communication Skills

How you, the dentist, and your team communicate between and among yourselves and with patients makes all the difference in the stability and effectiveness of a relationship. Each person on the team can make or break a relationship with a patient. Each interaction is vital, and no interaction is insignificant. Team members must understand this principle and have the communication skills to educate, motivate, and activate patients to accept the treatment that you are recommending.

In addition, creating a healthy, happy environment in which to work is essential. People choose to spend their valuable time in a dental practice where they enjoy the people and their working relationships. Communication is an important part of happiness in the workplace.

In this chapter the reader will learn the skills of listening, speaking, and problem solving. These skills are transferable to all situations in the dentist's practice. Nothing is more important than communication. It is the bottom line to the dentist's success.

Chapter 8: The Business of Bleaching and Tooth Whitening

Guidelines for successful whitening treatment are discussed. Success strategies are enumerated regarding how to build and organize the dentist's entire practice when preparing to undertake more whitening procedures.

The marketing and promotion of tooth whitening is discussed with specific recommended protocols that have proven to be effective in dental practices throughout the world. Through tooth whitening, many patients become more interested in the health of their teeth and mouth and request further aesthetic dentistry. The tooth whitening process provides minimally invasive, conservative aesthetic improvements which often stimulate the patients to make further changes to their smile. Tooth whitening is the beginning of the journey of making aesthetic improvements. This can help the patient to see the value of total oral health.

Chapter 9: Treatment Planning and Diagnosis of Aesthetic Dentistry

Gathering appropriate data about each patient includes not only the clinical data, but the personal data as well. Both elements of comprehensive diagnosis will be discussed. A thorough and workable way in which to create both a restorative and aesthetic treatment plan will be introduced. This critical time in the dentist's relationship with a patient will provide a vital roadmap for their treatment.

Chapter 10: Effective Case Presentation

The fulcrum of the dental practice is comprehensive diagnosis, complete treatment planning, and excellent case presentations. The patient first has to make the decision to receive the dental treatment before any appointment can be scheduled. People buy what they want long before they buy what they need. So, there's the dentist's ultimate challenge: helping people to want what you, the dentist, believe they need. How you present your recommendations makes all the difference.

Chapter 11: Developing the Role of Treatment Coordinator

The role of the treatment coordinator is to support the dentist's efforts to design excellent treatment plans in a timely manner. From direct discussions with the dentist, the treatment coordinator will know what the dentist is going to recommend, will help prepare for the actual presentation appointment, provide valuable third-party back-up support for the dentist, and follow up with any recommended treatments that are incomplete. The treatment coordinator will also perform the financial presentation.

Many patients do not make a decision to proceed the very first time treatment recommendations are presented to them. Following up may make the difference. If one person per month proceeds with aesthetic dentistry and a smile makeover, the dental practice takes a major leap forward. The critical role of treatment coordinator may make that kind of a difference. In addition, the dentist's level of patient care and contact can be elevated to a new and outstanding level.

Chapter 12: Financing Aesthetic Dentistry

Designing payment options that will make the financing of aesthetic dental care comfortable for the majority of patients is essential. Recent data from the dental industry (American Dental Association, 2004) indicate that the issue of cost is the number one reason why people do not go to the dentist or say yes to treatment once it has been recommended. Offer the very best treatment possible, make the financing of the dentistry comfortable, and get out of the way so that patients have a chance to say "yes!" to treatment. Through effective financial vehicles dentists can overcome the major barrier of cost.

Chapter 13: Scheduling Aesthetic Dentistry

Scheduling is the heartbeat of the dental practice. Scheduling aesthetic cases is unique unto itself. Providing and undertaking excellent aesthetic dentistry requires the appointment schedule to be well engineered. Attention to the utmost detail is essential and this requires longer appointment times in an unhurried manner. Allocating time in the schedule for providing excellent aesthetic treatment for patients while still managing a busy dental practice is discussed. In this chapter, the specific guidelines for establishing and managing this major system of the dental practice will be defined.

Chapter 14: The Hygienist's Role in Promoting Aesthetic Dentistry

One of the main responsibilities of any dental professional is to educate patients about recommended treatment and about the opportunities that are available for them. There is no one on the team who has a closer relationship with a patient than the hygienist. A hygienist spends long, quality appointment time with a patient, is able to converse during most appointments, has a confident level of trust with patients, and is qualified to be a dental educator. This is a good opportunity to maximize the talent of hygienists while enhancing the patient experience by introducing each person in a dentist's practice to the aesthetic opportunities available in dentistry today.

Chapter 15: The Use of Technology in Building the Aesthetic Aspect of a Dental Practice

The effective purchase and use of technology will be an asset to a dentist's case acceptance if training and integration are well planned and well performed. When appropriately designed, planned, and executed, a plan for technological advancement takes the dentist, the dentist's practice and the dentist's patient care to the next level.

In this chapter, various technologies are discussed that are an asset to an aesthetically-oriented dental practice. In addition to the details regarding the technology itself, methods of integrating the technology into a dentist's practice are also explained.

Chapter 16: Continuing Education

W. Edward Deming encourages businesses to be on a continual path of improvement (Deming, 1986): "Long-term commitment to new learning and new philosophy is required of any management that seeks transformation." In today's world of continuing education, a variety of courses are available such as lectures, workshops, and e-learning programs. Continuing education is a vital path of growth, both clinically and managerially. One goes hand in hand with the other. How do you, the dentist, plan for the continued education of yourself and of your team? How do you select the appropriate continuing education courses? Why is it important? How will your investment of time and money come back to you multi-fold? Learn the ways in this chapter.

Chapter 17: In Conclusion

When you get your mind focused clearly on that which you truly desire, your energy and confidence will move you forward.

"A great dental team is a group of leaders working cohesively towards a common set of goals" (Jameson, 2004). The ultimate challenge and perhaps the most rewarding is to develop your own leadership in order to maximize your own talent, the talent of your team and to lead patients towards decisions that are good for them, including receiving a beautiful smile.

The chapters that make up this book are built one upon the other. Every system in your dental practice is essential to the whole. Build on the foundation of mission, vision, and goal setting. Then, one system at a time, create a dental practice that epitomizes your "ideal" and create a work environment where the brightest and best will want to come to work with you, devote themselves to your aesthetic practice, and stay with you throughout time. The systems of your dental practice, as outlined in this book, are the pathway to that kind of success. Each chapter is a Success Strategy.

How to use the book to get positive results

It is the authors' hope that you, the reader, will truly put the success strategies that are presented in this book into practice. These systems will work, if you work the systems. What follows is a suggested method by which you can "use" the book as a learning/teaching vehicle to truly integrate the learning into practice. Become more than a reader: become a doer.

Bringing this book to life:

- Read through the book once.
- Use the Vision Worksheet (see Chapter 2) to get focused on what you are trying to build.
- Write goals that you passionately want to accomplish. Time activate your goals.
- Then read through the book again. Use the checklists to plan your practice, customize the checklists to make them specific to your unique dental practice. This will help you to plan each step along the way.
- Take one step at a time and master each step as you go along.
- Develop a protocol manual for your dental practice which addresses each system. How will it be set up? What are the end results you wish to accomplish? Who will do what, how, and why?

- Evaluate your plan of action (your goals or strategic plan) often. Make sure you are on track.
- Monitor your progress with respect to your goals. Celebrate the small victories along the way, but adjust when things are not progressing.
- Provide feedback for your team.
- Use the authors' websites for checklist updates, new information, tips for success, and contact with your colleagues.
- Learn from others.
- Read the recommended further reading books and resources.
- Enjoy the journey!

Action steps

At the end of each chapter, the reader will find a section called "Action steps." In this summary, action steps are recommended that integrate the principles proposed in each chapter. These action steps will help the reader continue forward. These are proven, effective steps of action that have been applied to thousands of dental practices throughout the world.

It is the authors' desire that you, the reader, do not become frustrated that you have "read another book", only to put it back on the shelf while doing nothing to make things happen. Detailed information has been provided not only of what to do but also of the action plans for how to do it. Knowing what to do is one thing. Doing it is sometimes another issue!

Take advantage of the action steps section of every chapter and be consistent in following up and following through with each one of the steps. You will be amazed and delighted with the results … and your dental practice will be great!

The chapters are designed to be both inspiring and practical. You have taken step one by picking up this book. Now take step two. Read it with commitment. This commitment, along with your own personal passion, will determine the measure of success you will obtain from the book. The authors provide you with their success strategies. The decision of what you do with the information depends upon you.

References

1. American Dental Association. 2003 Public Opinion Survey: Oral Health of the US Population. Chicago, IL: American Dental Association, 2004.
2. Deming WE. Out of the Crisis. Boston, MA: MIT Press, 1986.
3. Greenwall LH. Bleaching Techniques in Restorative Dentistry. An illustrated guide to bleaching teeth. London: Martin Dunitz, 2001.
4. Greenwall LH. The Business of Bleaching. e-learning program. Smile-on Ltd and Dr Linda Greenwall, 2007.
5. Jameson C. Collect What You Produce. Tulsa, OK: PennWell Books, 1997.
6. Jameson C. Great Communication Equals Great Production. Tulsa, OK: PennWell Books, 2004.
7. Jameson C. The Cosmetic Dentistry Workbook: A Step-by-step Program for the Dental Office Team. New York, USA: JF Jelenko, 1991.
8. Kwon S, Ko S, Greenwall LH. Tooth Whitening in Esthetic Dentistry. Chicago, IL: Quintessence Publishing, 2009.

2 The Foundation: Mission, Vision, Goals

Cathy Jameson and Linda Greenwall

> *To believe in the things you can see and touch is no belief at all: but to believe in the unseen is a triumph and a blessing.* Abraham Lincoln

Mission statement

A mission statement clearly communicates the purpose of your dental practice. Who are you? What do you do? Why? The mission statement rests on a foundation of the values that are of most importance to you, and it becomes the benchmark for every decision you make. Ask yourself, "If I do this will it help me to fulfill my ultimate mission?" If the answer is "yes," you are probably making a good decision. If the answer is "no" or "I'm not sure," then go back to the drawing board. The decision is not aligned with your mission. The answer must be "yes."

The following are examples of mission statements. These dentists have had their mission statements printed, matted, and framed. Then, they are placed in a location within the office where it can be seen by the team and/or patients. Every action of the dental practice and each member of the team must support this statement of purpose.

Dr John Jameson's mission statement: *"Our philosophy is to provide optimum dentistry for our patients in a loving and caring way with emphasis on function, aesthetics and prevention."*

Dr Linda Greenwall's mission statement: *"To provide advanced comprehensive dental care to our patients."*

Dr Charles Puntillo's mission statement: *"Dentistry – my chosen life's work, has but one aim: to help my patients keep all of their teeth for all of their lives. We can achieve this working together, while maintaining maximum comfort, function, health and beautifully natural aesthetics. We are always striving to accomplish this appropriately."*

Dr Mark Hyman's mission statement: *"Our mission: We are a team of compassionate, dedicated professionals who provide optimal dental care using state of the art technology. We are enthusiastic in our commitment to you, our patients, to excellence and to building relationships within our community."*

Your mission statement does not have a beginning or an end. It is the benchmark against which everything you do, all decisions you make, and all the activities and actions you perform are measured. The statement of mission is like the spine that runs down the backbone of your practice. It is the integrity, the strength, the character of you and of your dental practice.

Rick Warren (2002) said that "Living on purpose is the only way to *really* live. Everything else is just existing."

Vision

While the mission statement is your benchmark, the development of a vision moves you toward greater clarity of what you specifically want in your dental practice. What do you see as your "ideal" dental practice in your mind's eye? In other words, what does your "ideal" dental practice look like?

The first step to achieving the ideal is to define what that looks like to you (Fig 2-1). What you determine to be ideal is uniquely yours. Look deep within yourself and be true to your own vision. Ask yourself the following questions and write out your response. This becomes the beginning of your strategic plan. It is the pathway to your abundant success.

- What do you want?
- What kind of dentistry do you want to do?
- How do you want to provide your care?
- What do you want your patients to experience each time they encounter your dental practice? (Describe your ideal patient visit from the initial visit throughout their time with you.)
- What kind of team do you want?
- What are their characteristics and how do they interact with each other, with you, and with your patients?
- What is your facility like?
- What kind of technology do you have and how are you maximizing it?
- What is your gross and take-home income?
- What is your reputation in the community? When people are seeking aesthetic care, how will you establish yourself as the aesthetic dental practice in your area?

Once you have honestly answered these questions, then ask yourself two challenging questions:

- Do I have this now? Describe this.
- If you do not have this now, then ask yourself, "What do I need to do to make this happen?" Describe this.

You may find upon answering these questions that your existing systems are not functioning in a manner that supports your new vision. That will not be unusual. Nor is that catastrophic! You can implement healthy change in order to move toward your ideal. Do not let anything or anyone prevent you

VISION WORKSHEET

1. In my mind's eye – the vision of my ideal practice looks like this:
   Type of treatment I'm providing: ____________
   Doctor: ____________
   Hygiene: ____________
2. My ideal patient visit: ____________
   My Team: ____________
   Business Administrator: ____________
   Assistants: ____________
   Hygienists: ____________
   Laboratory: ____________
4. My facility: ____________
5. My equipment and technology: ____________
6. Number of days: ____________
7. Hours: ____________
8. Vacations: ____________
9. Amount of Production/Collection: ____________
10. Take-home salary: (Gross) ____________
11. Reputation in Community: ____________
    Now, ask yourself: How do I make this happen? ____________
    What's getting in my way? ____________
    What will I do to overcome my own barriers/obstacles? ____________
    Who do I need in my life to help me? Who do I need as resource person or company? ____________
    What's getting in the way of me inviting these resources into my life? ____________
    Why? ____________
    What do I need to do to overcome my own resistance? ____________
    What will be the benefits of having resources/coaches/helpers in my life? ____________
    Will I do this? ____________
    When? ____________

Fig 2-1 Dr Jameson's vision worksheet.

from having your ideal dental practice. You can have this and deserve it. But how can you or anyone who works with you strive toward the ideal if they are not sure what that means? The more clearly you describe your ideal and the more steadfastly you make an effort to move in that direction, the better your team will respond. This is excellent and effective leadership.

▶ *"After a few years of solo private practice, I realized that there had to be a better way to practice dentistry. I was basically performing the same kind of dentistry I had learned in dental school.*

"I wanted to learn how to practice more advanced dentistry. I began searching for high quality continuing education in areas where I could learn to practice better dentistry. I studied at the Pankey Institute and with Dr Pete Dawson and learned to perform comprehensive dentistry, which has been foundational in my aesthetic cases.

"I developed a vision for my practice which was to practice in a way that consistently provided excellent dentistry that exceeded our patients' expectations. For me it was professionally and emotionally satisfying and was necessary for me to become financially profitable and successful."

Dr Charles Puntillo (interview)

Change

As you build the aesthetic aspect of your dental practice, you may find that certain changes are appropriate. You or members of your team may feel nervous about those changes. Stepping out of the comfort zone can be frightening because the "unknown" may seem risky. Think of risk as a two-sided coin (Fig 2-2). On one side of the risk coin is the possibility that you may make a mistake. On the other side of the coin is the possibility of ultimate success. No successful person or business has reached the pinnacle of success without facing and mastering risk.

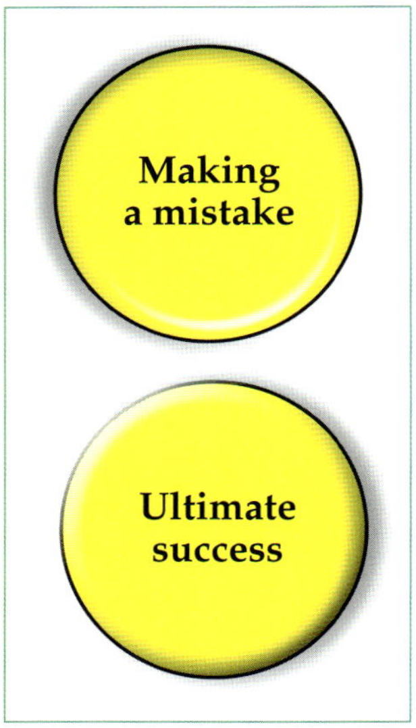

Fig 2-2 Facing change: risk coin.

Identify what you want. Then think about how you will feel if you *do not* work toward that which you truly want. How discouraging to work throughout a lifetime and never experience the joy and satisfaction that comes with accomplishing your ideal dental practice. Ask yourself what is the worst thing that could happen if you try to make necessary desired changes and hit a few bumps along the way? Even if you make mistakes, or things don't go the way you wish the first time, learn from your mistakes and you will gain strength on the other side.

According to Senge (2006), the key requirements of leading people through the change process begin with having a clear sense of purpose supported by a defined vision. Develop clear lines of communication so the vision is clear to all team members, as well as to patients. Your values will shine through in all that you do.

The leader's desire to change, grow, or expand will not come to fruition without the commitment of quality team members who share the vision (Senge, 2006). When the members of the organization join together as a closely functioning, focused group of compatible colleagues, the vision takes on life, and productivity increases (Jameson, 2010).

Once you have a commitment to your mission statement and when a clear vision has been written so that the team sees the possibility of accomplishing the ideal vision, a plan of action must be developed so that everyone sees a clear path. Otherwise, confusion and wasted energy result (Kotter, 1996). Continuous channels of communication are required. Each member of the team must know their responsibilities and be accountable for carrying out those responsibilities. No one on the team must be held back from fulfillment of their own tasks because another member of the team failed to perform (Kotter, 2008). To build the aesthetic aspect of your dental practice, team members must be willing to write and work toward goals that support the growth of the practice. The connectedness of one person to every other team member becomes obvious when strategic planning includes all team members and when each person's role is held in esteem and importance. Goals can then be reached.

Goal accomplishment

What

Tom Hopkins (2001) defines success as "the continuous journey towards the achievement of predetermined, worthwhile goals."

Your goals must be aligned with carefully developed management systems that support the attainment of these goals. In order for goals to become motivational and to become a reality, there must be solid teamwork and a congenial group of people working together toward reaching these predetermined goals (Jameson, 2000). These goals, supported by a set of efficient, effective systems are critical if excellent results are to be achieved. Durkheim (1982) found that without order, the energies of the people can be misdirected, resulting in chaos. Chaos will sap the energy from your team and your dental practice. Without energy and desire on the part of employees, nothing occurs. Inertia sets in. This inertia can stand in the way of progress, productivity, and organizational success (Fig 2-3).

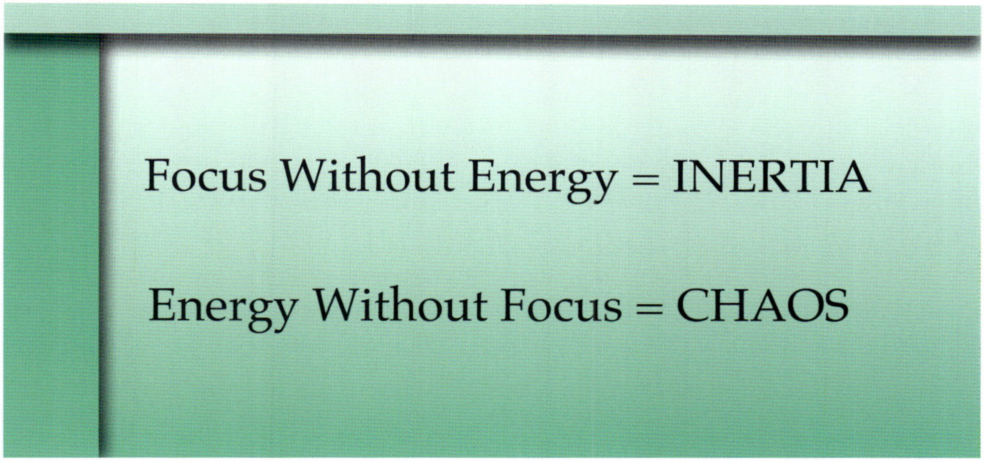

Fig 2-3 Energy and focus are required for success.

Individuals gain personal fortitude when they believe in the clearly defined goals of the dental practice and they feel empowered to provide a relevant contribution. The employee's ability to make a difference and to be acknowledged for that ability becomes ultimately motivational (Mullins & Devendorf, 2007).

Although technology has impacted every business, the need for careful and caring attention to customer service remains steadfast. A dental practice is built by serving patients, one person at a time. When team members feel valued and empowered, they transfer this goodwill to patients. Goal accomplishment supports this empowerment.

The process of goal accomplishment has been proven to produce the following results:

- increased production
- increased personal income
- motivation of team members, including the dentist
- improved teamwork
- enhanced decision-making
- reduced procrastination
- faster achievement of results.

How

Most people are not clear about their goals. They indicate that they may have some idea about their goals but have never written them down (Jameson, 2000). They go through their lives without the clarity of direction that accompanies a clearly written set of goals that evolve throughout time.

A goal does not truly become a goal until it is written down. The act of writing the goal in a specific format helps the mind to visualize the goal as if it were already accomplished. Then the human mind takes the lead. Write your goals in the affirmative and your actions will go immediately to work to bring that goal into a state of reality. "Whatever the mind of man can conceive and believe, so shall he achieve" (Hill, 1960).

You attract to you that which you think about (Byrne, 2006; Hicks & Hicks, 2008). Be careful not to wallow in negativity, which saps the life out of you, your team, and your dental practice. For example, "We set a goal of having 18 new patients per month but what a joke! We only get 12 new patients each month and nothing seems to work to change that." This kind of negative thought process and negative talk sets you on a path to attract more negativity to yourself and to your dental practice (Hicks & Hicks, 2008).

> *"In our aesthetically oriented practice, our team meetings are extremely important in monitoring our progress in achieving our goals. It gives the team purpose and responsibility but goal setting also gives us a sense of pride when we have been successful. We celebrate our victories!!"* ***(see Fig 2-4).***
>
> ***Cindy Butler (interview), Business Administrator and Treatment Coordinator for Dr Charles Puntillo***

This means that you set a goal and make note of every step you take that moves you closer to that goal. "We set a goal of enrolling 18 new patients per month and we enrolled 12 new patients this month. Great. What did we do to attract those 12 people and how can we continue to develop these processes?" Focus on the things that are going well. Celebrate each step taken toward the accomplishment of your goals and you will be moving yourself closer to fulfilling those goals.

In terms of your goal of building the aesthetic aspect of your dental practice, if you think of all the reasons why people in your area will never want or be able to afford aesthetic treatment, you will attract just that. If you believe in possibilities and imagine people saying yes to your treatment recommendations, including aesthetic treatment, more people will come to you and agree to treatment.

jameson

Celebrate the Victories!

(Even the small ones!)

It is very important that the team take the time and effort to reach around and pat itself on the back. If you wait for others to recognize your work, you may wait for a very long time. Too often, others are quick to criticize, but slow to praise. So, when you've accomplished a goal, improved your processes, installed a new system, or put a new service into effect, celebrate the event! Congratulate yourselves, throw your own party, give out gifts or simply bring in a pizza!

Many team members work behind the scenes. They aren't on the front lines getting immediate feedback from patients. They don't have the visibility and may not get "kudos". They keep the ship afloat by making sure that bills are paid on time, payroll is completed and checks go out, information is distributed accurately and in a timely fashion, etc. As the saying goes, no one ever calls to say "thanks for getting my check to me on time." It's just expected.

Think of examples of this in your own practice. How can you express appreciation for one another more effectively?

Have your own celebrations when certain milestones are accomplished. But remember to express gratitude for the every day activities that make it possible for you to perform excellently. Also, remember to be a role model, an example. If you pat others on the back, you set the tone for them to do the same thing.

Ways We Will Celebrate Our Victories:

1.

2.

3.

4.

Fig 2-4 Celebrate the victories worksheet.

When you follow specific steps in your dental procedures you do so because you want and expect to accomplish great results for your patients. When you follow specific steps in your management systems, you can expect great results as well.

Your vision illustrates a belief in possibilities. Now begin the process of making your vision concrete by planning and writing down your goals. Successful dental practices realize the importance of mission, vision, and goals.

▶ *"After creating and writing our mission statement, we defined our vision [see Vision Worksheet, Fig 2-1]. Then, realizing that I didn't want to do average dentistry, I defined one of my most important goals – to learn to do occlusal reconstructions and restorations by studying with the very best instructors. However, I realized that what I really needed was guidance for the entire team, for the whole office. We needed to develop people skills, communication skills, and practice management systems. As a team, we all needed to be on the same page in order to carry the practice forward. And so, I set a goal of finding a coach to work with us and teach us how to manage our office, how to communicate more effectively, and how to coordinate as a team for the betterment of the practice. This was the only way that my vision was going to become a reality."*

Dr Charles Puntillo (interview)

Why

Understanding the benefits of goal setting, learning the techniques of goal planning, and committing to the goal accomplishment process are all vital parts of self-actualization, both in your personal life as well as your professional life.

According to Merriam-Webster (http://www.merriam-webster.com/, accessed 19 Oct 2011), a "goal" is "the end toward which effort is directed." A goal focuses your attention on the result of specific actions or behaviors. Many people have a *vague* idea of what it is they want to achieve, but very few spend the time and energy necessary to plan for the successful achievement of goals.

Studies show productive results

Studies of motivation have shown that people or businesses that write and pursue goals become more productive than those people or groups who do not. Dr David McClelland and his research team at Harvard University studied motivation to determine the major attributes that characterize successful people. The researchers found that one of the key characteristics of successful, highly motivated people was that these people were goal oriented (McClelland, 1989).

These researchers discovered that this group was goal oriented but that only 3% *wrote down* their goals and participated in a goal accomplishment process. An expanded study of this group uncovered the fact that the 3% who began and followed a disciplined goal accomplishment process increased their own productivity by a minimum of 10% and increased their incomes by approximately 100%.

Yale University performed a similar study (Tracy, 2010). They surveyed a class of graduating seniors and asked if the individuals wrote down their goals. Again, 3% said "yes." The university tracked this group of graduates for 10 years. At the end of that 10-year period, they found that the 3% who had written their goals (and had continued to do so) had accomplished more than the other 97% put together!

Obstacles to goal accomplishment

You may be asking, "If this goal setting business is so great, then why don't more people do it? If the success rate of the 3% is so tangible, why don't more people take this step?" Good question! There are several reasons why people choose not to write their goals, and they are explained in what follows (Jameson, 2004).

Fear of failure

Many people hesitate to write a goal down, because if the goal is not accomplished, they will consider themselves or the project a failure. People fear failure, because they see it as a risk, and most people are not comfortable with risk. Facing a fear takes a great deal of courage. Thomas Gordon (Gordon & Edwards, 1995) said "Courage is not the absence of fear, but the willingness to act in spite of fear." The fact that you have faced something you have previously feared is a success within itself. Not ever facing an issue or a task that you fear takes away from your very being. This stifles your journey toward self-fulfillment.

The dental professional is often caught in the trap of believing that they must be perfect. The environment in which the dentist performs is extremely unforgiving and there is no margin for error. The dentist believes that he/she must meet the needs of all people, relate exceptionally well to all people, be a top-notch leader of the dental team, be the total provider for the staff and for family, and must not show any emotions that might be misconstrued as negative. They may feel that any conflict could be seen as a statement of ineptitude on the part of this "leader" and since most dental professionals are not taught how to effectively deal with conflict, they tend to just pretend that conflict doesn't exist. "Maybe if I ignore it, it will go away." This perfectionist misconception leads to incredible stress.

The only way to overcome a fear is to face that fear "head on." When you face that fear, deal with it, and survive, you take great strides in overcoming the fear. Once you discover that you can do something (and survive), the task will be more comfortable for you the next time.

However, if, in fact, you do not reach a goal that you have set, change your response. Instead of seeing this as a failure, look at the experience as an opportunity to learn. You have just learned a plan of action that does not work!

If you set a goal and you find that the strategies you have set forth don't work, don't quit! Learn from your experience. Learn to turn negatives into positives and your life will be a constant learning experience.

Low self-esteem

You may feel that you are not worthy of success. You have told yourself many times that "you can't" or "you wouldn't be able to" and your subconscious mind believes just that! Remember, you become what you think about. The subconscious mind doesn't know the difference between reality and non-reality. If your subconscious mind constantly receives messages about your lack of worth, it believes that this is true. Creating constant positive input about yourself, your abilities, and your desires or goals is essential for growth. You can overcome a feeling of low self-esteem by feeding positive thoughts and nutritional information to your mind.

Don't know how to write goals

Most people have never had instruction on the value of or the methods of writing goals. While an intricate study of this skill is recommended, this chapter will provide an introduction.

Start by letting your thoughts flow freely. Write down your every dream for the purpose of visualizing that which you desire. Think of what you want to *be, do,* and *have*. Do not stifle yourself by putting a lid on your thoughts and dreams. All progress starts with a thought.

While all progress begins with a thought, it does not become a goal until it is written down. The purposes of writing the goal down:

- it becomes something you can visualize
- it becomes tangible
- it becomes something you can refer to for evaluation and modification
- it evaluates your path towards reaching the goal
- it lends a sense of gratification and positive reinforcement for your work well done.

Don't see any reason

If you truly want to build the aesthetic aspect of your dental practice, follow the advice of people who have done so successfully. These are people who not only believe in goal setting, but perform this strategic planning methodology with commitment.

Adding aesthetics to the existing treatment mix requires goals to be set to follow that direction. This helps the whole team focus their energies to make this happen within the dental practice.

> *"Following the goal setting process allowed us to implement the changes needed in our practice so that we could add aesthetics to our treatment mix. This paved the way for us to focus the energies of the team so that we could make this possible."*
>
> ***Dr John Jameson (interview)***

Don't know what their goals are

Many people do not write goals because they are unclear about their goals. Think of the "ideal" dental practice, as has been recommended. Imagine the specifics of that dental practice. This is the beginning. The identification of what you want is step one. You do have goals – you just may not have identified them as goals.

Consider these questions:

- Who do you want to be? The best aesthetic dentist in your community?

- What dentistry do you want to do? Provide aesthetic care for more patients?
- What type of dental practice do you want to have? A practice that focuses upon aesthetics and is rewarded professionally, financially, personally and spiritually because of the difference you make in the lives of others?
- How will you make this happen? You will need a clear plan, setting down the goals, vision, and mission.
- Who will be on the journey? Have you got the best dental team that you can gather?
- Where are you at this present stage?
- Where will this happen? What will your dental facility look like in order to provide excellent aesthetic dentistry?
- When?

Think this through. This is your starting point.

The five-step process for goal accomplishment

Writing the goal is the first step to accomplishing the goal, however the specific process for goal accomplishment must be followed.

1. Write the goal

The first step of goal accomplishment is to write your goal in the affirmative, as if it has already been accomplished. Decide what you want, and begin the process by writing it down. For example, "We will do one more aesthetic case per month than we did last year."

Dr Ken Blanchard (2000), author of the *One Minute Manager* series, says that your goals need to be SMART:

S — Specific
M — Motivational
A — Attainable
R — Relevant
T — Trackable

What do these goal-setting parameters mean?

Specific: Write your goals as clearly as possible. Write the goal so clearly that you can visualize the end result. Avoid generalities. Remember that you are giving your mind direction so that your actions will proceed on the desired path. Once you have written a goal, pause and imagine playing a video in your mind of what it looks like to have that goal achieved. For example, visualize a completed case. Visualize the happy patient. Visualize yourself finishing the case to your satisfaction and feel the emotion that goes along with the successful case. Visualize your team enjoying the work you are doing. Visualize even the actual tooth preparation of the case and the end result.

Motivational: In his book, *GMP: The Greatest Management Principle in the World* (1985), Dr Michael LeBoeuf said "That which is rewarded is repeated." People's behavior and performance is driven by "what's in this for me?" That's not bad. That's just a reality. A reward doesn't have to be monetary.

While money is a motivator for people in the workplace today, it has been indicated that appreciation far outweighs money as a motivator. Of course, people need money in order to put food on the table, a roof over their heads, fuel into the car, etc. However, people will leave an organization over not feeling appreciated faster than they will leave a practice to make a bit more money down the street.

Involve your team in setting and working toward goals. Celebrate the victories along the way and integrate motivational principles into your dental practice (McClelland & Burnham, 1976). At the same time, eliminate factors within your dental practice that de-motivate the team. A motivated, involved team can transfer enthusiasm to patients.

> *"I find that every person must be empowered with the ability to control their own work environment. I have learned through the years to treat each employee as they need to be treated rather than use one particular management style with each person. People are individuals and want to be treated as such. It is important to give your team the room to be the best that they can be by encouraging and acknowledging a job well done."*
>
> ***Jacqueline Pastore (interview), Practice Administrator for Drs Larry Rosenthal and Michael Apa***

Be courageous enough to discover things that are de-motivational in your dental practice. It is only when problems are identified that solutions can be generated.

Attainable: W. Edward Deming (1986) encourages us to be on a continuous path of improvement. Set your goals so that they are attainable but also stimulate you to stretch, to become more than you ever imagined possible. Everyone has potential and talent that has not been tapped. Stretch.

Determine your "critical factors of the business of dentistry" (see Chapter 3). Where are you at the present moment? Where do you want to go? Then, set goals that will move you to that next level slowly, carefully and in a manner that is accomplishable, while at the same time challenging. For example, at the present time if you are doing one aesthetic case per month, set a goal of doing two aesthetic cases per month. Then, when you have done this for three months in a row (which indicates a business trend), take your goal up to the next level, if you so desire.

Relevant: Your goals must support your mission/purpose and must be congruent and relevant to you and to your values. Your long-term and short-term goals, as well as major and minor goals, are all important. Each must receive an affirmative answer to the question "if we do this will it help us to fulfill our ultimate mission/purpose?" Your mission has no beginning and no end. It is the life force of your dental practice. Your goals do have a beginning and do have an end. They are precise, specific, and finite. Once you see the completion of a goal on the horizon, you will be organizing for the next step – the next, progressive goal.

Trackable: Monitor your success. That which is not monitored cannot be measured. You cannot know if you are on track or off track if you do not have your goals specifically written and if you are not continually evaluating your progress. The tracking of your progress will let you know if you need to continue on the same path, or if you need to make alterations. If you are not making the desired progress, be an excellent leader and orchestrate the necessary changes. Do not keep repeating things that are not working! That is a waste of time, money, and energy. You will become frustrated and could stagnate, neither of which are healthy or support your path toward success.

2. Design the plan of action

Here are the nuts and bolts part of goal setting:

- What are you going to do?
- How are you going to do it?
- Why is every step of the plan significant?

Carefully detail your plan of action for reaching each specific goal. Identify necessary resources that you will need to make this happen.

- Carefully identify outside resources: books, online courses, continuing education courses, coaches, training, monies, advisors, and consultants who can help you. Your willingness to be coached will move you along more quickly and precisely.
- Identify the challenges or barriers that appear as roadblocks to your progress. Design a strategy to overcome these. Dr Michael Doyle (1982), in his book *How to Make Meetings Work*, said, "A problem is only a problem until it becomes defined. Once it becomes defined it becomes manageable."

3. Assign responsibilities to the appropriate person or persons

The next step is to determine who will be responsible for carrying out each aspect of your plan. If you do not assign responsibilities, nothing will happen. When you include your team members in writing the goals and designing the plan of action, you will find that they will be more enthusiastic about participating in the work of execution of the plan. Dr Doyle said, "If a person is allowed to be a part of a decision-making process, that person will be more likely to buy into that decision" (Doyle, 1982).

The more specific the description of position responsibilities, the more confidently and excellently your team members can perform. People want to be involved, respected, and challenged. Talented people will leave an organization if they are not challenged, so open this door to creative endeavor.

4. Time-activate each step of the plan

In order to offset procrastination, define the time frame by which each aspect of your plan is to be completed. Confer with the people who are going to carry out each task and make sure there is an agreement on the time frame. Expect to hold people accountable for meeting this agreement and expect individuals to hold themselves accountable.

Team members get frustrated because ideas are generated, plans are designed, but nothing happens. They lose enthusiasm if time is spent in creating a plan but then follow-up and follow-through is absent. This can become debilitating to individuals, to the team, and to the dental practice.

Do not think that team members will be frustrated or upset if they are held accountable. People in the workplace want to know what is expected of them and they want to perform well for their employer and clients. Feedback is essential and desirable.

5. Evaluation

Evaluation may be as important as any other step. This step allows you to follow up and follow through. If you find that progress is being made, celebrate even the smallest victory. However, if you find that something you planned is not achieving the desired results, change the plan!

Go back to the goal itself and ask whether you truly want to accomplish the goal. If the answer is "yes" but the plan is not working, alter the plan. You learn as much from things that do not work as you can from things that work immediately. Determine what is working well and keep on doing those things. Alter or refine those steps that are not getting positive results. That is how development occurs. That is a healthy evolutionary process.

Use a worksheet (Fig 2-5) during your team meetings, strategic planning sessions, or during brainstorming sessions to record decisions and track your progress. Make sure that each person who is involved in a project has a copy of the worksheet so that they can hold themselves accountable, and keep a copy in a three-ring binder that you bring to each team meeting so that you can continuously review progress. Remember, evaluation is as important as any other step of the process.

Goal Accomplishment			
Goal:			
Strategies	Person responsible	Time Frame	Evaluation
#1			
#1			
#3			
#4			
#5			
#6			
#7			

Fig 2-5 Goal accomplishment worksheet.

Three vital elements for a successful dental practice

The success strategies for building the aesthetic aspect of your dental practice depend on establishing three clear vital elements: mission/purpose, vision, and strategic planning or goal accomplishment.

▶ *"Set goals – daily, weekly, and monthly, etc. It is easy to get distracted by daily items, but you need to keep the big picture in mind. Write your goals."*
Debra Hamlett (interview), Office Manager for Dr Ken Hamlett

In summary

The first step to success is deciding to be a success. You have decided to build the aesthetic aspect of your dental practice. Give yourself an "edge:" **write your goals!** Work through any fear of failure that may have prevented you or your team members from writing your goals prior to this reading. There is a powerful reason to write your goals: you will accomplish more in a shorter period of time. The vision you have of providing more aesthetic treatment can become a reality. Start this journey now. Do not waste your time and talent by procrastinating. **Start now!**

Success

Successful people:

1. *Decide* to succeed. *Decide* to be happy. *Decide* to face the "goods and the bads" of life with a positive attitude. *Decide* to find the best in each and every situation so that learning can occur from *each and every* person and event.
2. Write their goals. Are highly goal oriented and have a burning desire to achieve their goals.
3. Combine their desire for success with a sincere caring for the people whom they serve.
4. Are willing to reach within themselves to "pull out" the potential that lies within. Are willing to risk.
5. Overcome barriers or fears by facing them with strength and perseverance.
6. Are willing to withstand the "pain" that sometimes comes with growth and change.
7. Write their plans – *daily!* Practice excellent time management.
8. Control their lives – rather than allowing the circumstances of their lives to control them.
9. *Get and stay fit – physically and mentally.* Nurture their minds on a regular basis by feeding them with positive data such as books, tapes, seminars, and people. Have a *positive mental attitude.*
10. Work at maintaining a balance in their lives – a balance between Worship, Love, Work, and Play (Aristotle/LD Pankey).

Action steps

1. Write or revisit your mission statement.
2. Complete the vision worksheet (Fig 2-1).
3. Write goals related to each aspect of your vision.
4. Follow the process of goal accomplishment using the goal sheet included in this chapter.
5. Celebrate each step that you take toward the accomplishment of a goal. Integrate positive reinforcement into the management and culture of your dental practice.

References

1. Blanchard K. The One Minute Manager Builds High Performing Teams. New York, NY: Blanchard Family Partnership, 2000.
2. Byrne R. The Secret. New York, NY: Beyond Words Publishing, 2006.
3. Deming WE. Out of the Crisis. Cambridge, MA: MIT Press, 1986.
4. Doyle M. How to Make Meetings Work. New York, NY: The Berkley Publishing Group, 1982.
5. Durkheim E. The Rules of Sociological Method. New York, NY: The Free Press, 1982.
6. Gordon T, Edwards S. Making the Patient Your Partner. Westpoint, CT: Auburn House, 1995.
7. Hicks E, Hicks J. The Law of Attraction: How to Make it Work For You. London: Hay House, 2008.
8. Hill N. Think and Grow Rich. New York, NY: Fawcett Crest Books, 1960.
9. Hopkins T. Selling. New York, NY: Hungry Minds Press, 2001.
10. Jameson C. Controlling Stress in the Dental Profession through Effective Communication. Oklahoma City, OK: JC Educational, 2000.
11. Jameson C. Great Communication Equals Great Production. Tulsa, OK: Pennwell Books, 2004.
12. Jameson C. The Impact of Training in Transformational Leadership on the Productivity of a Dental Practice [dissertation]. Minneapolis, MN: Walden University, 2010.
13. Kotter J. Leading Change. Boston, MA: Harvard Business School Press, 1996.
14. Kotter J. A Sense of Urgency. Boston, MA: Harvard Business School Press, 2008.
15. LeBoeuf M. GMP: The Greatest Management Principle in the World. New York, NY: Penguin Group, 1985.
16. McClelland D. Human Motivation. New York, NY: Scott Foresman, 1989.
17. McClelland D, Burnham D. Power is the great motivator. Harv Bus Rev 1976;54:100–110.
18. Mullins M, Devendorf S. Assessing goal-directed attention as an indicator of self regulation: A comparison of two approaches. N Am J Psychol 2007;9:229–250.
19. Senge P. The Fifth Discipline. New York, NY: Doubleday, 2006.
20. Tracy B. Goals: How to Get Everything You Want – Faster Than You Ever Thought Possible. San Francisco, CA: Berrett-Koehler Publishers, 2010.
21. Warren R. The Purpose Driven Life. Grand Rapids, MI: Zondervan, 2002.

3 The Critical Factors of the Business of Dentistry

Cathy Jameson and Linda Greenwall

> *Objectives are not fate; they are direction. They are not commands; they are commitments. They do not determine the future; they are means to mobilize the resources and energies of the business for the making of the future."*
>
> *Peter Drucker (2002)*

Successful systems: successful business

One of the challenges that many dental professionals face is balancing their commitment to being a healthcare provider with being a successful businessperson. There is no question that your main purpose is serving your patients. You went into dentistry because you wanted to be a healthcare provider and you wanted to make a difference in people's lives. Then, you realized that running a dental practice takes a different set of skills beyond performing dental procedures. Business and personnel management are unique skills that are required for an excellent dental practice to be realized. Most dental schools do not teach business skills and the skills required to manage a successful dental practice, and most dentists reluctantly acquire these skills on an informal need-to-know basis rather than planning to learn them.

Mastery of clinical skills requires dedication, study, a pathway of continual improvement in aesthetic dentistry, along with hands-on and academic knowledge. The same commitment must be given to the business aspect of your dental practice. This requires dedicated time, study, and investment in learning how to effectively run a successful dental business. The management systems in the dental practice need to support your mission, vision, and your goals. If appropriately applied, the investment you make to improve both clinical and management skills will pay for itself quickly and manifold. There will never be a day when you "arrive" at your journey's destination; you will always be "arriving."

Many dentists say that they just want to come into their practices and do the dentistry. They do not want to run or manage the business or their personnel. They feel that this is the most stressful part of the dental practice. Some dentists say that they would love dentistry if it weren't for the challenges and responsibilities related to business, practice management, and personnel. However, these responsibilities are a part of owning a business and must be handled with excellence if the dental practice is to be successful.

Ultimately, if you don't run your business as a healthy and profitable one, you won't be able to stay in business to serve and treat patients. As a dental practice owner, you are expected to be a master of these advanced business and management skills, even though you have not had formal training in these areas. Great people and great businesses reach out to advisors and coaches who are experts in various fields to receive assistance and training in skills that are necessary but heretofore not mastered. Advanced training in the complex area of management is imperative if you are to realize your "ideal" dental practice. Great athletes, performers, leaders, and dentists seek the coaching, support, and encouragement of valued advisors. Do the same.

Write down what you see as the "ideal" dental practice and give yourself permission to pursue that "ideal" (see vision worksheet, Chapter 2). There is no reason why you should not have your "ideal" dental practice, however you define the "ideal." Life is too short and too valuable to settle for anything less. Study the critical factors of the business of dentistry to ascertain the appropriate benchmarks for your dental practice. Define where you are at the present time, where you wish to go, and what or who you need in your life to help you get there. Identify any barriers that might be getting in your way and eliminate those barriers. Don't let anyone (including yourself) or anything prevent you from being all that you can be and from fulfilling your career goals.

Success strategy

Establish your dental practice systems, have outstanding people who administer those systems, and put monitors in place to measure progress to see if you are hitting the benchmarks. If you are not reaching desired goals, be a good leader and take proactive steps to improve systems or performance, or both. This is the only way to assure continuous growth and goal accomplishment.

The critical factors

The following is a look at the major "critical" factors in your dental practice. These are not all of the critical factors, but are major ones: "The Dominant Dozen."

As you review these systems, ask yourself, "What are we doing well?" Then make sure to keep on doing those things. Give positive feedback to your team. Then ask yourself a more difficult question, one that leads to growth: "How can we do everything we are doing a little bit better?" That is the critical and productive question.

The top 12 critical factors. The Dominant Dozen are:
1. Production
2. Collection
3. Accounts receivable
4. Patient financing programs
5. Overhead
6. Scheduling
7. Broken appointments and no-shows
8. Case acceptance
9. Hygiene
10. Practice building: external and internal marketing
11. Team
12. Attitude.

1. Production

Determine your production goal carefully. Don't just pull a figure out of the air. Analyze (perhaps with the help of your accountant or consultant) the monthly costs of running your dental practice. Then add to that the dentist's required and desired salary and compensation (obviously, this is for the dentist's confidential information). This should be your minimally acceptable goal. Add to this figure a margin of profit that you wish to accumulate for an emergency fund, continuing education, or future purchases. As the owner of a business, always be willing to invest in the development of your business and your people. This production goal will go up every year or as your own costs of operation climb.

Schedule toward these predetermined production goals on a daily, weekly, monthly, and yearly basis.

2. Collection

Establish a goal of collecting a minimum of 97 to 98% of production. Some months will exceed this minimally acceptable goal due to pre-payments or collection of past due accounts. However, a 97 to 98% collection benchmark is desirable. The chapter on financing (Chapter 12) explains this in more detail.

According to American Dental Association (ADA) surveys (2010), the national collection average in a dental practice in the United States is 96%. Four percentage points of lost revenue! That 4% loss is enormous. Multiply 4% times the total amount of your production and you can see the magnitude of your loss. This loss impacts the dentist significantly. Staff members are paid, the dental laboratory is paid, suppliers are paid, etc., but whatever you calculated as your lost revenue due to uncollectable revenue comes directly out of the dentist's pocket.

You work too hard to absorb those kinds of losses. Monitor this carefully. If your collection ratios are not in alignment with this recommended benchmark, investigate the reasons behind this "glitch." Then develop specific protocols directed toward correction of the problem. Collection experts will tell you that an account is considered uncollectable if it is 120 days past due and if the person who owes you money has made no effort to pay. Plus, carrying an account on your own books is expensive and time consuming (Jameson, 2005). Low collection ratios will drive your overhead percentage out of proper alignment.

This is your money. You worked hard to produce it. Be committed to collecting all that you produce unless you are doing charitable dentistry by choice, which we advocate.

Note that if you are involved with managed care programs, your collection percentage will be lower. Add your collections with your adjustments to see if you are collecting all that you *can* collect.

3. Accounts receivable

When asked, many dentists do not know (for sure) the total amount of their accounts receivable, nor do they know the percentage of accounts that are 30, 60, 90, or more days old. Accounts receivable means that you have performed the dentistry and that a patient owes you money for that treatment. You may or may not have made a financial agreement, but the balance of the account remains on your books.

One of the reasons that collection percentages are low in the dental industry is because many dentists do not pay attention to the accounts receivable nor do they have a protocol in place for the collection of past due accounts (Jameson, 2005).

Consider moving out of the banking business. Instead of carrying accounts on your own books, which means that you are "loaning" money to your patients, consider getting involved with a patient financing program. Let financial experts manage the credit portion of your dental practice so that you can focus on patient care.

Your accounts receivables should be no more than half of your average monthly production, and that is only if you are accepting assignment of benefits of insurance. That's your benchmark. If you are not accepting assignment of benefits, then you should have no accounts receivable. Zero! Assignment of benefits of private indemnity insurance means that you file the insurance as a service to your patient and the insurance pays you directly. This is relevant to certain countries more than others.

Recent financial information from the ADA (2010) indicates that the average dental practice in the United States receives approximately half of its income from insurance checks. So, if you offer the payment options that we recommend in Chapter 12, you will see that you will have no accounts receivable other than a one-month rollover (or less) of insurance payments. Thus, you should have no more than half of your total monthly production in accounts receivable and that half will be insurance, but only if you are taking assignment of benefits. If you are not taking insurance on assignment, you should have no accounts receivable.

If assignment of benefits of insurance is not applicable in your country, you should have no accounts receivable if you follow the recommended protocols in Chapter 12.

4. Patient financing programs

The issue of cost is the main reason why people do not come to the dentist or do not accept treatment once it has been recommended (Linhart, 2010). Therefore, become involved with a patient financing program. If you are already involved with a program, consider using the program more extensively in your dental practice. Providing a convenient, comfortable payment method is a great service to your patients and is good for the practice as well.

When a dental practice uses a patient financing program to the fullest degree, revenues increase substantially. Increases occur when you introduce the program to your patients, offer it during financial discussions, note the offering of comfortable financing in all of your marketing materials, both internal and external, and communicate effectively about the program to your patients.

Patients will benefit in the following ways:

- They will be able to receive recommended treatment. They will not have to "put off" needed or desired care due to financial constraints.
- They can spread their payments out over a period of time and keep the payments small enough to fit into their family budget.
- They will not owe you any money.
- They will understand their financial obligation and responsibility.
- They can afford to take better care of all members of their families on a more regular basis.

The dental practice will benefit in many ways:

- You will receive your monies in a timely fashion.
- You will gain a much higher level of case acceptance.
- You will be able to do the dentistry that you love to do.
- Your costs of operation will reduce because professionals can run the credit portion of your business at a much lower cost than you would incur if you were running a banking business in your own dental practice (Jameson, 2005).
- Patients will feel better about you because they won't owe you money.
- You will be able to perform procedures that are more costly, such as aesthetic procedures, because patients can spread the payments out over a period of time and not have to come up with the full amount at one time.

5. Overhead

Overhead control is an ongoing "critical factor" for any business. Obviously, when overhead is held in an acceptable alignment, profit margins are also acceptable. Expansion of the profit margin makes it possible to provide increases in salary and/or benefits when and where appropriate. Without an increase in profit margin, these distributed dollars come out of the dentist's pocket rather than from healthy increases in available profits. If and when the entire team begins to work cohesively toward the control of overhead and the increase of profit margin, then increases in salaries can occur for the dentist and for team members.

There are three ways to increase profit margin and lower the percentage of overhead:

- increase production
- decrease costs
- increase fees.

Any of these three entities will increase profit margin. By incorporating all three of these measures, your profit margin increases substantially.

6. Scheduling

Scheduling is a complex and multi-faceted "critical factor" and system within your dental practice. In Chapter 13, we will discuss specific strategies for scheduling aesthetic cases. In some dental practices, being too busy can get in the way of a profitable practice and can be a barrier to scheduling aesthetic cases expediently and properly.

Scheduling methodology must respond to production needs for the dental practice, physical needs of both the patients and the dentists, and the challenges that come with today's busy patients.

Scheduling carefully and succinctly in an organized and streamlined fashion will allow the dentist to reach predetermined production goals most of the time, allowing patients to be treated in a timely fashion. Stress relief and business stability will result.

> You need to control your appointment book rather than having the appointment book control you.

In evaluating the effectiveness of your scheduling system, ask the following questions.

- How far out are we solidly booked into the future?
- When can we schedule a new patient?
- When can we schedule a long aesthetic or comprehensive restorative case?
- When can we schedule a hygiene patient?
- Can we see a periodontal patient quickly and regularly?
- Do we run behind schedule?
- Are we delegating responsibilities when and where possible according to the laws of our state or country?
- Are we exhausted at the end of the day because we have seen so many patients?
- Are our days smooth flowing as well as productive?
- Do scheduling difficulties cause stress on a regular basis?

There is no reason not to have excellent and effective control of your appointment book. It is a difficult and challenging system but one that can be mastered. It is one of the most critical factors.

7. Broken appointments and no-shows

Along with scheduling comes the challenging "critical factor" of managing broken appointments and no-shows. Are you monitoring the number of broken appointments, changes of schedule, or no-shows on a daily basis? You will never know if this is a problem that is impacting your productivity and profitability if you do not track the number of these occurrences. Also track whether or not patients are being rescheduled and if voids are being filled. Do this for both no-shows and canceled or changed appointments.

No-shows and broken appointments can be debilitating for a dental practice. Be clear about what is happening in the practice so that a corrective plan of action can be developed and implemented.

You may have a well-scheduled day that meets your predetermined production goal, but find that the day falls apart for numerous reasons. If voids in the schedule are not filled, or not filled with appointments of similar productivity, your days will fall short of the financial requirement. This becomes stressful for everyone.

While you will never eliminate broken appointments and no-shows, you can reduce them by applying the strategies outlined in Chapter 13. Be interested in reducing broken appointments and no-shows. Do not be complacent regarding this critical factor. You have more control over this than you might realize.

8. Case acceptance

One of the most important critical factors of your dental practice is gaining high levels of case acceptance (see Chapter 10). Be as interested in increasing your case acceptance ratio as you are interested in attracting new patients. As we will discuss in the chapters on marketing, it does you no good to attract new patients into the dental practice only to have patients walk out the door not saying yes to treatment recommendations and not staying actively involved in your hygiene program. If you are losing as many patients each month as you are attracting as new patients, your dental practice will plateau. Growth becomes difficult if you are working so hard to simply maintain your existing dental practice.

Perform a comprehensive diagnosis and design a treatment plan for all patients. Enter these treatment plans into your computer. Then, carefully and regularly follow up on all patients who have dentistry diagnosed and treatment recommendations that have not yet been performed. You will be evaluating several aspects when you begin monitoring this critical factor of your dental practice.

- You will be determining how well you are presenting the cases in the first place. Are patients accepting your recommendations? Or do you need to improve your case presentations?
- How well are you following up on untreated diagnoses? How many of those patients are moving ahead with treatment recommendations?

The fulcrum of your dental practice is comprehensive diagnosis, complete treatment planning, and excellent case presentations for each patient. When you have carefully documented data on every patient, only then is follow-up possible. These three systems are intricately tied together. Everything else will springboard from the following systems:

- thorough diagnosis
- comprehensive treatment planning
- well planned, prepared, and presented consultations.

9. Hygiene

The hygiene department is the lifeblood of your dental practice. This is where you help people achieve oral and dental health and maintain excellent oral hygiene. This is where much of your patient education will take place; not just education about how to brush and floss, but education about periodontal concerns and re-education about diagnosed but incomplete restorative treatment. The hygienist, who usually has a very close bond with patients, can begin talking to a patient about new areas of concern since the last visit. It is here that many aesthetic opportunities can be introduced and discussed with the patient. Many of your aesthetic cases will come right out of your hygiene department when your active patient family discovers what is possible in aesthetic dentistry today (see Chapter 14).

Within your hygiene department there are multiple systems and critical factors:

- What is the hygiene production daily, monthly, yearly?
- What percentage of the overall production of the dental practice is coming from hygiene? Your benchmark should be to have approximately one third of your total practice productivity coming from the hygiene department.
- Hygiene retention: What percentage of your active patients is participating in your hygiene program? Your benchmark is to have approximately 85 to 90% of your active patient family actively involved with hygiene. An active patient is someone who has been to the dental practice to receive treatment within the past 2 years (and this is a generous number).
- If someone has not been in the dental practice within 2 years and you have made a conscientious effort to schedule them for an appointment without success, he/she would be an inactive patient. They may come back to see you one day; perhaps for an emergency or some other need. However, this patient's record can be inactivated. Your marketing efforts that focus on reactivation would be appropriate.
- What percentage of your hygiene production is non-surgical periodontal therapy? Use your procedure analysis report to obtain accurate information on this critical factor. Make note of the number of periodontal procedures you provide on a monthly and yearly basis and the amount of productivity generated by these procedures. Divide this by your total relative hygiene production number. This will give you the percentage of hygiene production coming from periodontal procedures. Your goal should be that approximately 50 to 60% of your hygienic procedures are periodontal in nature.
- How much restorative treatment is coming out of hygiene? Your benchmark is to have 40 to 60% of your restorative treatment and aesthetic cases coming from hygiene patients.

- How many aesthetic procedures or smile makeovers are being scheduled out of your hygiene department? Track this. Depending on how many cases were scheduled last year out of hygiene, set new goals that expand this number. Are you providing educational materials, videos, before and after photography, cameras, etc., for your hygienist so that she can explore aesthetic opportunities with patients? She can open the door for this kind of discussion, evaluation, and/or consultation with your patients.

10. Practice building: external and internal marketing

Develop a strategic plan for marketing and building your dental practice. You want and need to attract an appropriate number of new patients to your dental practice every month and stabilize your existing patient family at the same time. Be interested in both of these vital areas for practice growth and consistency.

Marketing is an ongoing part of your dental practice. Everything you do is marketing and marketing is a part of everything you do. Implement a strategic marketing plan. Educate patients about what is happening in dentistry today and what you are doing to stay on top of the latest and best of dental opportunities (Jameson, 2004). Marketing is practice building.

New patients: Generating *new* business is a critical factor. New patients bring not only themselves to your dental practice but, in many cases, the entire family. The number of new patients you need to generate per month depends on many factors. For example:

- What type of treatment are you providing?
- If you are doing large aesthetic/cosmetic, implant, or reconstruction cases, you will not need as many new patients to fulfill production goals as you would need if you are a general family dental practice.
- How many dentists are in your practice?
- How far out are you already booked? Pre-block your appointment book for new patients. Establish these reserved times according to the number of new patients you are seeing or would like to see. Hold these pre-blocked appointments until about 1 week in advance. If you have not filled those reserved time slots 1 week in advance, you can let them go and fill those spaces with other types of treatment.

Set a goal of seeing your new patients within 2 to 3 weeks from the time they call (or sooner). Having respected pre-blocked appointments will make that possible.

Develop a carefully organized and impressive new patient experience. Determine what you believe would be the best new patient experience. Then, provide this each time a new person enters your dental practice.

Existing patient family: The purpose of your internal marketing program is to help more patients say yes to treatment, stay actively involved in your hygiene program, and refer others to you because of the excellent service and care they received. Track the amount of recommended treatments being diagnosed and presented, and how much is being accepted and scheduled. Develop a program of follow-up on any patient who leaves the dental practice without scheduling an appointment. Not every person says yes the first time they are presented with your recommendations. That does not mean that they will never accept. Follow up and follow through. That's the key. For many people it takes several contacts, substantial education, and time to accept treatment. That's fine. Be there to educate and follow up. You never know who will accept your recommendations.

11. Team

No critical factor, system, or protocol in your dental practice can work effectively if you don't have a great team working together to accomplish the goals that have been established for your practice (see Chapter 4).

Having a great team established and working cohesively together can be the key to productive, fulfilling, fun days. On the other hand, a team that doesn't get along, or that is in constant conflict, or that is just there for the paycheck can be the most stressful part of dentistry (Jameson, 2000).

Do whatever it takes to establish an environment that fosters healthy teamwork. Answer these questions:

- Are you well staffed? Do you have the appropriate number of team members in the right positions so that patient care doesn't suffer, production is not limited, and stress is controlled?
- Do you have current, well-defined, workable descriptions of position responsibilities? Do these descriptions focus on key responsibilities, expected results, and accountabilities?
- Do you have a current personnel policy manual? Has everyone read and agreed to this manual?
- Are your team meetings and daily meetings productive and effective?
- Do you have equitable salary, benefit, and incentive programs in place? Are these healthy for the dental practice as well as for team members?

▶ *Dr Charles Puntillo makes a poignant statement regarding the value of outstanding teamwork.*

"As I go home every evening, the most rewarding feeling that I have from my practice is the fact that all of our team members are going in exactly the same direction, saying the same message, working together as a unit. When we bring new patients into our practice, or treat existing patients, they are absolutely amazed that the practice runs so smoothly. They appreciate the professional quality of all the team members. We do a lot of laughing, a lot of joking around. Our practice is fun. But our commitment to provide quality care extends to every encounter a patient has with any member of our team and excellent dentistry is our benchmark. Our team is proud of that."

Dr Charles Puntillo (interview)

12. Attitude

Hire attitude over any other characteristic. Hire people who have a willing spirit and a positive attitude. Then, provide (1) instruction for the skills required for a position, (2) induction into the systems of your dental practice, and (3) integration of the new person into the culture of your dental practice. A person with a great attitude brings harmony and joy into the day-to-day activities of the workplace while a person with a negative attitude will "bring down" the enthusiasm and energy of everyone else, including patients.

Life is too short not to be surrounded by people who are excited about the dental practice, who are interested in excellence, and who are willing to walk the extra mile to make sure that things go well. Do not let anyone pull you away from your dreams or the pursuit of your ideal dental practice. Life is all about choice. Make a choice to surround yourself with people who have a positive attitude and who are on the same path as you. This is the key to a harmonious and healthy work environment.

Reflect on these questions and answer them honestly:

- Is your team cohesive?
- Is your team goal-oriented?
- Is your team supportive of practice building and practice development? Or, are they comfortable with the status quo?
- Does conflict among your team members cause stress for you or any other member of the team?
- Is communication effective among team members?

Self evaluation

Analyze your own attitude. What are you, individually, doing to lift the morale of your team and of your dental practice? What kind of energy are you bringing to each day? Are you being a leader of yourself, a leader of your team members, and a leader of your patients?

You are a critical factor of the dental practice in your own right. Each member of the team can make or break a relationship with a patient. Each member of the team is as important as every other member of the team. Make a decision each and every day to be an asset to your dental practice. Bring your best self to the dental practice each day. Put out positive energy and positive energy will come right back to you. Your life is a reflection of your thoughts and energy.

25 management systems

There are 25 major systems in your dental practice and many other subsystems. Included here is a listing of those systems that Jameson Management, Inc. has defined as the major systems of your dental practice (Fig 3-1). While there are many critical factors in the dental practice related to these systems, the 12 systems that have been identified here as the "critical factors" are foundational to the health of your practice: The Dominant Dozen. Take the time to evaluate these systems. Monitor them regularly. Certainly, you will want to establish monthly monitors to measure your ongoing progress (see Fig 3-2). How effectively are your systems functioning? Remember to ask two questions: "What is going well?" Make sure you keep doing those things. Then ask yourself, "How can we do this better?" Plan on improving each and every one of these critical factors/systems on an ongoing basis. Being on a path of continuous improvement is the "road to success".

jameson
ADVISORS FOR YOUR DENTAL CAREER

25 Management Systems

"The success of your practice is in direct proportion to the success of your systems" -Cathy Jameson

	☹ ☺
1. Teamwork	1 2 3 4 5 6 7 8 9 10
2. Effective Communication	1 2 3 4 5 6 7 8 9 10
3. Mission / Vision / Goals – Strategic Planning	1 2 3 4 5 6 7 8 9 10
4. Personnel Management	1 2 3 4 5 6 7 8 9 10
5. Organizational Meetings	1 2 3 4 5 6 7 8 9 10
6. Financing	1 2 3 4 5 6 7 8 9 10
7. Insurance Management	1 2 3 4 5 6 7 8 9 10
8. Collections	1 2 3 4 5 6 7 8 9 10
9. Scheduling	1 2 3 4 5 6 7 8 9 10
10. Overhead Control / Fee Analysis	1 2 3 4 5 6 7 8 9 10
11. Monitors	1 2 3 4 5 6 7 8 9 10
12. New Patient Experience	1 2 3 4 5 6 7 8 9 10
13. Diagnosis / Treatment Planning/ Consultations	1 2 3 4 5 6 7 8 9 10
14. Treatment Coordination and Acceptance	1 2 3 4 5 6 7 8 9 10
15. Full Use of Technology and Equipment	1 2 3 4 5 6 7 8 9 10
16. Patient Education	1 2 3 4 5 6 7 8 9 10
17. Clinical Efficiency / Ergonomics	1 2 3 4 5 6 7 8 9 10
18. Documentation	1 2 3 4 5 6 7 8 9 10
19. Advanced Hygiene Program	1 2 3 4 5 6 7 8 9 10
20. Hygiene Retention	1 2 3 4 5 6 7 8 9 10
21. Sterilization / Infection Control	1 2 3 4 5 6 7 8 9 10
22. Marketing / Practice Building	1 2 3 4 5 6 7 8 9 10
23. 5-Star Customer Service	1 2 3 4 5 6 7 8 9 10
24. Building the Cosmetic Aspect of the Practice	1 2 3 4 5 6 7 8 9 10
25. Leadership	1 2 3 4 5 6 7 8 9 10

For more information, contact Jameson at 877.369.5558 or info@jamesonmanagement.com

Fig 3-1 25 systems worksheet.

12 critical factors checklist

1. Production
   - ☐ Determine your production goal daily (calculate this hourly, weekly monthly, and yearly).
   - ☐ Get your accountant to analyze your monthly costs of running a dental practice.
   - ☐ Analyze the required salary and compensation.
   - ☐ Add profit, emergency fund, investment fund for education, equipment.
2. Collection (benchmark: 97 to 98% of production).

MONTHLY MONITOR REPORT
for
JAMESON MANAGEMENT, INC.

Month/Year: ______________________

Dentist/Practice: ______________________

Totals for Practice

Production: ______________________
Days Scheduled with Patients: ______________________
Average Production Per Day: ______________________
Total # of New Patients: __________
# of Comprehensive Evaluations (Code 00150): ______________________

Collection: ______________________
Write Offs: ______________________
Collection %: __________
Accounts Receivable Total: __________ Current: __________

Totals Per Provider

	Dentist A		Dentist B		Total Dentist
Dentist Name:	________		________		
Dentist Production:	________	+	________	=	________
Dentist Days Worked:	________	+	________	=	________
Dentist Avg. per Day:	________		________		________

	Hygienist A		Hygienist B		Total Hygiene
Hygienist Name	________		________		
Hygiene Production:	________	+	________	=	________
Hygiene Days Worked:	________	+	________	=	________
Hygiene Avg. per Day:	________		________		________

Fig 3-2 Monthly monitors report.

3. Accounts receivable (benchmark: no more than half of your average monthly production).
4. Patient financing programs.
5. Overhead.
6. Scheduling.
7. Broken appointments and no shows. Monitor:
   - ☐ The number of broken appointments.
   - ☐ Changes of schedule, no shows on a daily, monthly basis.
   - ☐ Are patients being rescheduled.

- Voids in the schedule that are open and ones that are being filled.

8. Case acceptance
   - Perform comprehensive diagnosis and treatment planning on all patients.
   - Are patients accepting your recommendations?
   - Do you need to improve your case presentations?
   - Follow up on any treatment recommendations not accepted.
   - How many of those patients are moving ahead with treatment recommendations?
   - The target is to have 100% accept recommended treatment.
9. Hygiene
   - What is the hygiene production daily, monthly, and yearly?
   - What percentage of the overall production of the dental practice is coming from hygiene? The target is to have approximately one-third of your total practice productivity coming from the hygiene department.
   - Track how many aesthetic procedures or smile makeovers are being scheduled out of your hygiene department?
   - Hygiene retention: What percentage of your active patients are participating in your hygiene program? The benchmark is to have approximately 85 to 90% of your active patient family actively involved with hygiene.
   - The benchmark for periodontal therapy is to have 50 to 60% of your hygiene procedures be periodontal treatments.
10. Practice building
    - Develop and implement external and internal marketing strategies.
    - Determine how many new patients per month you attract.
    - How many new patients do you actually need?
    - Pre-block your appointment book for new patients.
    - Ensure that you see new patients within 2–3 weeks from when they called the dental practice.
    - Develop a carefully organized and impressive new patient experience.
    - Establish retention systems to make sure that your existing patient family remains actively involved with the dental practice.
11. Team
    - Develop a great team that work together to accomplish the practice goals.
    - Are you well staffed?
    - Are the appropriate number of team members in the right positions so that patient care doesn't suffer, production is not limited, and stress is controlled?
    - Do you have current, well-defined, workable descriptions of position responsibilities? Do these descriptions focus on key responsibilities, expected results, and accountabilities?
    - Do you have a current personnel policy manual? Has everyone read and agreed to this manual?

- ☐ Are your team meetings and morning meetings productive and effective?
- ☐ Do you have equitable salary, benefit, and incentive programs in place?

12. Attitude
    - ☐ Analyze your own attitude.
    - ☐ What are you, individually, doing to uplift the morale of your team and of your dental practice?
    - ☐ What kind of energy are you bringing to each day?
    - ☐ Are you being a leader of yourself, a leader of your team members, and a leader of your patients?
    - ☐ Analyze your team attitude.
    - ☐ Hire people that have a willing spirit and a positive attitude.
    - ☐ Provide instruction for the skills required for a position.
    - ☐ Induct the team member into the systems of your dental practice.
    - ☐ Integrate the new person into the practice culture.

Action steps

1. Define your ideal aesthetic dental practice:
   - ☐ Where are you at the present time?
   - ☐ Define where you wish to go.
   - ☐ What or who you need in your life to help you get there?
   - ☐ Identify any barriers that might be getting in your way.
   - ☐ Eliminate those barriers and obstacles.
2. Review the 12 critical factors as a team: The Dominant Dozen.
3. Determine how you are measuring the success of these 12 factors. If there are areas that need to be more carefully measured, design a plan of action to do so.
4. Evaluate where you are at the present time in these 12 areas and set new goals for the intentional improvement of each area.
5. Spend time reviewing each of the 12 critical factors, one by one. Schedule a series of team meetings related to each individual critical factor. Read and study the chapter or chapters related to each of the 12 critical factors. Develop a plan of action, even if it is one thing, for the purpose of improving each of the 12 factors.
6. Perform the evaluation of your practice using the 25 systems form in this chapter. Have each team member complete the form, assigning a number to each system with 1 being the lowest and 10 being perfection. Then, add up all the numbers and divide by the number of team members who have completed the survey. Determine a plan of improvement for each system that is rated a 7 or less. If a system rates as 8 or higher, keep on doing what you are doing, but be willing to make improvements along the way.
7. Become astute students of each area of the business of your practice and commit to continuous improvement. Do not become complacent or satisfied with the status quo.

8. Determine what is going well. Make sure you keep doing those things. Ask yourself, "How can we do this better?"
9. List improvements that can be made to each of these critical factors/ systems on an ongoing basis.
10. Be on a path of continuous improvement along the "road to success."

References

1. American Dental Association. Survey of Dental Practice – Income from the Private Practice of Dentistry. Chicago, IL: American Dental Association, 2010.
2. Drucker P. The Effective Executive. 4th ed. New York, NY: Harper Collins, 2002.
3. Jameson C. Great Communication Equals Great Production. Tulsa, OK: Pennwell Books, 2004.
4. Jameson C. Collect What You Produce. Tulsa, OK: Pennwell Books, 2005.
5. Jameson C. Controlling Stress in the Dental Profession Through Effective Communication. Oklahoma City, OK: JC Educational Services, 2000.
6. Linhart J. 5 Reasons Why People Do Not Go to the Dentist. New York, NY: Castle Connolly Medical Ltd. EZineArticles, 2010.

4 The Most Critical Factor: The Team

Cathy Jameson and Linda Greenwall

> *"When employers, managers, and supervisors genuinely honor, respect, and trust their people first, they create a nurturing atmosphere that inspires individuals to 'fall in love' with their job. Through this connection, employees become more enthusiastic about their contributions and far more interested in advancing the organization beyond their own level of need."*
>
> *Risa Simon (2006)*

The team

A great team is a group of leaders working cohesively together toward a common set of goals (Jameson, 2004). This cohesive group of leaders realizes that dental practice success is dependent upon each person functioning in a productive manner. Figure 4-1 shows the Jameson Management Team and Figure 4-2 shows Dr Galip Gürel of Istanbul, Turkey working side-by-side with his team. As a group of leaders, each person supports the achievements and successes of other team members and is proud rather than jealous of the accomplishments of teammates. By nurturing the strengths of individuals, the whole organization is strengthened. Positively reinforcing strengths will overcome weaknesses (Jameson, 2010). An outstanding leader identifies the strengths of team members and acknowledges, reinforces, and develops those strengths. Limitless success results from the nurturing of individual talent.

▶ *"My senior associate has been with me for 20 years and my senior assistant has been with me for 23 years. This longevity produces a family atmosphere, which we like and our patients like. Every member of my team has started his/her working life in my practice. This special condition helped me to create my own concept of a practice and to infuse my own working style to my team members.*
Personally I am a dynamic, innovative person whose aim is to discover

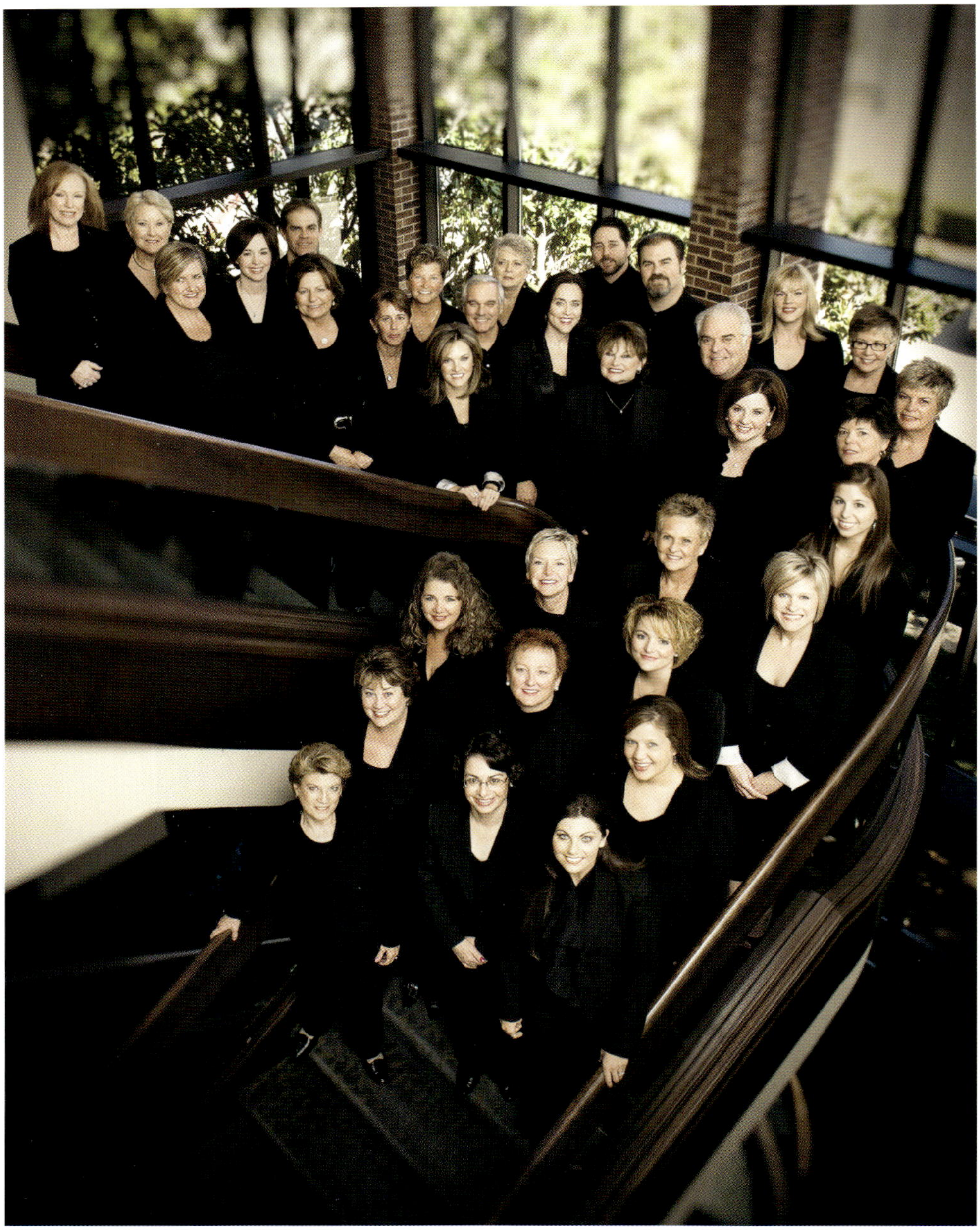

Fig 4-1 Jameson Management Team.

Fig 4-2 Dr Galip Gurel with a member of his clinical team.

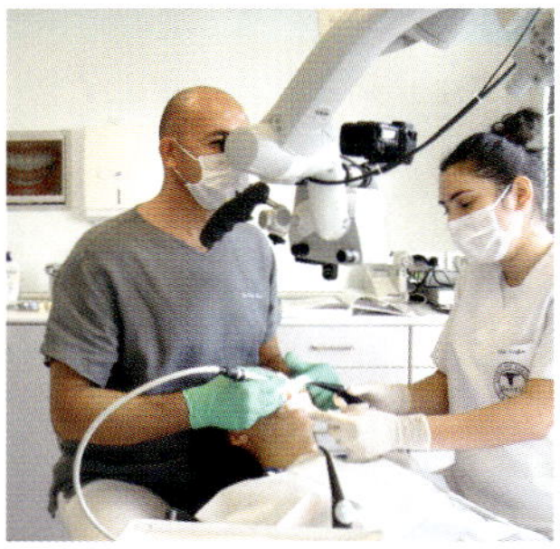

and use new techniques, obtain better and more beautiful results and to never forget treating the patient as a human being and not only as a client [Fig 4-2]. This approach is approved and very well applied by my team members who care about the practice as if it were their own business."

Dr Galip Gurel (interview)

Characteristics of an outstanding team

There are 14 specific characteristics of those teams that perform at a high level, work well together, and are enthusiastic and dedicated to their dentist, patients, and practice. An outstanding dental team:

1. is made up of the right team members

2. possesses a positive attitude
3. is one that works well with different personality styles
4. has a clear sense of mission and purpose
5. is goal focused
6. supports accountability
7. has clear, constructive lines of communication
8. supports a trusting climate
9. has the ability to face and solve problems
10. can make decisions
11. has productive, dynamic team meetings
12. welcomes a network of outside resources
13. is rewarded for work well done
14. has focus and energy.

1. An outstanding team is made up of the right team members

In the research for his book, *Good to Great* (2001), Jim Collins discovered that getting the right people in place is the number one characteristic of companies who are ultimately successful. Collins (2001) writes, "We thought that people were a company's greatest asset. We were wrong. The right people are a company's greatest asset." Once the right people are in place on a team, investing in the development of those people becomes some of the best money a dentist can authorize.

> *"As a leader, working to develop and support my team is one of my greatest joys and one of the most productive things I do."*
>
> *Dr Charles Puntillo (interview)*

The first challenge is to hire correctly, which is easier said than done! Hire slowly and hire correctly. When you have a change of staff, the departing team person needs to be replaced. If your dental practice is growing, new positions will need to be established.

Before you start looking for a new team person, sit down individually or as a team, and write a description of the person you would like to add to the team. What characteristics will this person possess? Describe the attitude you desire. What skills are necessary? Hire characteristics and attitude first. You can always teach the skills.

Once you have defined the characteristics of the ideal team member, write a job description. Be very specific about what you want this person to do. The description of the position responsibility will be critical during the hiring and training phases. The job description should contain not only what a person is to do, but the expected end results of his/her performance.

Now you are ready to go to the world with your invitation for employment. There are numerous places to find applicants. Here are a few suggestions:

- recommendations from other team members
- people in your community or dental practice

- dental society magazines
- dental society employee listings, dental assistant or dental hygiene schools
- website placement services
- newspaper ads
- employment agencies.

Your advertisement should be interesting, punchy, abbreviation-free, enticing, and authentic. Encourage the candidate to email a résumé. Call your top choices to schedule the initial interview and complete an application. The person making these calls should spend a few minutes on the phone with the candidate, taking notes about the person's telephone etiquette and vocal quality.

Have the candidates come to the office for a brief interview with a qualified team member and a brief interview with the dentist. They must complete an application (one that follows all appropriate legal specifications). Assess:

- Did they think on their feet?
- Can they write well, spell, and punctuate?
- How was their personal appearance?
- Did they prepare well for their interview?
- Were they well groomed and manicured?
- Did they make a professional presentation of themselves?

If they do not come to their interview well-prepared, do not think they will change and come to work in any better condition. You are building an aesthetic dental practice. Your personnel must be a reflection of your commitment to excellence, quality, and professionalism. Everything you do makes a first and lasting impression on every patient, and that includes the professional appearance of your team. Do not expect people to trust your words about aesthetics if everything and everyone in your office does not present the same message (Fig 4-3).

From these applicants, select your top two or three candidates, and ask them to return for a final interview. This interview will be a bit longer, more detailed, more specific about the position responsibility, salary, benefits and all pertinent details. The interviewer should do about 30% of the talking, which leaves the remaining 70% to the interviewee. This is true in both interview one and two. Ask open-ended questions, ones that put the person at ease and invite conversation. An open-ended question cannot be answered with a yes or no.

Each person on the team has the opportunity to make or break a relationship with a patient. Therefore, excellence on the part of each team member is essential. Kindness, grace, poise, and professionalism are mandatory.

▶ *"I hire individuals that have a warm caring demeanor and natural people skills. There are some people that you are drawn to because they have that way about them. They have an excellent communicative ability both*

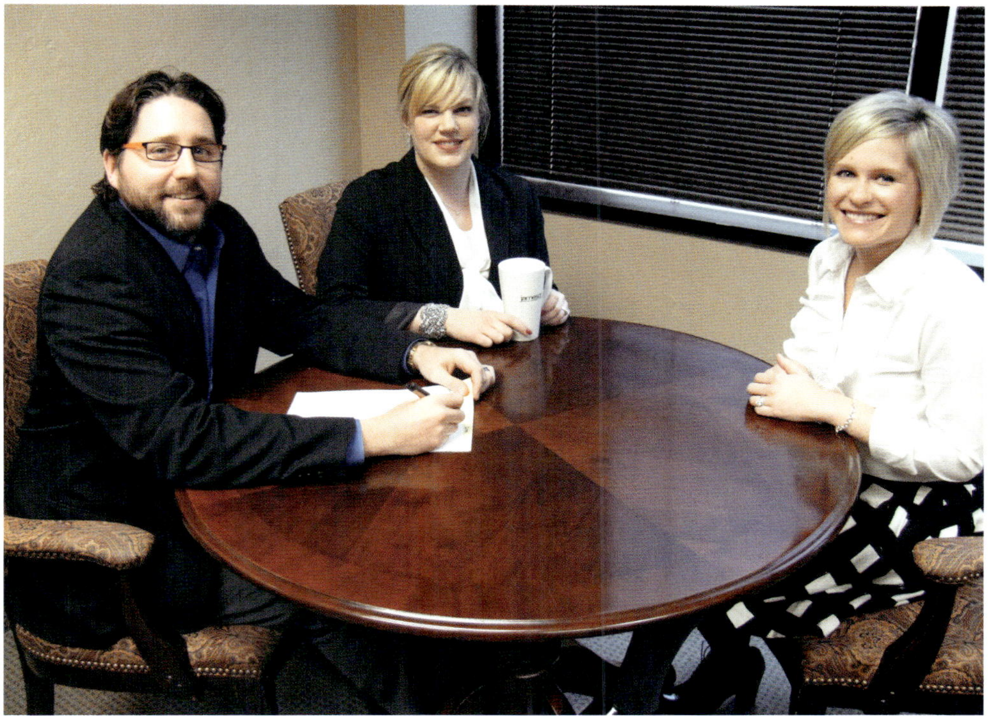

Fig 4-3 Conducting an effective interview.

verbally and non-verbally and bring a great attitude to work every day. If I can find somebody like that, no matter what kind of work they have been in historically, I try to hire that person and then place them on a developmental path that supports their growth."

Dr Charles Puntillo (interview)

2. An outstanding dental team possesses a positive attitude

Do not accept negativity. Negativity will sap the energy out of your dental practice and before you know it, one negative attitude spreads to two, then three, and so on. Attitude truly is everything.

Risa Simon, founder and CEO of Simon Says Seminars, made the following observation regarding attitude in the dental practice: "Having an 'ill-fit' among the group exacerbates the 'error factor' and heightens emotionalism by literally 'contaminating' team effort. A great core team is sabotaged by 'ill-fit' newcomers; or conversely, newcomers are sabotaged by 'ill-fit' long-timers. These types of dysfunctions damage the health of any organization. When these dysfunctions are ignored by management, they can spread like an infectious disease, causing irreversible damage to the entire organization. Likewise, their residual effects can lie dormant for years and suddenly emerge when least expected" (Simon, 2006).

As you develop your vision, make sure that you communicate that vision to your team members and that everyone is on board. They cannot get on board with you if they are unsure what is going on, the direction you are taking, and how their role fits into the development plan. Make sure that you have "the right people on the bus, the wrong people off the bus, and the right people in the right seats" (Collins, 2001). It is better to have the right people in the right seats doing the right things in the right way and with the right attitude.

3. An outstanding dental team is one that works well with different personality styles

Each member of the team has a unique personality. One of the challenges faced in the workplace is to learn how to work effectively with others, in spite of personality differences. In fact, a great team is actually made up of a combination of each of the different personality styles. The strengths of one person may support an area of need in another person. People are not going to change their personality. They can, certainly, develop areas of weakness and nurture areas of strength. People can work to modify mannerisms, but a personality is established early on in life. A key element for cohesiveness in the team is to learn about and appreciate the differences of the individuals and learn how to work with each.

The ability to work well with different personalities applies to patient relationships as well as team relationships. Each of your patients has their own unique personality and the better you learn to adjust and flex according to their personality, the better your relationship with those patients will be (Jameson, 2004).

4. An outstanding dental team has a clear sense of mission and purpose

This was covered extensively in Chapter 2 on Mission, Vision, Goals. Integrate these principles into your team development. Stephen Covey writes in his book, *Principle-Centered Leadership*: "A personal mission statement based on correct principles becomes a personal constitution, the basis for making the major life-directing decisions, the basis for making decisions in the midst of the circumstances and emotions that affect our lives. It empowers individuals with timeless strength in the midst of change" (Covey, 1992).

5. An outstanding dental team is goal focused

The guidelines for becoming goal focused are outlined in Chapter 2. Read and reread this section for the purpose of integrating goal setting into your personal and professional life.

People in the workplace today want to be involved. They want to know the goals of the dental practice so that their performance can support those goals. They will be more vital to the organization if they can participate in the creation of goals. The activities required to carry out tasks that are a part of the plan of action will make more sense if individuals on the team are clear as to how their role impacts the whole. This is an essential element of motivation.

The connection between one person and every other person on a team becomes obvious when the responsibilities of goal fulfillment include all team members and when each person's role is held in esteem and importance. Teamwork and leadership are connected to the overall productivity of the organization (Kotter, 2008).

6. An outstanding dental team supports accountability

People in a productive organization hold themselves accountable and hold each other accountable, as well. Certainly, if someone on the team does not fulfill the obligations of their position, this could have a negative impact on everyone else. A person may not be able to fulfill their role responsibilities if a teammate does not do what they are supposed to do. One person is not isolated in the dental practice. Each person's activities are connected and intertwined with the activities of everyone else.

Job descriptions need to be revised and updated on a regular basis. These descriptions of position responsibility will give people the guidelines they need to perform well and to realize the end results they are expected to accomplish. Someone cannot really be held accountable if they are not clear about expectations and if the results of their work are not monitored.

7. An outstanding dental team has clear, constructive lines of communication

Most of the interpersonal problems that occur among dental personnel relate to poor or missing communication. A study of communication is worthwhile, including communication within work relationships. These relationships are made or broken by the effectiveness of communication. Good communication translates to good relationships with patients. Study and practice good communication with each other and your communication with patients will improve proportionately.

"Communication is the bottom line of success within a dental practice" (Jameson, 2007). Communication includes listening with respect rather than with judgment. It includes speaking your mind in a way that gets your message across while honoring the other person.

8. An outstanding dental team supports a trusting climate

Team members must feel safe. The basic requirements of a person are safety and security (Maslow, 1998). Team members must know that they will not be reprimanded in front of other team members or patients. They must know that if there is a problem, there will be an honest discussion of the problem with the goal of developing a solution. People will dive into a well of fear if they are unsure about the security of their job. Dentists need to speak to the team about areas of needed improvement so that the team member has a chance to develop with appraisals, assessments, and general discussions. Continuous feedback will prove valuable in this process.

9. An outstanding dental team has the ability to face and solve problems

Good communication also supports problem solving. Every business encounters problems. Most relationships encounter problems at some time. The difference between being successful or not in these relationships is the ability to identify and solve the problem. Ignoring a problem and hoping that it will go away can lead to the dissolution of the relationship. Relationships are honored when honesty and commitment support a willingness to face and solve problems. Communication skill is an asset in this process.

While you may not always agree with a member of your team and you may hold a difference of opinion, in a respectful manner listen to another person's ideas without criticizing them for that idea. Criticism of a person's thoughts and ideas will squelch creativity and stop people from participating. Trust evolves from open honest discussion.

10. An outstanding dental team can make decisions

The ability to make decisions in a timely manner is a characteristic of an outstanding team with an outstanding leader. It is important to gather the facts related to a decision that needs to be made, but know when enough is enough! Zig Ziglar (1991) says that most people are stifled due to "paralysis by analysis."

Bossidy and Charan (2002), in their book entitled *Execution*, identify the inability to make decisions "quickly enough" as one of the major reasons that CEOs fail. Be an outstanding CEO or leader by learning the skills of clear decision making. Be willing to "pull the trigger" when the time is right.

Some of the reasons why people avoid making decisions are as follows (similar to the reasons people do not write their goals):

- fear of failure
- attitude
- perfectionism
- fear of hurting someone
- lack of confidence.

Think about your own ability to make decisions. If you procrastinate in this area, study the above listed barriers to decision making and make effort to overcome those factors that may keep you from moving forward as quickly as you desire. You will have many decisions to make as you progress on this journey of building your aesthetic dental practice. Get your mind ready. Build your own confidence. Make decisions. Your leadership is dependent upon your ability to do so.

11. An outstanding dental team has productive, dynamic team meetings

When our audiences are asked if they hold team meetings, most participants answer in the affirmative. However, when asked how many think their team meetings are dynamic, productive, and fun, rarely does a hand go up! Certainly, holding effective meetings is also system based.

There are different types of meetings that are relevant to your dental practice and that will support your growth goals: (1) daily huddles (morning meetings), (2) regular team meetings, and (3) quarterly brain trust meetings where you take time away from the dental practice to do strategic planning and where you practice new skills or work on the improvement of systems.

Place regular team meetings on your schedule and honor those meetings. These meetings are times you reserve to communicate with each other, discuss ideas that may arise related to the development of the dental practice and where solutions to challenges can be developed. Encourage the participation of all team members and honor each person for their idea, even if it differs from yours.

> *"To maintain the team spirit, the internal communication is really important which is why once in a week we set a meeting with our entire team and discuss and evaluate the issues of the week and to keep the dynamism of the work."*
>
> *Dr Galip Gurel (interview)*

12. An outstanding dental team welcomes a network of outside resources

In the sophisticated world of aesthetic dentistry, it is impossible for any one person or any one team to know everything. You will surround yourself with a team of professionals who will support you on your path to building the aesthetic aspect of your dental practice. As a wise business owner, invite coaches in the various areas of your dental practice to provide training and education for you and your team.

You will need clinical, technological, marketing, communication, and management coaches. Take responsibility for building dynamic relationships with these coaches and advisors. Develop interactive relationships with your ceramic specialists and product experts. Some of these coaches will come to you in your office and work one on one with you and your team. Some of your coaches will be a part of a continuing education organization, including universities. Access people in your life who can be a part of your progress and growth. These will be people who possess expertise beyond your own.

> *"Learn from people who have mastered a skill and know more than you."*
>
> *Dr Ron Goldstein (interview)*

This network of resources will be a part of your team. They are only a phone call away.

13. An outstanding dental team is rewarded for work well done

In a study by Dr Lawrence Lindahl (1949), which is a study that has been duplicated over time with the same results, participants rated money as a motivator, but not the top motivator (please see further discussion in the following section, "What team members want most"). Appreciation is rated as the number one desired aspect of a job in order for a person to find and retain fulfillment in the workplace. Identify what your team considers appropriate rewards for the accomplishment of goals. They may set goals that are rewarded with bonuses, time off, trips, dinner together, gift certificates. As a leader it is important to remember that feedback and positive reinforcement are considered the most important reward by people in the workplace today. People will leave your dental practice for a lack of appreciation long before they will leave to make more money down the street.

Identify what you consider a motivator. Then, identify what motivates your team. Integrate the principles of motivation into your dental practice and know that people feel honored when their work is acknowledged and appreciated.

"We set high standards in our practice. We want our team members to function independently, and we want them to function cohesively as a team. We respect our team members. We give them feedback all the time, feedback for needed improvement and positive reinforcement for each step they take toward predetermined goals. We want them to be successful and to develop a sense of co-ownership for the practice. Being recognized for their good work is motivational. Being a part of a team that provides a great service is motivational. Being rewarded financially for work well done is motivational. We have a team bonus system through which everybody shares when we work together and reach and exceed our goals."

Dr Charles Puntillo (interview)

14. An outstanding team has focus and energy

When a team is clear about the mission and vision of the "ideal" dental practice, the practice goals, the plans of action that have been developed, and when they are confident that their role on the team is as valuable as anyone else's role, energy is exuded.

Focus the energy and talent of the individual members of the team on a common set of goals and watch your dental practice stream ahead. There is no limit to the goals that you can reach when your talents and those of your team are focused on a common set of goals. Work becomes play when people on your team, including the dentist, are excited about those goals and find personal fulfillment and joy not only from the reaching of the goal but also from the journey toward the goal. People don't dread going to work. They look forward to it. Focus and energy: two key elements of an outstanding dental team.

Integrating the right team members

Once you have hired the right person, spend quality time integrating this new team member into your dental practice and to his or her job responsibilities. No matter how long someone may have been in dentistry, if they change dental practices, everything they are used to doing may change. This does not mean that experience is useless. Not at all. However, every dental practice is unique, and the new person must be allowed to understand what you do, how you do it, and why you do it a certain way.

In the first few days of a person's employment, go over the personnel issues: how and when payroll will be distributed, specifics about the benefit package, hours of work, attire, etc., all of which will be documented in the policy manual and employee handbook. The new employee should sign a form stating that he or she has read the manual and agrees to cooperate with the given protocols. Create a personnel file, and add it to the other files of all employees.

Now, begin the training by reading the job description and prioritizing each responsibility. Then, design an induction training program. Decide what will be studied first. Schedule non-patient time for instruction. On-the-job training will only go so far. If you have a busy dental practice and do not schedule non-patient training time, you are asking for trouble.

A new person should know what is expected of them, how each system should be managed and the acceptable time frames for the completion of tasks. With this knowledge, the new person will work more confidently, will make fewer mistakes, and will be productive more quickly with carefully orchestrated training. They will appreciate the orientation, training time, and your effort to integrate them gracefully into the team.

Don't wait until 3 months have passed to give the new employee a performance review. Give one on a daily or weekly basis. Ask what things are going well. Then ask what areas create confusion or uncertainty. Give further instruction, ask how you can help, and answer any questions. It is critical that the new employee understands that asking questions is encouraged. Otherwise, things will keep being done the same way, and that way may not be correct.

During this initial phase of employment, make a special effort to integrate your new person into the team. Go to lunch as a group. Have a meal at someone's house, and invite the families. Have a retreat where you go over the dental practice vision/mission, the practice goals, communication skills, and communication avenues, etc. Orientation, training, and integration can make the difference as to whether or not a person stays on board with you. People want to know what they are to do, how they are to do it, what you expect of them, what they can expect of you, all financial issues, and that they are accepted and valued.

Keeping those good employees, and keeping them happy!

According to Frederick Herzberg (1999), there are two sets of factors affecting an employee's performance. The first set relates to the work environment itself. Usually, an employee's dissatisfaction will occur due to discontent about one (or more) of what follows below. Complaints will be centered on these issues:

- company policy and administration
- supervision
- interpersonal relations with peers, supervisors, and subordinates
- working conditions
- salary
- status
- job security.

The second set of factors, according to Herzberg, are motivators and deal with the issues of job satisfaction and job fulfillment. These are the factors that increase productivity in an employee and encourage longevity:

- achievement
- recognition
- the work itself (interesting and challenging)
- advancement
- responsibility.

Herzberg found that workers might remain in an environment with only the first set of factors in existence, but these workers experienced reduced job satisfaction, which resulted in lowered productivity. Unless motivating factors such as challenge, interest, and recognition were introduced, performance did not excel. Staff members who receive sizable challenges and motivation must be rewarded commensurate with their work and the success of the dental practice. These two sets of factors go hand in hand to establish satisfied workers. There is a need for reward, motivation, and/or challenge in order for a person's skills and talents to be maximized in the workplace (Herzberg, 2007).

Another factor that affects productivity is an individual's character. Does this person possess an inner drive to succeed? Does this person want and need achievement? Is this person a self-starter? One of the conflicts we see in the workplace is when a person lacking the inner drive for achievement is placed in a highly challenging position. Conversely, the opposite scenario can breed dissatisfaction if a self-starter, who thrives on and needs challenge, is placed in a stifling environment. If this person, talented and ambitious, is not allowed to create and is not given responsibility, discouragement and frustration result. This is often the person who leaves dentistry for a more fulfilling career.

As is often the case within a dental practice, a person may be misplaced for peak performance. In other words, a person who does not excel in one position might be excellent in another position within the dental practice. Thus, misplacement can negatively affect performance and job satisfaction.

An excellent leader/manager of a dental team will give individual team members a chance to grow both financially and personally. In *In Search of Excellence*, Peters and Waterman write "Get the incentives right, and productivity will follow. Incentives can take many forms, ranging from monetary reward to a pat on the back to self-esteem from task responsibility" (Peters and Waterman, 1982).

Motivating your team

Synonyms for the word "motivation" from *Roget's Thesaurus* (2011) are "helpfulness, support, assurance, encouragement, comfort, urging, enlivening."

Motivation comes from within. A person must have both the aptitude and the attitude that make performance excellence a possibility and a probability. Then, in an environment of positive reinforcement, open communication, camaraderie, creativity, and appreciation, people can flourish.

Psychologists and educators have discovered that people learn and thrive in an environment of positive reinforcement. Positive reinforcement acknowledges or rewards constructive behavior. Simply defined, positive reinforcement means to note behavior (or performance) that exemplifies the desired outcome or behavior that is moving in the direction of the desired result.

Dr Michael LeBoeuf (1985), in his bestseller *The Greatest Management Principle in the World*, writes "That which is rewarded is repeated." The goal needs to be to identify those behaviors you desire and make a point to reinforce those. Thus, you will see those behaviors being repeated.

How do you apply the principle of positive reinforcement?

The following summarizes many of the concepts previously introduced. These steps will make it possible for you to integrate or more fully develop these proven motivation principles into your dental practice.

Step 1: Make sure that people on your team are clear about performance objectives. Everyone needs to be crystal clear about job descriptions: what they need to do, how they need to do it, time parameters for completion of tasks, and why their performance is crucial to the performance of other team members and to the health and well being of the dental practice as a whole.

Step 2: Monitors should be developed for team members, dentists, and business managers to assess and evaluate progress. These monitors are like a thermometer that takes the temperature of any particular "system" in your dental practice. Goals and objectives need to be clear so that team members who are administering the various systems will be able to see where they are in relationship to the desired goal.

Step 3: Make sure that you get together with each team member on a regular basis to review these monitors, the system, and their performance. (This can be done at team meetings or during one-on-one meetings with various members of the team, during performance appraisals.)

Step 4: Acknowledge progress of any team member, no matter how great or small the progress. Behavior that has accomplished a goal or behavior that is moving toward that goal is worthy of a compliment and a sincere acknowledgement. When you take the time to note that forward movement, you will solidify that performance modality. "That which is rewarded is repeated."

Dale Carnegie's (2009) definition of a compliment is, "A statement of appreciation backed up by evidence." When you compliment someone in this manner you give positive reinforcement and acknowledge your pleasure with a certain performance result. This will give the recipient of the compliment clear direction about what pleases you. Remember, people want feedback. This will give them incentive to continue in the same manner.

Step 5: There can be physical rewards for the accomplishment of a goal, if you decide on this strategy. This can be done individually, or the entire team can be rewarded for the accomplishment of a team-defined goal. If you choose to develop this type of system, take the time to think it through carefully. Make sure that any reward system is fair and equitable, both to the individuals and to the dental practice. Be sure that no system, including a reward system, pits one person against another.

Step 6: There are benefits to a specifically defined reward system, one that people can work toward. But there are also benefits to intermittent rewards. Immediate reinforcement for work well done is proven to be powerful in motivating people.

What do team members want most?

Dr Lawrence Lindahl (1949) conducted an enlightening study of motivation, mentioned previously, in which he and his research team performed a two-sided study to determine (1) what team members want most, and (2) what employers think their employees want most.

Table 1 Studies conducted by Dr Lawrence Lindahl (1949)

	Leaders/managers	Employees
Good wages	1	5
Job security	2	4
Promotion/growth opportunities	3	7
Good working conditions	4	9
Interesting work	5	6
Personal loyalty to workers	6	8
Tactful disciplining	7	10
Full appreciation for work done	8	1
Sympathetic to personal problems	9	3
Feeling in on things	10	2

Table 1 contains the results of the study. While Dr Lindahl's study was originally performed in 1949, it has been repeated with the same results (Richardson, 2003).

Notice that employers (leaders/managers) thought money was the number one motivator and appreciation was number eight. However, employees said that appreciation was number one, and money was number five. Money is important, but not nearly as important as appreciation.

Positive reinforcement can take on many faces. However, no reinforcement, no reward, no bonus, no physical gift is more valuable than your sincere acknowledgement of excellent performance. People would rather have a "pat on the back" than almost anything else. Show someone on your team genuine appreciation and they will walk the extra mile time and time again. Money is important and is a motivator. However, money is not usually the major motivator of people on a dental team. Feeling appreciated far outweighs any other type of reward and is the ultimate motivator.

Study the aspects of motivation that are outlined in this book and determine what and how these motivators are impacting your dental practice. In order to move your practice into a higher level of sophistication and to develop it into a highly acclaimed aesthetic dental practice, you want a committed team to work alongside you toward the vision you have designed.

In summary

Cindy Butler, Business Administrator and Treatment Coordinator for Dr Charles Puntillo, epitomizes the principles of teamwork taught in this chapter.

▶ *"First, we truly make a commitment to this office and take ownership of it. We do not work here just as employees working for a paycheck. I, as the office manager, started taking more and more continuing education to learn the necessary skills of business and personnel management to be able to carry out my responsibilities more effectively. The best decision we ever made was to bring Practice Management advisors into our office: Jameson Management. Once we put the 25 Management Systems of Jameson into place, our office productivity and collections skyrocketed and stress was greatly reduced. [See Chapter 3, The Critical Factors of the Business of Dentistry.]*

"Dr Puntillo and I realize the value of a positive, constructive attitude on the team. It is important to hire enthusiastic, motivated people with positive attitudes. One negative person can bring the whole team down, as we have learned the hard way. Working well as a team takes a long time and a lot of hard work so we don't want a team member leaving because they don't feel appreciated or feel that they are in a dead end job. We want them to feel invested in the practice and respected for the professionals that they are. We do not tolerate gossip. That does nothing to promote a healthy environment.

"We have written very specific job descriptions and expect every team member to become an expert in their responsibilities. We insist on continuing education and goal setting. Our office meetings are extremely important in monitoring our progress toward the achievement of our goals. It gives the team a sense of purpose and responsibility, and also gives all of us a clear sense of pride when we have been successful. We celebrate our victories."

Cindy Butler (interview), Business Administrator and Treatment Coordinator for Dr Charles Puntillo

Action steps

1. Evaluate the size and the roles of your team. Discover whether or not you have the appropriate number of team members to (a) see patients in a timely fashion, (b) provide optimum customer service and patient care, and (c) have control of stress. If you are either under- or overstaffed, make necessary changes.
2. Study the art of hiring and integrating a new team member into your dental practice and use these skills any time a new team member is hired.
3. Review the 14 characteristics of an outstanding team. At a team meeting, conduct your own evaluation of the 14 characteristics. Ask yourselves the following questions: "Which of these characteristics do we epitomize? Which ones could benefit from improvement?" Then, design a plan of action (goal activation, Chapter 2) of how you will work on improving these areas.
4. Study the motivation section and determine which motivational factors are in place in your dental practice. Then, identify ways in which your team can experience intensified motivation. Put these into effect.
5. Practice giving positive reinforcement as a part of the culture of your organization. Write out at least one note of appreciation, as defined by Dale Carnegie (2009), and give this note to your teammate.

1. Bossidy L, Charan R. Execution: The Discipline of Getting Things Done. New York, NY: Crown Business, 2002.
2. Carnegie D. How to win Friends and Influence People. New York, NY: Simon and Schuster, 2009.
3. Collins J. Good to Great. New York, NY: HarperCollins Publishers, 2001.
4. Covey S. Principle-Centered Leadership. New York, NY: Fireside, 1992.
5. Gurel G. The Science and Art of Porcelain Laminate Veneers. London: Quintessence Publishing, 2003.
6. Herzberg F. Motivational Theory: Hygiene Theory and Motivation. Available at: http://westrek.hypermart.net/maslow/od_hr_06.htm. WesTrek Webs, 1999.
7. Herzberg F. The Motivation to Work. New Brunswick, NJ: Transaction Publishers, 2007.
8. Jameson C. Great Communication Equals Great Production. Tulsa, OK: Pennwell Books, 2004.
9. Jameson C. Leadership Symposium. Oklahoma City, OK: JC Educational, 2007.
10. Jameson C. The Impact of Training in Transformational Leadership on the Productivity of a Dental Practice [dissertation]. Minneapolis, MN: Walden University, 2010.
11. Kotter J. A Sense of Urgency. Boston, MA: Harvard Business School Press, 2008.
12. LeBoeuf M. The Greatest Management Principle in the World. New York: Penguin Group, 1985.
13. Lindahl L. What makes a good job? Personnel, 25 January 1949.
14. Maslow A. Maslow on Management. New York, NY: John Wiley and Sons, 1998.
15. Peters T, Waterman Jr R. In Search of Excellence. New York, NY: Warner Books, 1982.
16. Richardson M. Rewards, recognitions that make cents. California CPA 2003;71.
17. Roget PM. Roget's Thesaurus of English Words and Phrases. Niche Edition, 2011.
18. Simon R. TeamFirst! Scottsdale, AZ: Simon Says Solutions, 2006.
19. Ziglar Z. Ziglar on Selling. Nashville, TN: Oliver-Nelson Books, 1991.

5 Internal Marketing

Cathy Jameson, Linda Greenwall, and Misty Absher Clark

> *"Implementing internal marketing strategies in your practice on a regular basis will not only help patient retention, but will also increase case acceptance and encourage existing patients to refer friends and family to you."*
>
> *Misty Absher Clark,*
> *VP of Creative Services, Jameson Management, Inc.*

Building your dental practice

Proper internal marketing and promotion is vital to building an aesthetic dental practice. This is where trust is built, seeds are planted, and the groundwork is laid to prepare patients to hear your message. Patients need to hear, see, and experience your message five to seven times before they will act upon it. That message is learned externally (referral from a friend, an advertisement, website, etc.) and continues to spread internally. What patients have learned about you from external sources, including personal referral, must match what they actually experience with you once contact has been made with the dental practice. Then through hard work and by implementing the systems laid out in this book, the message will continue, because your patients will want to refer their friends, family, and colleagues to you based on their own positive experience. Without strong and consistent internal marketing, your dental practice will never meet its maximum potential.

If you do not have your internal marketing working properly, your external marketing will not matter. Patients may come to you because of external marketing protocols, but if their experience with you is not excellent and does not meet their needs and expectations, they will not say "yes" to treatment, will not stay with you, and certainly will not refer.

Your goal should be to access 70% of all new patients from personal referrals. As such, you can see why your internal marketing is so important. You want people to come and to stay. You do not want people to come into your practice only to fall through the cracks. If you are losing as many people each month as you are receiving as new patients, your productivity will plateau. You want the marketing and management of your dental practice to create what follows below. A comprehensive checklist for your internal marketing is shown in Appendix 5-1. The ideal dental patients:

- come to you as new patients in the appropriate numbers for your dental practice
- accept treatment
- agree to the fee and pay willingly
- schedule and keep appointments
- stay actively involved through your hygiene department
- refer others to you.

Dr Ken Blanchard, in his book entitled *Raving Fans*, teaches that having satisfied clients is not enough. Rather, he encourages businesses to create "raving fans," people who receive everything they expected from you, and a little bit more, every time they have an encounter with you, your team, and your business (Blanchard & Bowles, 1993). The six steps above reflect the creation and maintenance of a raving fan in your dental practice.

You need your patients. The good news is that they need you, too. They need you to take care of their oral health and to make their smiles radiant. To make this relationship work, internal marketing protocols need to be in order.

What defines internal marketing?

Internal marketing is geared towards your existing patient base and the activities that you undertake inside your dental practice. Everything you do in the practice is an aspect of internal marketing. Taking care of your patients is the most important thing you do. Providing quality care and excellent customer service is good marketing. Always remember that the first step of good marketing is a well-managed dental practice.

There are seven key areas on which you can focus your internal marketing efforts:

- job descriptions
- new patient phone call
- welcome packet
- smile evaluation
- the greeting area
- photography
- internal marketing campaigns.

Job descriptions

A well-managed dental practice has all systems set up to run smoothly and effectively and has team members who consistently administer those systems. Each member of the team must know exactly what they are supposed to do, how they are to perform each task, what results are expected, and what is expected of them (see Chapter 4).

In Chapter 3 on "Critical Factors," we included a list of 25 major management systems (see Fig 3-1). In the "Action steps" section, you were encouraged to complete an exercise. Review the assignment and determine the team rating of your systems. This is a good time to evaluate what you are doing, clarify goals, and develop new strategic plans for practice development.

Make sure that everyone is clear about the goals that have been set for each of the critical factors. Then, review your job descriptions or, as we prefer to call them, position responsibilities. Who is doing what and how? Is everything being done that needs to be done? Does someone have the ultimate responsibility for each system? Are there too many "hands in the pot?" Do people "assume" that someone else is going to complete a task or do people understand their own individual responsibilities within each system?

Job descriptions do not remain stagnant. They change as the dental practice changes. As you add more aesthetic cases to your dental practice, the responsibilities of each team member will change and evolve, just as your systems will do. "Tell your team what you are doing as you develop company mission and value statements and ask for their ideas and feedback. If employees don't feel that they shape the mission of the company they will become resentful" (Erickson, 2004).

Managers benefit from defining job descriptions and role responsibilities in order to reduce the "cognitive, emotional, and physical strain" that some employees experience. Extreme stress, extensive overload of responsibility, and ergonomic challenges can all lead to job dissatisfaction. Managers need to encourage the improvement of skills for employees so they can develop a sense of confidence and fulfillment in their work and realize their value to the organization. This value to the organization must be realistically outlined, detailed, and accomplished so that positive feedback on effective performance is a reality (Van Vianen & Fischer, 2002).

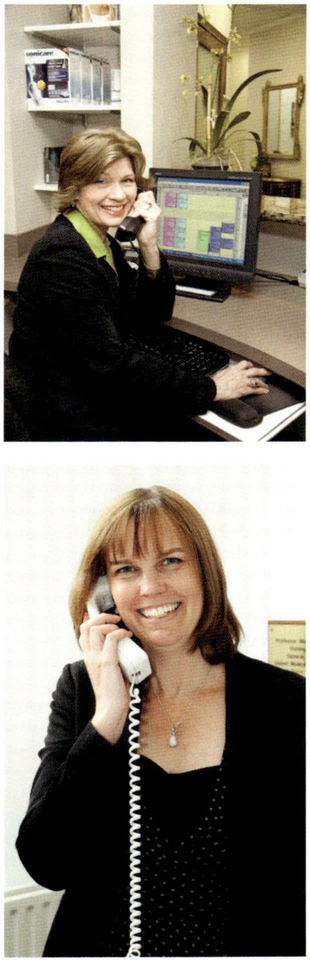

Figs 5-1a and 5-1b New patient phone call: have a smile when greeting on the telephone.

New patient phone call

The new patient phone call is one of the most critical marketing tools in your dental practice (Fig 5-1). All of the effective marketing in the world does not matter if you can't schedule those patients for an appointment. That is why phone skills have to be impeccable. The first goal of your new patient call is to build a relationship and the second goal is to schedule an appointment. Your third goal is to prepare the patient for what they can expect during their time in your office. Everything you do is marketing. Remember the value of repetition in the learning process. If you want your patient to say "yes" to treatment, they need to hear your message five to seven times. The "message" may begin with the referral source or with your external marketing. It continues with the initial phone call. In Chapter 10 on "Case Presentation," telephone etiquette is reviewed again as an integral part of the new patient experience and the entire case presentation system.

The key elements in a productive and successful new patient phone call are:

1. the greeting
2. listening
3. taking accurate notes
4. building value in the dental practice and the new patient appointment
5. scheduling the appointment.

1. The greeting. The call needs to start with the right tone and the right greeting. Answer the phone with a smile and say, "Thank you for calling Dr Greenwall's office. This is Nicola, how may I help you?" What you do *not* want to offer as an initial greeting is "Doctor's office, can you hold?" (With no pause for the patient to respond before they are actually placed on hold!) Before the phone is answered, take a deep breath, smile, and focus attention on the caller.

After the greeting, which includes a question regarding the purpose of the call, begin gathering vital information. The very first thing to ask for is the patient's name, correct spelling, and a phone number where he/she can be reached in case you are disconnected. Knowing your patient's name allows you to use it throughout the conversation. People like to hear the sound of their name. By using the patient's name, you are showing him/her that you care, thus further building the relationship (Jameson, 2004).

2. Listening. Here is the most important part of your telephone call, listening. Ask questions and listen. In this initial phone call you have the opportunity to begin developing a relationship of trust and confidence. Determine the patient's purpose for calling. During this time you will be taking notes. Repeat to the caller what she has told you to make sure you are hearing her accurately.

"Jane, to make sure I am clear, you want to learn about your options to replace a missing tooth and how to improve the overall brightness of your smile. Do I have this correct?"

Repeating what you have heard helps ensure that you heard the caller correctly. It also signals to your prospective patient that you are listening and genuinely care.

3. Taking accurate notes. Make sure that the elements of the call are documented carefully. When the patient arrives for her initial appointment, she does not have to repeat everything. This is another way to show the patient that you are organized, professional, and caring. This is good customer service.

4. Building value in the practice and the new patient appointment. The goal of your telephone call is to encourage a person to schedule an appointment and to keep that appointment. You will be reserving time in your schedule for this new patient and you want them to not only agree to the appointment but to show up.

The value of the appointment must be built on this initial phone call. The patient needs to understand the importance of the initial appointment, the initial evaluation. This is your chance to present the practice philosophy and to graciously begin demonstrating that they can expect something special in your dental practice.

5. Scheduling the appointment. Once you have listened to the patient, ascertained his/her purpose in seeking care, built value in your dental practice and in the appointment itself, now schedule the appointment. To make this transaction go smoothly and to position the patient to say "yes", present a series of "alternative of choice" options. First, find out if mornings or afternoons are best.

Business Administrator: *"Jane, do mornings or afternoons work best for you?"*
Jane: *"Mornings."*
Business Administrator: *"Thank you, Jane. Do you prefer Tuesdays or Thursdays?"*
Jane: *"Thursdays."*
Business Administrator: *"Great. Dr Greenwall has an available appointment at 8:30am on Thursday, the 15th, or at 9:00am on Thursday, the 22nd. Which of these times works best for you?"*

Find out what works for the patient. Then find the times that are available to accommodate him/her.

Welcome packet

Now that the new patient appointment has been scheduled, it becomes important to bridge the gap between this phone call and the actual appointment. Connect and reconnect. Stay in front of the patient so that a sense of urgency remains. You do not want the patient's enthusiasm or commitment to waver, so stay in touch with them. Sending a welcome packet serves this purpose.

Here is what should be included in an effective welcome packet (Figs 5-2 and 5-3):

- new patient letter welcoming the patient and giving them a motivational introduction about what they can expect
- brochure that matches the look and feel of the office
- smile evaluation form
- latest copy of your newsletter
- appointment card confirming the appointment
- map to your office
- patient financing information, including a brochure and an application
- any other educational materials that support the patient's goals, such as aesthetics
- all required medical/health history forms as well as patient information forms
- folder with your logo in which everything is placed.

Because people are utilizing the web for information and resources, you may choose to eliminate sending a physical welcome packet. Instead you may request that new patients go to the web to download forms. This may seem to be easier for the patient and seem to save money for the dental practice. However, in reality, the opposite is true. Yes, having the welcome packet presented digitally on your website is beneficial. But we encourage you to offer both. Direct the patient to the website and then also send a full welcome packet for these reasons:

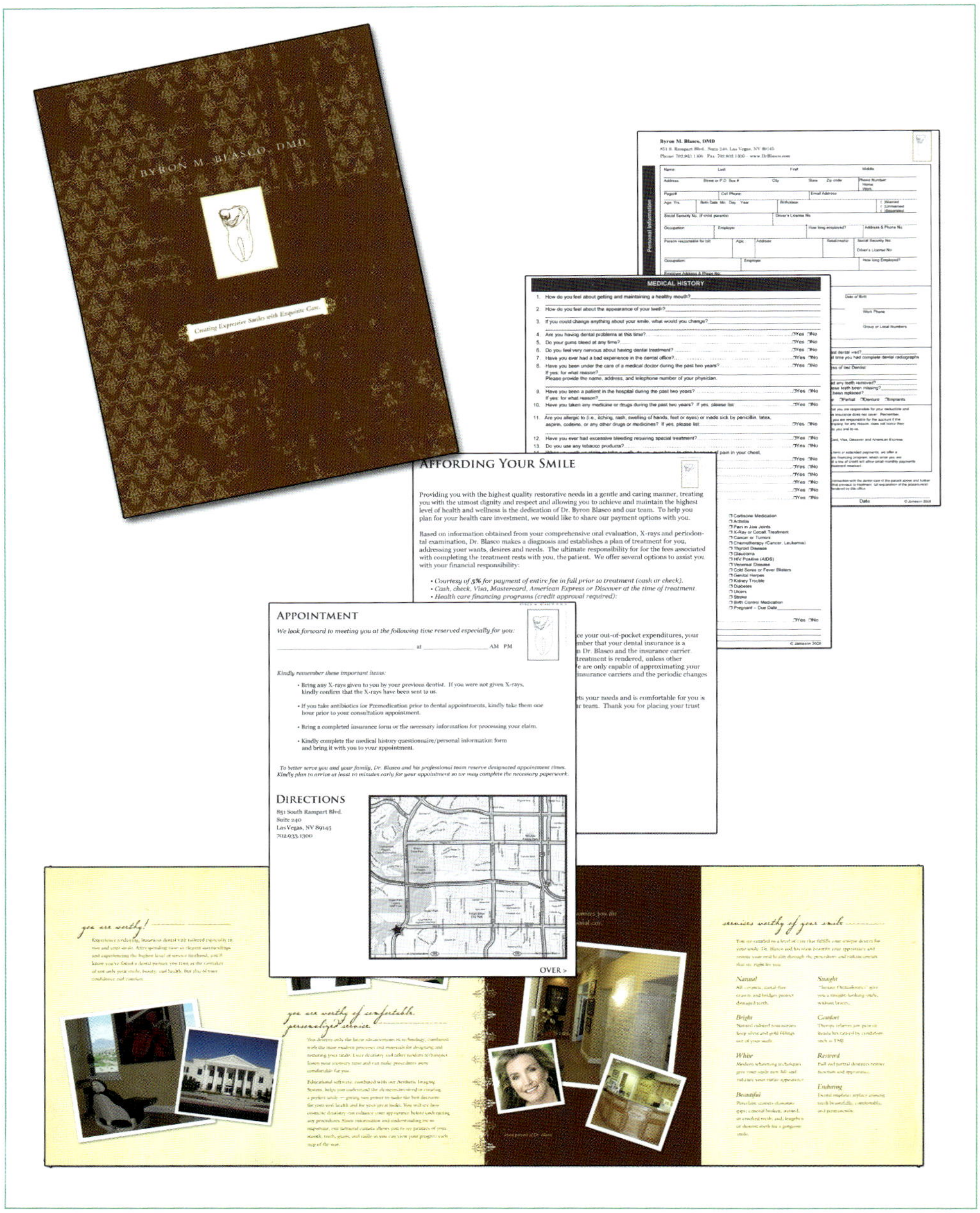

Fig 5-2 Welcome packet, Dr Byron Blasco.

- The patient may see the digital option as requiring more work. Plus, there is some risk to you. You are relying on the patient to find time in his/her schedule to go to the website, find the forms, download, print, complete, and mail. It may or may not happen. Some people are not comfortable with the Internet. Age and generation may affect this. Give the patient the choice and let them decide which method of providing the information works best. Your chances of receiving compliance will be better if you give them the "alternative of choice."
- Sending a physical packet to the patient gives him/her something tangible to touch and feel. It is another element that makes the appointment more real.

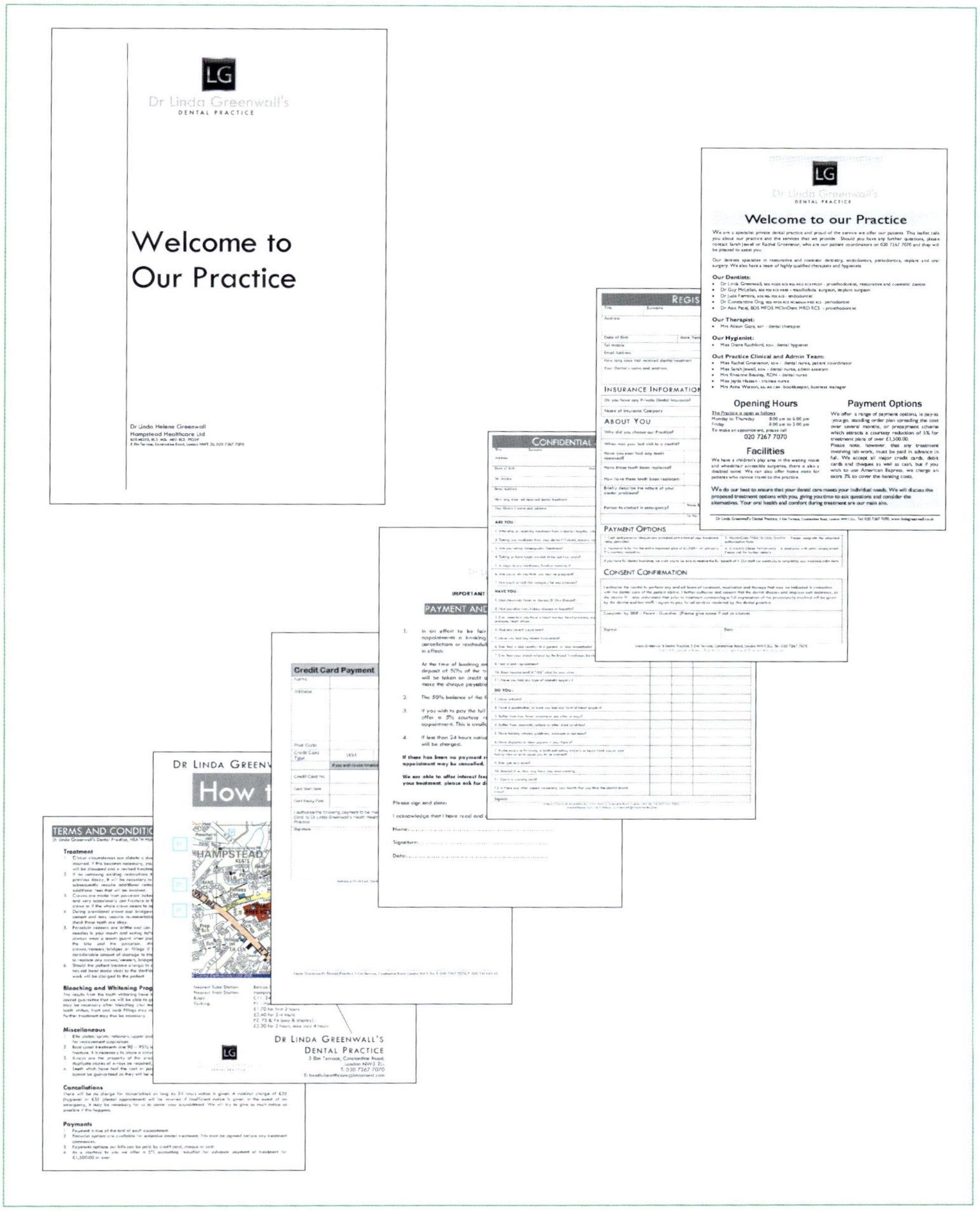

Fig 5-3 Welcome packet, Dr Linda Greenwall.

- It gives you the opportunity to include additional information about services the patient mentioned.
- The welcome packet helps to set the tone for the initial appointment. It gives the patient an idea of what that experience will entail. If the patient receives a brochure that was printed on the office ink jet and hand-folded, he/she will associate that unprofessional feeling with the dental practice and expect lower fees. If she sees a nicely developed and printed brochure, she will expect a nicer visit in the office.

The result from offering *both* the electronic version and the paper version will be a reduction in broken appointments and no shows, as well as an increase in case acceptance.

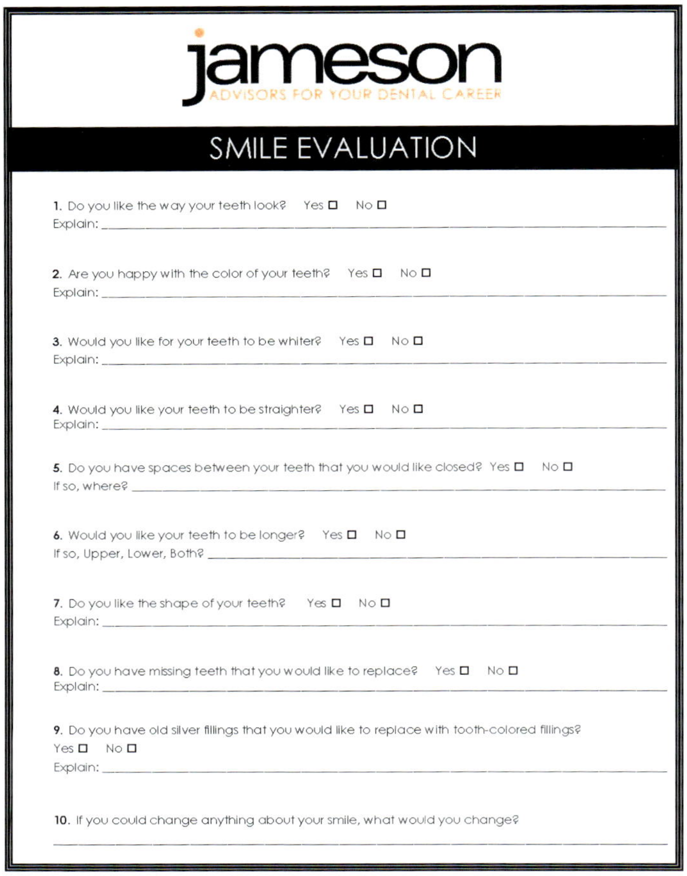
jameson
ADVISORS FOR YOUR DENTAL CAREER

SMILE EVALUATION

1. Do you like the way your teeth look? Yes ☐ No ☐
Explain: ______

2. Are you happy with the color of your teeth? Yes ☐ No ☐
Explain: ______

3. Would you like for your teeth to be whiter? Yes ☐ No ☐
Explain: ______

4. Would you like your teeth to be straighter? Yes ☐ No ☐
Explain: ______

5. Do you have spaces between your teeth that you would like closed? Yes ☐ No ☐
If so, where? ______

6. Would you like your teeth to be longer? Yes ☐ No ☐
If so, Upper, Lower, Both? ______

7. Do you like the shape of your teeth? Yes ☐ No ☐
Explain: ______

8. Do you have missing teeth that you would like to replace? Yes ☐ No ☐
Explain: ______

9. Do you have old silver fillings that you would like to replace with tooth-colored fillings?
Yes ☐ No ☐
Explain: ______

10. If you could change anything about your smile, what would you change?
______

Fig 5-4 Smile evaluation form from Jameson Management, Inc.

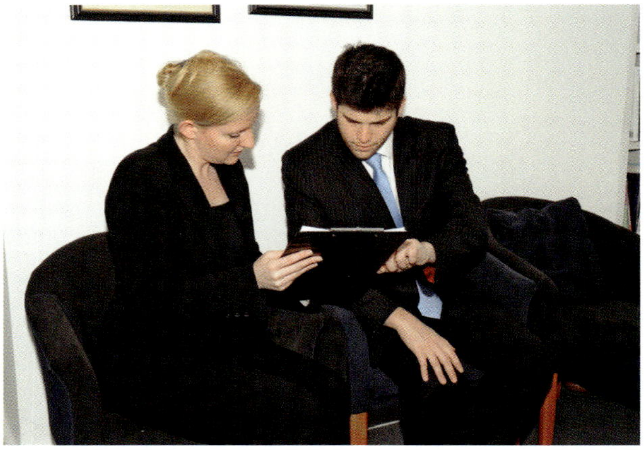

Fig 5-5 The patient completes paperwork including a comforts checklist with the business administrator.

Smile evaluation

A smile evaluation may open the door for people to ask questions or for you to do the asking. People may not ask questions related to aesthetic dentistry because they simply do not know what is available. They may not have ever thought they could be a candidate for smile enhancement or given themselves permission to even think about an aesthetic improvement. A patient's circumstances may have changed, and therefore they are looking at their smile differently. How do you reach these people or even plant a seed for future treatment? The answer is a smile evaluation.

A smile evaluation is a simple form used to ask the patient to evaluate his/her smile (Fig 5-4). It goes through a line of questioning intended for the reader to think about his/her smile differently. Once the patient completes the forms, go over it with him/her (Fig 5-5). Ask permission to address those areas of concerns listed on the form. This form should be used with all new patients and existing patients. It is a great way to start a conversation regarding aesthetics and advanced restorative treatments.

The greeting area

The greeting area or reception area is where you will first meet the patient face to face (Fig 5-6). This is where the patient will continue evaluating *you*

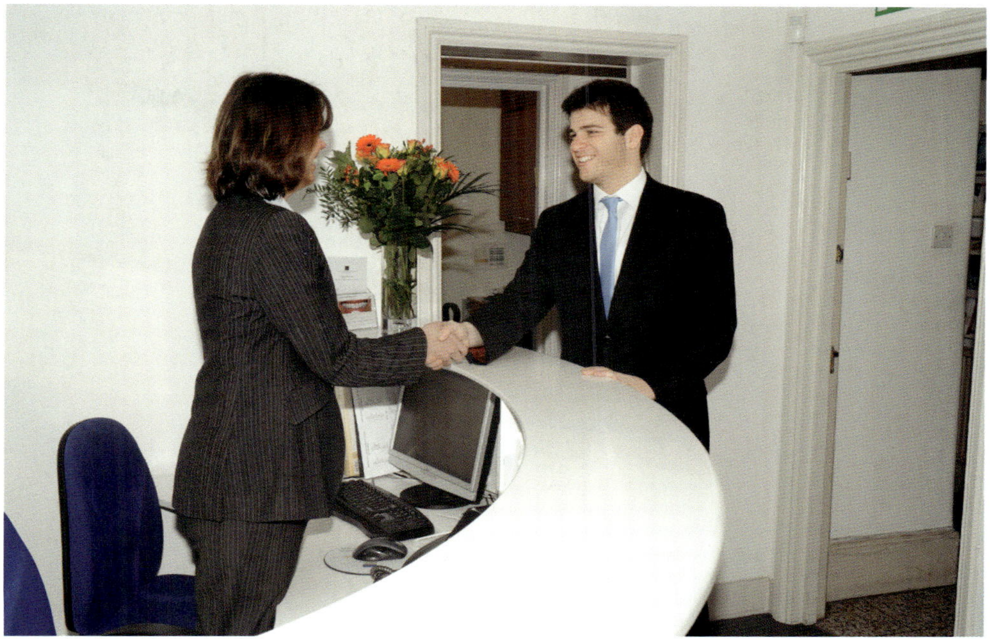

Fig 5-6 The patient is greeted warmly as they enter the dental practice.

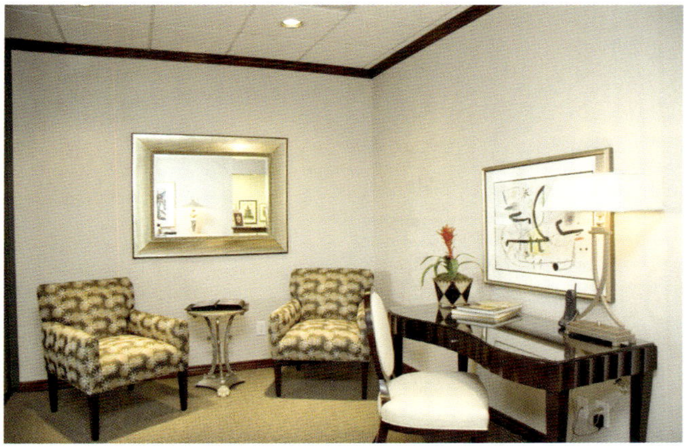

Fig 5-7a Dr Ken Hamlett's greeting area.

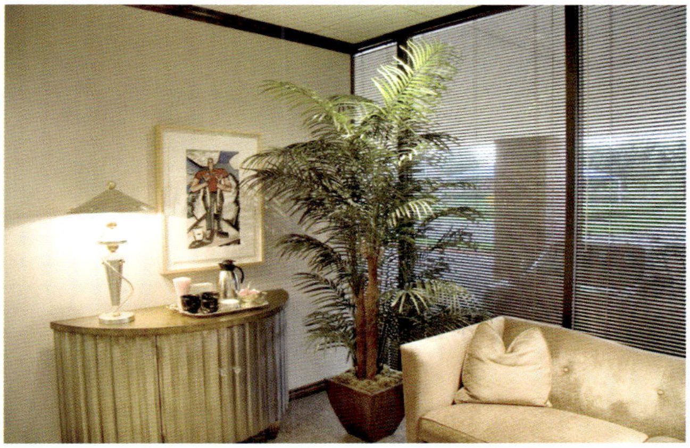

Fig 5-7b Beverages and snacks in a greeting area.

and your dental practice. Your patient does not know quality dentistry and cannot tell if the margins on your crown are appropriate. They may make a decision about the quality of your dentistry based on almost everything but the dentistry. Give yourself the edge. When a person first enters your practice, it must be clean, welcoming, well kept, and orderly (Fig 5-7).

In addition, if you are marketing aesthetics, your facility must be aesthetic as well. No stains on the carpet, fresh paint, up-to-date furniture, art, and literature. Ask yourself if the facility matches your desired image.

The greeting area is also a place where patient education continues. Often dentists will place magazines and other reading materials in the greeting area to occupy the patient's time and to ease any anxieties about an upcoming appointment. As the patient peruses the magazine, she may be reading negative news on the economy, viewing ads trying to sway her to spend

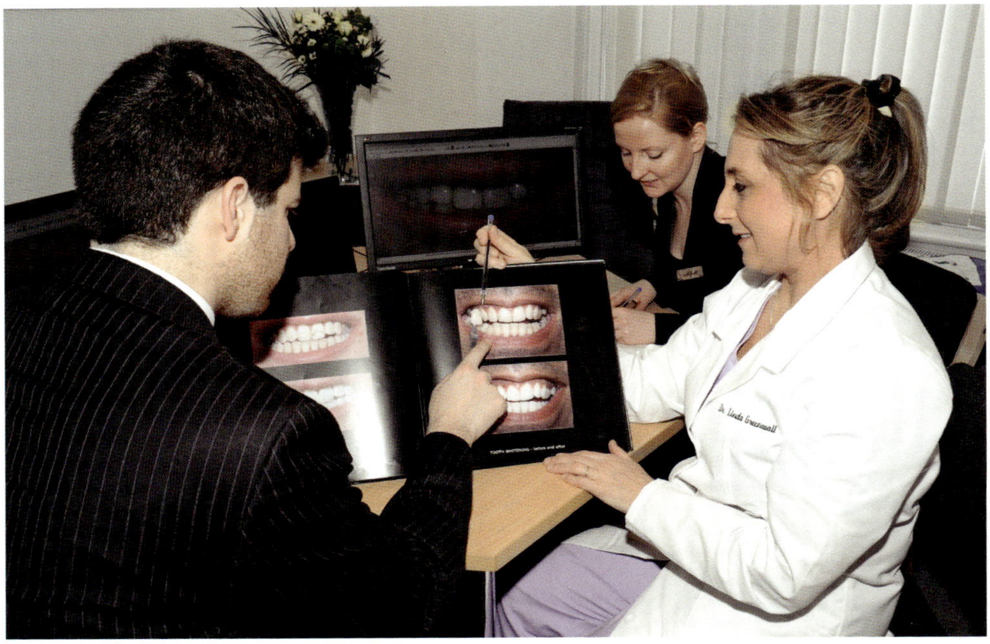

Fig 5-8 Dr Greenwall presenting a smile book to a patient.

money on numerous products, or articles that may present the opposite image you desire. The end result is a patient who is not focused on what you can do for them.

Instead, offer reading materials on why a beautiful smile is important. Take before and after photos and place them into nice leather-bound albums (Fig 5-8). Letters that patients have written to you should be used as testimonials and highlighted in a brag book along with any articles mentioning you, your service, charitable events, continuing education, and so on. Books on aesthetic dentistry, such as Dr Ronald Goldstein's book *Change Your Smile* (Goldstein, 1997; Fig 5-9), provide information, as well as beautiful before-and-after photography, and can stimulate questions and conversations about opportunities for smile enhancement.

These types of materials build value in you and in the treatment you provide. For your existing patients, it can be used to plant a seed and open the door to further conversations regarding advanced treatment opportunities, such as aesthetics.

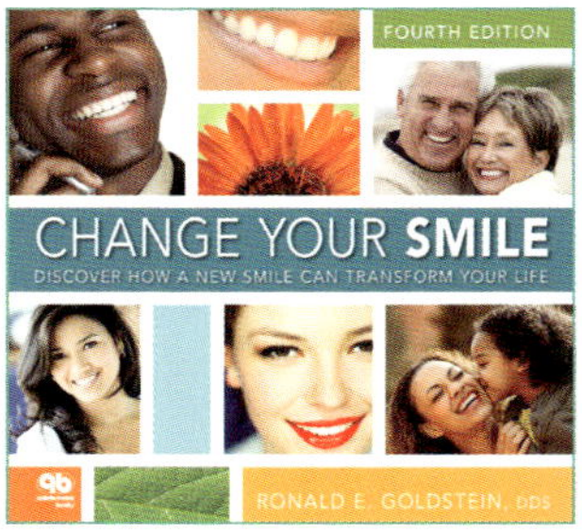

Fig 5-9 Dr Ronald Goldstein's book, *Change Your Smile*.

Make the greeting area a place that is welcoming and comfortable. Offer bottled water, hot tea, or coffee. You may consider having snacks available as well. Your greeting area should be kept clean, nice, and organized at all times. Offer comfortable individual seating. After each patient leaves, check the room to make sure a cup or napkin was not left behind. If you have fresh flowers in the office, make sure that they are indeed fresh and not partially dead. These are all internal marketing elements that create an impression. You want it to be the right impression!

Customer service is at the heart of internal marketing. No matter what you do to encourage a person to come to your office, the way they are treated in each and every encounter will ultimately make the difference.

The New York City dental practice of Drs Larry Rosenthal and Michael Apa epitomizes extraordinary customer service. Jacqueline Pastore, the Practice Administrator of the Rosenthal Apa Group, shared in an interview examples of customer service protocols that they provide for their patients.

"We have always believed that you only get one chance to make a great first impression. We want to create a memorable first experience that patients will rave about, setting us bars above any other dental practice they have ever visited. Our legendary New Patient Experience was created in 1987 to assure that each patient who visits our office has an exceptional new patient experience and leaves our practice with the best possible first impression of our office, our doctors, staff, and their clinical excellence. They will spread the good word, acting as ambassadors for our practice.

"We aim to exceed our patients' expectations and cater to our patients, anticipating their needs in a warm, caring, and comfortable environment. Our patient's comfort and satisfaction are of paramount importance to our entire team. Every patient in our practice fills out a "Comfort List" and it becomes part of their record. This enables our team to properly anticipate each patient's needs and make their dental experience more enjoyable and less stressful. These items include cozy blankets, iPods to listen to music of their choice, a selection of movies, scented candles, flavored lip balms, neck and back rolls. We also have a beverage bar in our new patient consult room and do offer our patients coffee, tea, espresso, cappuccino, and lemon-scented water. Every patient in our practice has the opportunity after their visit to complete an online survey and rate their personal experience in our office.

"To provide the finest customer service for our patients, they are escorted around the office and not left to roam around by themselves.

"We use excellent telephone etiquette. We always answer the phone within three rings, never putting a patient on hold in the middle of a conversation and, if there is an issue, we always try to address and resolve it so that our patient is satisfied with the outcome.

"Our entire team takes pride in the appearance of our office. We like to pay attention to every detail starting with the cleanliness of our office, to the beautifully appointed floral arrangements, to the highly polished floors and immaculate treatment rooms and cleanliness of our lavatories.

"Each new employee is given a copy of the Ritz Carlton Credo that we have adapted to our practice. We want our employees to learn to take pride in their work environment."

Jacqueline Pastore (interview), Practice Administrator for Drs Larry Rosenthal and Michael Apa

Excellent patient communication is essential in building a good relationship. In Figure 5-10, the dental assistant or hygienist is delivering the verbal and written postoperative instructions and/or take-home products. She gives the patient a copy of her business card for him to call her if he has further questions. It is here she can ask the patient for referrals.

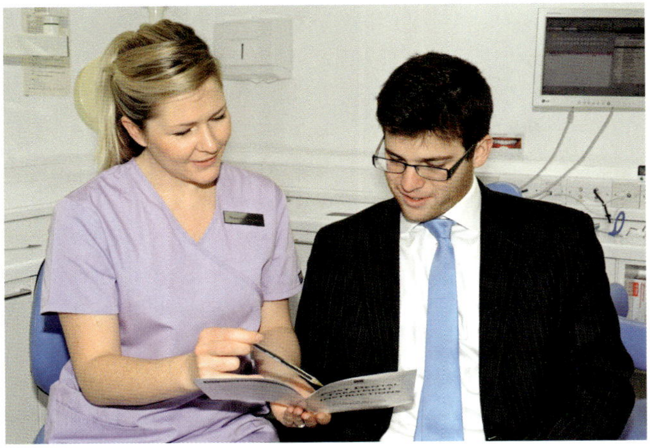

Fig 5-10a Example of excellent communication with the patient in Dr Greenwall's office. Patients are given written postoperative procedures for aesthetic treatments so they can have a copy and remember the home care instructions. The dental assistant has an important role in building excellent communication with the patient. At the end of treatment the assistant will give the patient her business card to assist with any clinical questions that the patient may have after treatment.

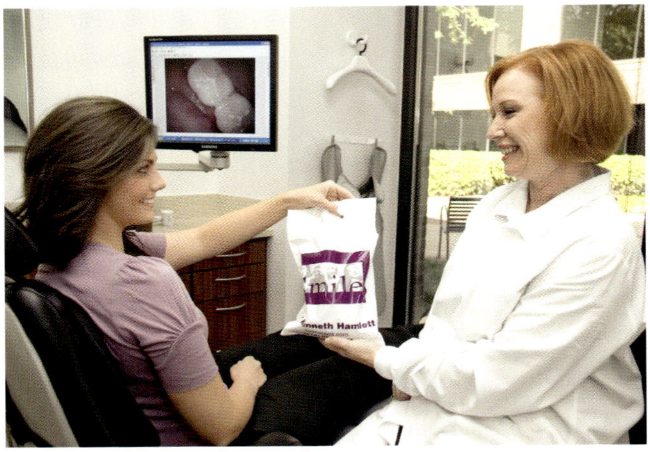

Fig 5-10b Example of excellent communication with the patient in Dr Hamlett's office in Dallas, Texas. Postoperative or home care instructions are given and home care supplies are provided.

Quality digital photography

Recognizing the value of good photography and being able to actually take excellent photographs are two different things. These are specific and difficult skills, but are imperative for an aesthetic practice. Hands-on training with this intricate skill is required. Take before-and-after photographs of each of your cases and develop a library of those cases so that you can easily access them for consultations and patient education (Figs 5-11 to 5-13).

Pictures are powerful. Photographs evoke emotion and tell a story without words. They can tell a story about your patient and their mouth.

A retracted image properly taken of your patient's mouth may show signs of wear and tear, stains, neglect, or, in your mind, an opportunity to improve someone's life. Your hygienist may look at that photograph and notice symptoms of periodontal disease. Your financial coordinator may look at the same smile and see that the financial investment is going to be large, so she needs to be prepared for objections. Your patient may look at the photograph and simply think, "Ugh. That's gross," and then completely shut down, not understanding what she/he just saw. Keep in mind, when your patient looks in the mirror every day, what your patient sees is a person with hair, lips, a nose, and a full face, as opposed to a smile with the lips pulled out of site. Retracted images are scary to many patients. We know how powerful that image is and we need the patient to see what we see. Therefore, the photographs are shown "with dental supervision only." Show the retracted images to your patient while you are there to explain what it means. If you

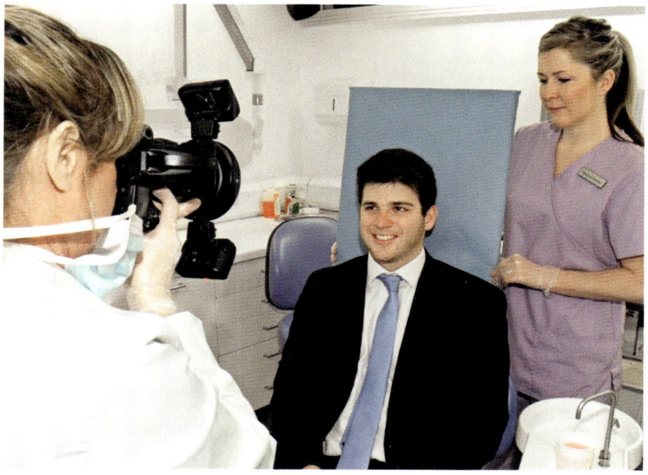

Fig 5-11a Taking digital photographs: portrait shots are taken first, in this instance with a blue photographic paper background to block out operatory detail.

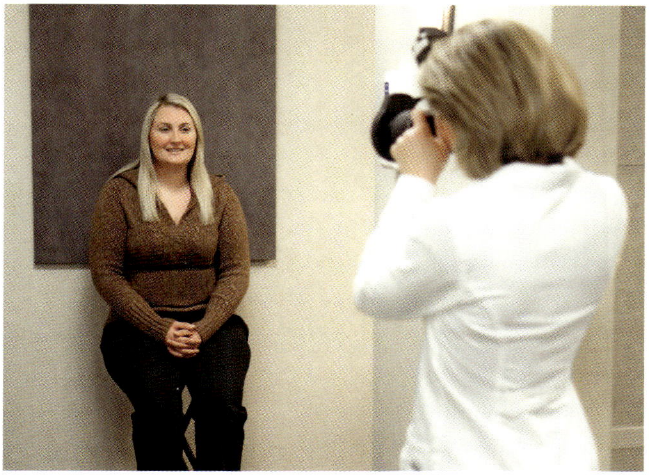

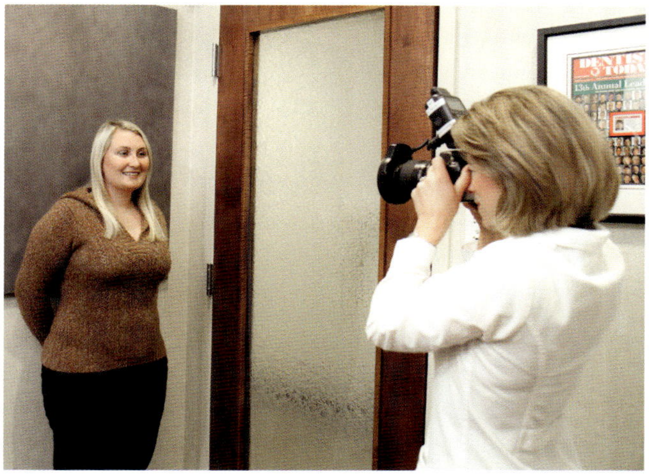

Figs 5-11b and 5-11c An excellent alternative is to have the patient stand or sit in front of a gray background hung on the wall, as seen here in the office of Dr Mark Hyman.

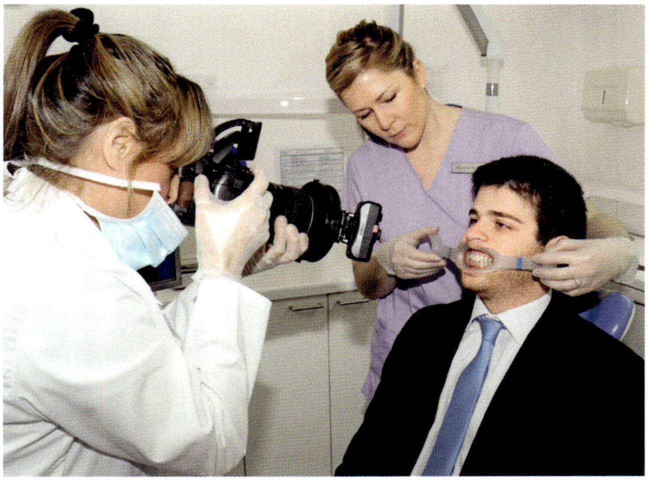

Fig 5-12a Taking digital retracted views.

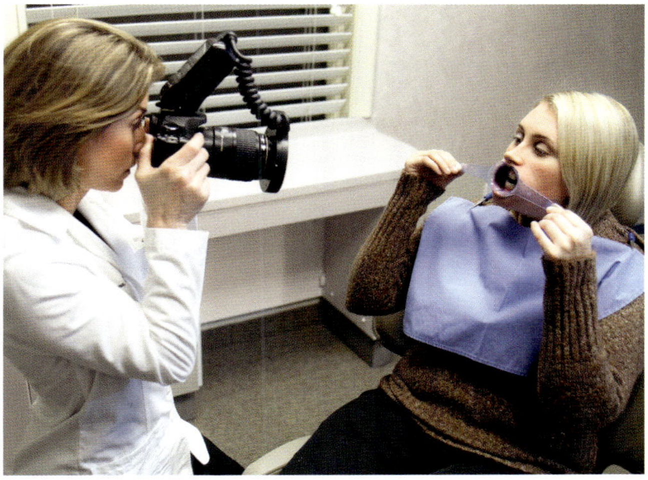

Fig 5-12b Alternatively, patients could hold the retractors themselves.

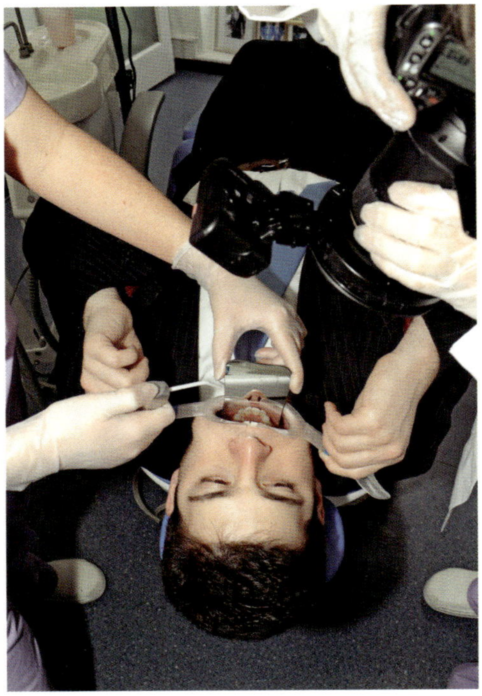

Fig 5-13a The palatal mirror view is also photographed. The patient may need to be positioned in the supine position to get a good palatal mirror view.

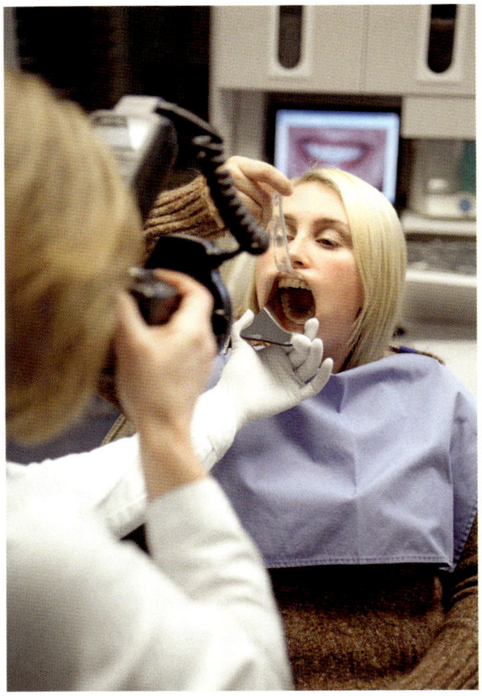

Fig 5-13b Have the patient sitting up when you are taking the upper occlusal view and laying down when you are taking the lower occlusal view. Dr Hyman's team illustrates another alternative, which is to use the Retract-EEZ retractor to pull back the lip (not the cheek retractors). The patient can hold both the Retract-EEZ retractor and the mirror. Note that this latter option eliminates assistant (nurse) time so that only one person needs to take the pictures.

detect that your patient is emotionally flooded, listen and reflect back her/his concerns. Then talk the patient through the image so that she/he hears that important message you have to share.

Photographs can tell stories about the condition of a patient's mouth and can tell a story about you and the kind of dentistry you perform. Quality photographs project an image of excellence. When your photographs are taken properly and are crystal clear, it allows the patient to focus on what you want them to see, the smile. However, when the photographs are crooked, grainy, or fuzzy, it sends a negative message. Remember that your patients cannot properly judge quality dentistry. They make decisions about the quality of your work by judging things they do know, such as your photography. If the images are crooked and time is not spent on taking a good photograph, the patient may wonder if the dentist is going to take time on their teeth. This goes back to trust. Any break in that trust is one more obstacle to overcome.

Invest time into your photographs. Learn how to take them properly. If you do not know how to do this, seek help. The result must be clear, consistent images that showcase your stunning results and that allow the patient to focus on what matters in the image. Distraction related to poor-quality photography serves no one.

A smile book of your own aesthetic dentistry cases is a good internal marketing tool. These can be uploaded and designed online and printed into a professional book of your own before and after cases (see Fig 5-8).

Internal marketing campaigns

Good marketing recommends that you stay in contact with your clients (patients) at least once per quarter. You can introduce them to new services being offered in your dental practice, reconfirm the benefits of existing treatment options, keep your name in front of them so that when they think of the dentist, they think of you, and always let them know how much you appreciate them. In addition, you can encourage them to refer their friends, families, and colleagues to your dental practice.

An internal marketing campaign is a way to effectively educate your patients. For example, let's say you recently started using a new dental laser. Your patients need to know about this. So you put together a campaign to educate them on the benefits and why this will make their future appointments more comfortable. The traditional way dental practices have shared a message was by sending out a letter or putting up signage. However, there are now numerous effective methods to get that message across and to fulfill the marketing truism that repetition is the key to effective marketing.

There are many ways you can do this both traditionally and non-traditionally. Here are 12 ways to get the message out:

- Send an email to your patients.
- Send eNewsletters.
- Post on your website.
- Place signage about a new product, service, or technology in the office.
- Send a letter with an insert.
- Place an insert into the hygiene bags (Fig 5-14).
- Have your team verbally communicate new information to patients.
- Mention it in your on-hold system.
- Post it to Facebook and Twitter.
- Have your team take a video with a Flip camera of them using the product. Then upload it to YouTube.
- Mail a postcard or a series of postcards.
- Write a press release and send to local newspapers and publications.

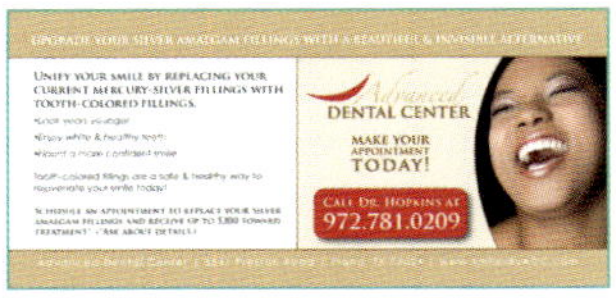

Fig 5-14 Hygiene bag insert.

All of these are ways to send out the message. Several of these require little, if any, monetary investment.

To be as effective as you can be, make a plan *before* you begin your internal marketing campaign. Spread out the campaign over three months to get traction. Implementing your campaign will require time. The plan includes not only what you are going to do but the time frames that are allocated to each project. Spread your plan out over several months. Reasonable time allotment will allow for the gathering of resources and the creation of various marketing pieces, and keeps your team from feeling overwhelmed.

A deliberately, coordinated campaign that is timed appropriately with a single message will educate your patients and show them that you are staying at the forefront of the services you are promoting. It also helps to plant the seed with patients you have that could benefit from aesthetic dentistry. You want your patients to know what you offer so that they do not seek that service somewhere else. Here are some ideas for internal marketing campaigns:

- Segment out patients who have had whitening. Market to them the benefits of aesthetic dentistry. Many patients who have had whitening return requesting further cosmetic dentistry services.
- Introduce a new technology or service.
- Target adults over the age of 50 and share advancements in materials, eg, no more dark lines at the margin of the crown with all-porcelain crowns.
- Market whitening to all patients.
- Replace amalgam fillings with tooth-colored material.

Asking for referrals

Your number one source of new patients is personal referral.

> *"Create and maintain dental missionaries for the practice. Dr Hamlett personally thanks patients each and every day for coming to the practice. We know they have many choices, and we thank them for choosing Dr Hamlett and our team. We give the patients business cards to give to their friends. We always ask for referrals."*
>
> *Debra Hamlett (interview), Office Manager for Dr Ken Hamlett*

This is the number one thing you can do in your dental practice to increase your new patient flow. This is something you can start doing today. Based on years of information gathered by Jameson Management and our Creative Services division, we have determined that approximately 70% of your new patients come from personal referrals. The easiest way to get your patients to refer is simply by asking them (Fig 5-15). A great time to do this is when they are paying you a nice compliment.

"Thank you for your kind words, Mr Jones. We build our practice on patients just like you. If you have friends, family members or colleagues who need a dental home or who might benefit from treatment such as we provide, please tell them about us. We will take care of them in the same way we have taken care of you."

Then give them some cards. If you do not ask, they will not refer. We can assume that patients will tell others about us, but that does not mean they will. Your patient may think you are not accepting new patients. When you ask someone to do something, they are much more likely to act on it.

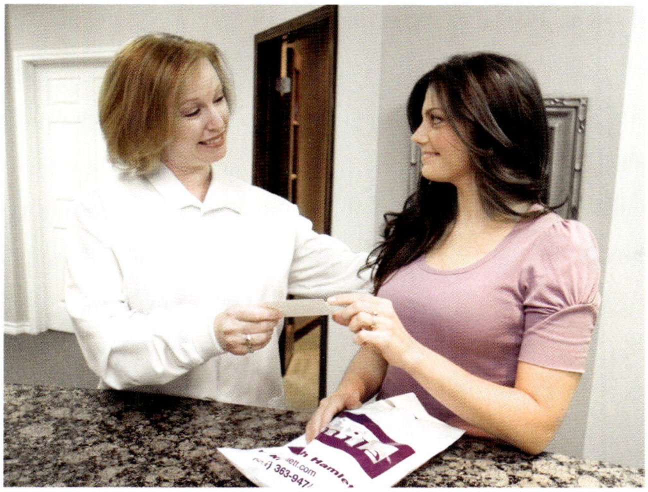

Fig 5-15 Team member asking for referrals.

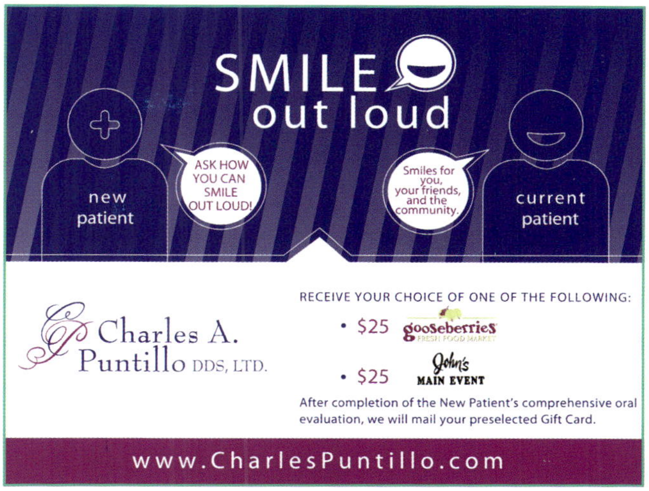

Fig 5-16 Smile Out Loud© card.

▶ *"The best way to generate new patients from your own area or from around the world is word of mouth. Most of my major cases and most of my new patients come from the referral of satisfied patients. I create dental missionaries. My patients are my best advertising. New patients can see friends with beautiful smiles that I have done and they are almost sold before they walk in the door. Also creating a fantastic website and networking with specialists makes a big difference."*

Dr Ken Hamlett (interview)

Not all patients are accustomed to referring and sometimes need encouragement. In those cases, it is beneficial to aid them by equipping your patients with the tools to talk about you. A program that we have effectively used in multiple practices is Smile Out Loud©. This is a program that rewards both the existing patient and the new patient. It gives both patients a choice of a gift card from two different stores or restaurants. This alternative of choice allows both parties to have a gift from a place they like, a place of their own choosing. During the patient's dental or hygiene appointment, he or she is presented with a fold-over card detailing the program (Fig 5-16). On the card there is a place for both the existing patient and the new patient to place their names and choose the gift card they want. When the patient comes in for his new patient appointment, he will hand the card to the business administrator. After the appointment, the gift cards are mailed to both patients. Of course, the use of this program should only be done in conjunction with your state or province's governing dental body.

Through appropriate approaches, excellent verbal skills, and beautifully designed pieces, this program will generate improved new patient numbers for dental practices. One of Jameson Management's consulting clients in Minnesota, a five-dentist practice in a town of 5,000, generated 436 new patients and nearly a half a million dollars in dentistry in just 10 months.

They employed the program exactly as instructed and received phenomenal returns.

▶ *"To date, this has been the most successful marketing program our office has experienced. I made sure that our team was thoroughly trained in promoting this program to our patients and others in the community and we even executed an employee incentive program to keep the momentum going. Smile Out Loud© has brought an astonishing amount of new patients to our practice along with an incredible amount of production and has truly encouraged team building among our employees."*

Shana Munson (interview), Treatment Coordinator/Director of Marketing, Soft Dental

The program works and it works because the message is sent five to seven times. It gives the existing patient a way to recommend you that feels good to him/her because their friend will also win. The physical fold-over card is stunning, matches the practice look and feel, and equips your patient with a tool to talk about you. This combination of activity turns a referral program with average results into one with phenomenal results.

The manner in which you choose to ask for referrals in your dental practice is something that you and the team need to discuss. Make sure that the program or method you choose is followed every day. Discuss possible referral sources in your daily meeting. Designate who is going to speak to which patient. Be consistent. Communicate with your patients. Reap the rewards from referrals.

▶ *"It is always nice to acknowledge a patient who refers another patient to the practice. Oftentimes I will personally call a patient to thank them and also offer them a complimentary cleaning or complimentary service. The doctors [dentists] also thank patients personally and we encourage our patients to send their friends and family to us for treatment."*

Jacqueline Pastore (interview), Practice Administrator for Drs Larry Rosenthal and Michael Apa

In summary

Marketing is an integral part of everything you do. Your internal marketing sends a clear message about who you are and what kind of dentistry you perform. In building your aesthetic dental practice, you must have good internal marketing to help patients say yes, stay with you, and refer their friends and family.

Action steps

1. Marketing is everything you do and say in your dental practice. Outline each step of your system protocols and determine the message being sent by your methods of management.
2. Record a new patient phone call. Then, analyze the call. Continue to do the things that you feel are effective. Work together to improve any aspect of the call that can be improved.

3. Create an excellent, comprehensive welcome packet consistent with the look and feel of your office. Then, design a plan as to when and how you will use it.
4. Have every patient complete a smile evaluation every year.
5. Make your greeting area welcoming and focused on you and your message. Step out to the greeting area and sit down. Analyze the area and, as a team, identify ways to make it more aesthetically pleasing, promote smile makeovers, and reflect comfort and class.
6. Ensure you have quality, consistent digital photography in the dental practice by engaging a specialist or dental photography expert to come to your office for personal coaching.
7. Design and implement internal marketing campaigns effectively on a quarterly basis.
8. Ask for referrals.

References

1. Blanchard K, Bowles S. Raving Fans. New York, NY: Blanchard Family Partnership and Ode to Joy Limited, 1993.
2. Erickson F. Raising the Bar. San Francisco, CA: Jossey-Bass, 2004.
3. Goldstein R. Change Your Smile. Chicago, IL: Quintessence Publishing, 1997.
4. Jameson C. Great Communication Equals Great Production. Tulsa, OK: Pennwell Books, 2004.
5. Van Vianen A, Fischer A. Illuminating the glass ceiling: the role of organizational culture preferences. Journal of Occupational and Organizational Psychology 2002;75:315–337.

Checklist for internal marketing

Appendix 5-1

The facility

1. The facility should be aesthetically pleasing
2. Floor coverings should be clean, with no stains
3. Walls should have fresh paint, and art should be well framed
4. Include up-to-date furniture, art, and literature
5. The facility should match your desired image.

Greeting area

1. Welcoming
2. Clean
3. Flowers are fresh
4. Well organized
5. Comfort menu
6. Patient information
7. Smile books are well presented and have well bound albums
8. Beverage selection
9. Team business cards
10. Patient testimonial book.

Patient restroom

1. Selection of toothpaste samples and brushes to use before the appointment
2. Samples of floss to use prior to the appointment
3. Good soaps
4. Clean towels
5. Perfumes to refresh
6. Hand cream
7. Toilet cleanliness checklist to show care and attention to detail in cleanliness of restroom.

Treatment rooms

1. Cozy blankets
2. Two ipods to listen to music of their choice
3. Ipads to watch a selection of movies
4. Scented candles
5. Flavored lip balms
6. Neck and back rolls
7. Paraffin hand wax.

Staff appearance

1. Attire is neat and tidy
2. Name label/tag
3. Hair is neat
4. Shoes are clean
5. Uniform/scrubs are spotless.

Patient aftercare

1. Written and verbal instructions given of procedure
2. Heated hand towel to pamper immediately after treatment
3. Lip balm placed at end of procedure
4. Patient escorted to greeting area
5. Patient testimonial given to complete at desk
6. Good cross-linkage communication to prepare for check out
7. Team business card given to patient
8. Ask for referrals
9. Patient called the next day for follow-up
10. Patient emailed to ask to complete online patient care survey.

6 External Marketing

Cathy Jameson, Linda Greenwall, and Misty Absher Clark

> *External marketing is a critical part of the growth of your practice allowing you to engage with your past, present and future patients in a significant way.*
> *Amy Logan Parrish (interview), Executive VP of Development, Jameson Management, Inc.*

What is external marketing?

When people define marketing, most think of external marketing, such as radio advertising or placing a classified advertisement. However, marketing is related to everything you do. As you are developing a comprehensive marketing plan or strategic marketing plan, conferring with experts will help you to combine a thorough internal and external program: one that works. While your internal marketing plan supports the retention and reactivation of your existing patient family, your external marketing plan relates to marketing directly to people who are not yet your patients. Some common external marketing strategies are participating in health/bridal fairs, speaking to local groups and organizations, as well as advertising in traditional mediums such as radio, TV, and print. The web also plays a vital role in your external marketing. Social media are used by dental practices as an effective new, inexpensive way of reaching a larger audience.

Your brand/ your message

As you elevate your marketing to include the marketing of aesthetic dentistry, you need to be clear in your own understanding of who you are and what you do. This knowledge starts with you and then transfers to marketing to potential patients. The two have to be compatible. The writing of your mission, vision, and goals has given you a head start on this requirement. Take this further as you design your external marketing plan. Ask "What is it that makes us unique from other dental practices?" This may be a difficult question, but it is an important one. Ask yourself that question. Ask your team members. Ask your patients who chose you as the dentist who performed their smile makeover. Find out what they say about you when they refer you to their friends and families. You want to find out what was most important to them and what left the longest and strongest impression. You may be pleasantly surprised. The answers will vary depending on the person or situation. Most patients will acknowledge the smile itself, but will also refer to numerous personal interactions that were especially important to them. The most imperative needs and desires of your patients will be transferred and translated into your marketing plan.

This was such the case with one of our clients. When we interviewed her patients, they stated that they had a positive dental experience in her practice, and that their life had been changed for the better. Her team members said the same thing. Therefore we packaged all of her marketing as "Positively Changing Lives." This critical element was of uppermost importance to her patients and her team. So, that became the theme or the brand of her marketing.

Fig 6-1 Dr Brock Arms has a practice that focuses on giving a percentage of the practice profits to support missions and charities across the globe. This logo captures that desire.

You should have one consistent message throughout everything you do. For Ritz Carlton, that message is great customer service. For you, it could be customer service too. The key message that you wish to send to potential patients, as well as existing patients, will be unique to you. Ensure that you are consistent with the message.

If you choose your message to be the premier dental studio for smile makeovers and your logo has an icon of an extracted tooth, you may have conflicting messages here. You are interested in restoring teeth to health and creating beautiful smiles. Extraction is not your message. Ask if the messages you are "sending out" are in alignment with a premier aesthetic dental practice. Or are you presenting an image of a general dental clinic where extractions are performed daily for dental care? Choose your logo wisely so that it reflects your desired image, rather than a photograph of your facility, your favorite hobby, a local landmark, or an extracted tooth. It has to be unique to you. It needs to set the stage for the image and preferred message of your practice. Examples of logos are shown in Figures 6-1 to 6-4.

Fig 6-2 Drs Gregg and Bradd Testerman own a father–son dental practice. The logo captures the two generations, as well as their approaches to dentistry.

Once you have identified your intended message and have designed a logo to match that message, continue to be consistent in delivering the message. Remember, your message must be seen, heard, or felt five to seven times before someone will act on it. It is not enough to say you are a premier aesthetic dental practice if you never mention it again. Your message has to be stated through words, design, and everything you do. Consistency and repetition are the two primary elements of effective marketing.

The wheel of marketing

Effective marketing requires that you send out one identified, consistent message through multiple different methods. Think of your marketing as a wheel. In the center of the wheel is your message. For each place where you are marketing your message, add a spoke. For instance, if you participated in a bridal fair, add a spoke. If you advertise on the radio, add a spoke; and so on. The more spokes you have, the better supported your message is.

Fig 6-3 Dr Charles Puntillo needed a logo that would appeal to his bread-and-butter dentistry while appealing to the high-end aesthetic dentistry of his practice. The logo shows tradition, artistry, and royal treatment/customer service through the graphics, fonts and colors used.

Fig 6-4 The new logo for Dr Greenwall's aesthetic dental practice. It was designed to be clean and simple to reflect the new aesthetic image.

The result will be a greater number of new patients who come to you and who are aware of the kind of care you provide.

For example: Jane is looking for a good dentist. She asks Bob for the name of one. He recommends Dr Greenwall. Jane decides to wait to see the dentist. In the meantime, she receives a direct mail piece from Dr Greenwall, she sees an advertisement in the newspaper, she goes to a health fair, and she sees her friends "liking" Dr Greenwall' s Facebook page. She finally decides she needs to go see the dentist. So she does a search and easily finds Dr Greenwall's website. She goes back to Bob and asks, "Now who is your dentist?" To which Bob replies, "Dr Greenwall." Jane replies, "You know, I see her everywhere." Finally she calls the practice and schedules her appointment. When asked what led her to the practice, she states, "Bob," when in fact it was many exposures that reinforced her decision to see Dr Greenwall.

The alternative is that Dr Greenwall is not marketing. Jane asks Bob for the recommendation. He recommends Dr Greenwall, but she forgets Dr Greenwall's name and sees someone else in marketing pieces. She does a search on the Web and Dr Greenwall's name does not appear. Dr Doe's name appears. She likes what she sees. Once more, Jane asks Bob who his dentist is. This time, when he says, "Dr Greenwall," she doesn't recognize the name. Instead she decides to go see the person she found on the Web and has seen in multiple places.

Figures 6-5 to 6-7 show some samples of different marketing wheels. The more spokes in the wheel, the more supported your message is. The goal is to be in multiple places so that you can reach your audience five to seven times with the same message, increasing the likelihood that they will act.

Tips for creating successful advertisements

When advertising, whether it is in a magazine, newspaper, direct mail, etc., you want it to be successful. The investment can be substantial and, therefore, you want to make sure that investment pays for itself over time. While all ads vary in creativity, message, and design, there are certain elements that should always be at play in your advertisement. Your advertisement should have the following elements (Fig 6-8):

- "you" focused content
- one single, consistent message
- call to action statement
- offer
- phone number.

"You" focused and action-oriented content

The simplest of changes in your marketing can make the most dramatic shift in results. "You" focused, action-oriented content is one of those recommended changes. Your ad only has a moment to capture someone's attention. Failing to do so, moves the viewer on to something else. Living in this "me" centered world, your prospective patients are not interested in what you do. Instead, they want to know what's in it for them. So when your

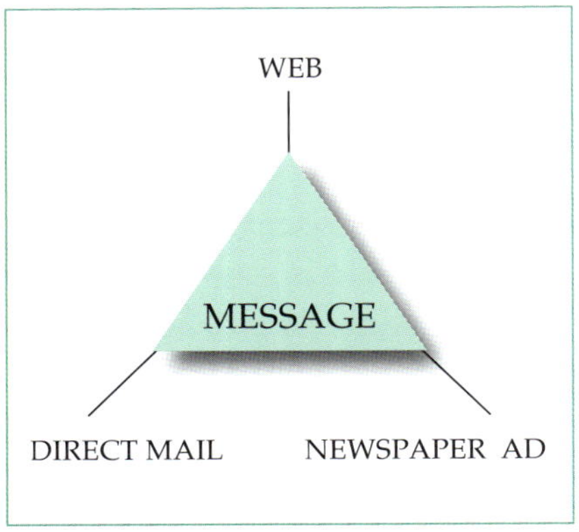

Fig 6-5 Non-ideal wheel of marketing (© Misty Absher Clark for Jameson Creative Services).

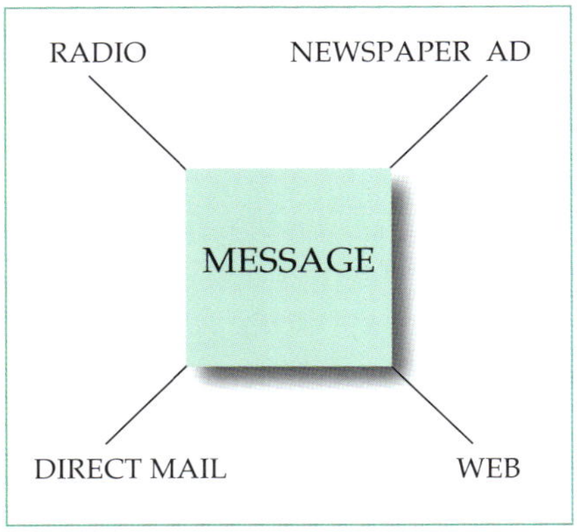

Fig 6-6 Non-ideal wheel of marketing (© Misty Absher Clark for Jameson Creative Services).

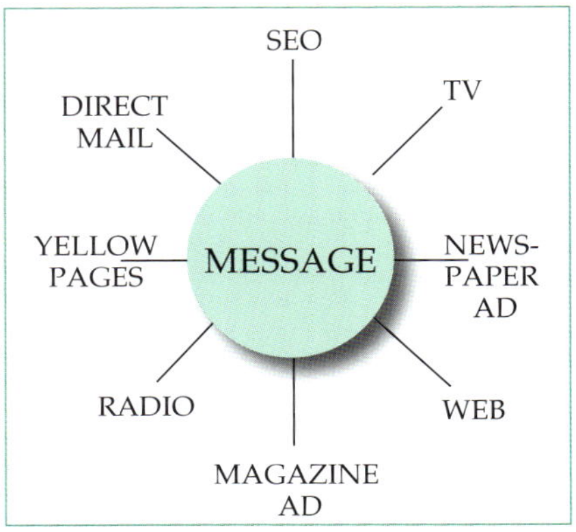

Fig 6-7 Example of an ideal wheel of marketing (SEO, search engine optimization) (© Misty Absher Clark for Jameson Creative Services).

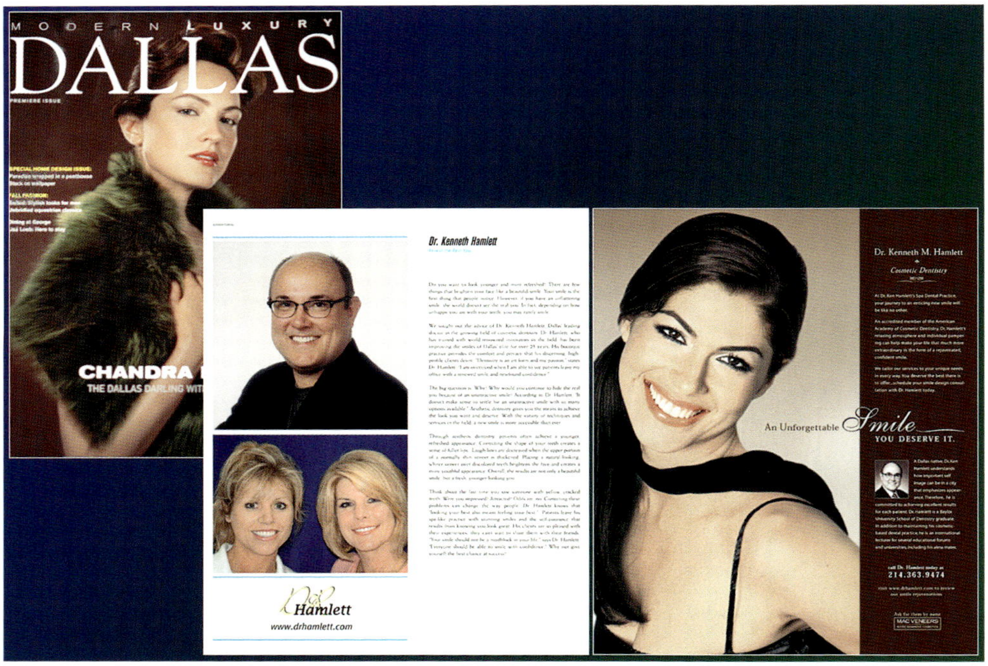

Fig 6-8 External marketing advertorial piece featuring Dr Ken Hamlett.

reading material is focused on the dental practice, you will lose the patient's interest and he will stop reading.

To make your copy "attention grabbing" and to make sure it is read, adjust the content so that it is focused on the patient. Take a look at this sentence: "We strive to make your visit as comfortable as possible." You may look at that sentence and think that it is talking about the patient's visit. In fact it is talking about what "we" are going to do. "We are going to make your visit…" A patient reading that sees the "We" and stops. "We" at the beginning of the sentence is talking about the dental practice. Instead, rewrite the sentence to say, "Your visit will be made as comfortable as possible." Now "you" is front and center, the focus of the sentence. It directly talks to the patient. You don't have to say that your dental practice is the one making the visit comfortable. It is assumed because it is your ad, your website, and your marketing materials that you are delivering that service. Writing content that is focused on your patient makes the prospective patient want to read more.

You can even make the content more powerful, which is often needed in the headline of an ad, by making it action-oriented. While the above sentence is appropriate and acceptable to use, it can be more powerful. Your sentence now becomes, "Enjoy your stay in our office." This simple phrasing asks the potential new patient to do something, to participate. By including the patient as an active participant, you are now greatly increasing the likelihood that he will read more and ultimately call the practice. A good marketing piece has a great combination of "'you' focused" and "action-oriented" content.

One single and consistent message

The message you identified earlier for your practice is the message you want to send in your marketing. It should be clear, concise, and most importantly consistent. If your message changes with every marketing piece, then it is more difficult for people to grab hold of it and remember it. Your audience needs to hear, see, and experience your message five to seven times before acting on it. When your message oscillates from one message to another, it confuses the viewer. If your message is the "premier cosmetic dental studio," then that is your message. It would not benefit you to design an advertisement that then says, "cosmetic and family dentistry." The messages are conflicting. If you send out a direct mail piece to a home, and then 6 weeks later send another direct mail piece that looks different and presents a different message, the people receiving your marketing pieces will be confused. Between the first time you sent out the direct mail piece and the second direct mail piece, did people receive different advertisements with different messages? The confusion may impact a person's decision to call you. Avoid confusing your potential patients by sending different or conflicting messages. Send the same or similar pieces multiple times before you change the design or message. Repetition is key.

Call to action

If you do not tell people to call you, they won't. You cannot assume that by simply placing your telephone number and website address in an advertisement that the viewer will act. You have to tell people to "Call today!" Or "Call today to schedule your appointment." Asking them to do something involves the patient and increases the likelihood a call will be made. This is true with any written marketing pieces and, certainly, with your website addresses. Be sure to ask the potential patient to "visit" your website.

Include an offer in the advertisement

The goal of your advertisement is to get people to respond. Do this by including an offer. The inclusion of an offer helps to create a sense of urgency and a reason why someone needs to contact you today. It is an incentive to get the patient to act earlier than he/she might have done without encouragement.

Phone number

This is an easy one. Make sure you have your correct phone number in the advertisement. Make it large and bold. If the patient were to only see one thing, it should be your phone number. The most appropriate place for your phone number is in the lower right-hand side of the advertisement. People read in a "C" format, and therefore your most important elements need to fit on the "C" inside the advertisement (Fig 6-9). As the advertisement is read, the viewer's eye is drawn to the end of the "C" (the lower right-hand side). This is where their eyes land and end. This is where you want your contact information easily found.

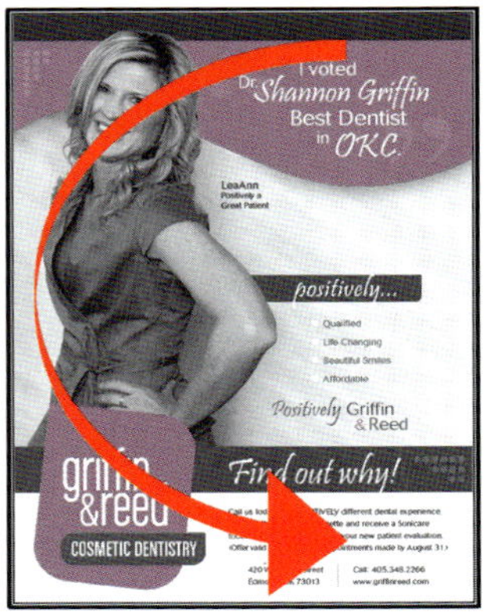

Fig 6-9 Example of the "C" format to be used in advertisement design.

Social media

Social media is a profound marketing medium that has entered the arena. It is a great medium for dentists, including those who choose to build the aesthetic aspect of their practice. Social media is effective for dentists who want to spread the message, retain patients, and have patients say "yes" to the beautiful treatment they provide. The two most common social media networks are Twitter and Facebook.

Have a presence on these sites. This is where your patients and prospective patients are gathering together to have conversations. Up until now, the World-Wide Web was a one-way conversation, a step above a brochure. The web was a place where patients went to read information about you. Now, with the advent of social media, it is a place where people are engaged, asking questions, and talking with others. These patients or potential patients are involved with Facebook, Twitter, etc. and are talking about you and about dentistry. Be in these places to have an opportunity to answer questions and provide relevant information.

Facebook, Twitter, and blogging are great platforms on which to get started. These services are free. What is required of you is an investment of office resources. Facebook is a platform that fosters better relationships with your patients. Twitter is a medium that moves quickly. The focus of Twitter with dental practices is to get small pieces of useful information (140 characters) to your patients. Facebook is slower-paced and sets the stage to build relationships. Because Facebook is not as rapid as Twitter, and your posts are not as limiting, we recommend practices first start with Facebook and then move into Twitter.

When posting on your social media pages, 80% of the posting should be giving/relationship building and 20% selling. That means 80% of your posts should be giving information such as inspirational smile quotes, comments about community events (ie, the results of a local sports event, news event, etc.), fun facts on the practice (eg, today is Dr Greenwall's birthday), information about dentistry, etc. The other 20% should be focused on selling your services and promotions. Make sure you are also posting, at a minimum, once per day.

Social media is a forum where you can post before-and-after cases, patient testimonials, and any other pertinent information. After you place veneers on a patient, pull out the Flip camera and video your patient's reaction. You can video patient testimonials, comments from the team, and your response to a recent CE course you attended. Take these videos and upload them to your social media sites. (Only upload patient photos and testimonials if you have your patient's written consent.) Let your patient know that it has been posted. Send a link to that patient. The result is a patient sharing that link with friends and family, thus encouraging the patient to refer. In addition, you are helping to plant the seed with patients who are visiting these multiple sites to visit your website and, eventually, your practice.

To keep up with your social media, put one person in the dental practice directly responsible for making the daily posts and for checking your sites every day. If someone makes a post or tweet, the dental practice should be responding to this within 24 hours. If you are not responding, then you are losing the two-way conversation part. Instead it becomes one-way. Know that your marketing is a set of systems and social networking is a division of your marketing system. Attention to detail will be imperative, as will timeliness.

Social media is a great way to get your message out, to be creative, and to participate in marketing in an innovative manner. You are reaching people in a new way and engaging them in conversation. This active participation will result in another lead source for your website, as well as to further build your brand so that you can increase your new patients. Plus, your potential patients will see that you are up-to-date, current, and "cutting edge," just like your dentistry.

Networking events

Participating in networking events is a way to spread your message of aesthetic dentistry. Choose groups that would be interested in aesthetic dentistry and speak of your services with enthusiasm. "When we are truly passionate about something, it's contagious. Our passion draws other people to who we are and what we care about" (Ferrazzi, 2005). Speak to these groups and demonstrate how their appearance and their lives can be improved through aesthetic dentistry. To make the event a powerful and strong "spoke" in your marketing wheel, make a plan. The networking event itself is actually the least important piece of the puzzle. What you do with this event before and after will determine its success. The event itself is a reason to promote your services.

When you participate with a group, follow these steps:

1. Before the event
   - Determine your message for the event.
   - Decide on an offer to present to the participants.
   - Mention your appearance on your Facebook, blog, Twitter, and website.
   - Discuss your pending appearance with your patients.
   - Send a letter to the participants before the event if the organization will provide you with a list.

2. During the event:
   - Focus the presentation on the patients and the benefits they will receive.
   - Raffle a gift (free whitening).
   - Leave something behind such as a brochure and a mirror bearing your logo.
   - Promote your offer.
   - Take photos.
3. After the event:
   - Follow up on any leads with a phone call. Interested leads are the potential patients who expressed a strong desire to move forward with aesthetic dentistry.
   - Add all participants to your email and mail lists.
   - Send a follow-up email to all participants.
   - Send a follow-up letter to all participants.
   - Write a handwritten thank you note to participants if it is a smaller group.
   - Write a press release and send it out to all of the local publications.
   - Post photos to the website, Facebook, and Twitter pages.
   - Place photos in a brag book in your greeting area.
   - Talk about the success of the event to your patients.

Follow these steps and your event will be successful. It is a way to build a buzz about you and your practice. It is another spoke in the marketing wheel. If only two people show up to your speaking engagement, it is still successful when you use that event as a way to effectively promote yourself.

Tracking the results

As there are multiple spokes in your marketing wheel and there is consistency throughout all messages, tracking the results is essential. The more information you have, the better you can tell how your marketing is working and what needs to be modified. Parts of your marketing system that need improvement can be identified through excellent tracking or monitoring.

To be effective you need to track or monitor the following (Fig 6-10):

- Every new patient telephone call into the practice (whether or not the patient schedules).
- Did the patient schedule the appointment?
- Was the patient a no-show or broken appointment, or did they show up for their scheduled time?
- How much treatment was presented?
- What treatment was accepted?

New patient call tracking

By tracking every call into the practice, even if the patient doesn't schedule, you can begin to see if your marketing is generating calls. If the phone is ringing but no one is scheduling, what's happening? Does the new patient call need improvement? If so, modify the verbal skills and try again. If after

Marketing Tracking Log for:

Patient Name	Referral Source	Date of Initial Call	Appt. Sched.	Show Y/N	COE	Tx Diag	Tx Accept	Date of Accept	Type of Patient
Jane Doe	Google Search	3/1/2009	3/15/2009	Y	Y	$15,250	$5,500	4/7/2009	Cosmetic
John Doe	At the Lakes Magazine	3/12/2009	3/21/2009	N	N				General
Jerry Doe	WBL Radio Spot	3/12/2009	4/1/2009	Y	Y	$7,500	$7,500	4/1/2009	Denture

Fig 6-10 Jameson new patient tracking log.

modifying the verbal skills, patients do not schedule, then it is time to look at the marketing message as well as the placement of that message.

Broken appointments and no-shows

If your new patients are consistently breaking their appointments, this bears analysis. One reason could be the new patient phone call (see Chapter 5, Internal Marketing). As we said earlier, the telephone is the most important marketing tool in your practice. It doesn't matter how well you market if people are not calling and scheduling appointments. Telephone skills can be learned and can always be improved. The initial call is a "sales" call, inviting the potential patient to consider your practice. It has to be good. If after modifying your initial phone call, the results stay the same, then the next step is to analyze your welcome packet. Are you sending one? If so, is it sending the right message and is it "you" focused? With eyes wide open, evaluate every piece in your welcome packet. Ask yourself what you think is good and presenting the right message. Then ask that challenging question, how can you do everything you are doing a little bit better? Remember that it is the little improvements that add up to make a big difference.

Treatment presented and accepted

After tracking your results, you may find that patients are calling, they are scheduling, and they are showing up to their appointment. However, people may not be saying "yes" to the aesthetic treatment you are recommending. Are you opening the door to aesthetic possibilities through your marketing and initial contacts? From there, the internal systems of new patient experience and consultation become critical. By tracking all appropriate and desired data, identify key areas that need improvement. Place the Google Analytics free web analysis tool on your website. You will be able to coordinate an increase in visits with particular marketing activities. If there is not a spike after your direct mail drops, then you know that the piece needs work. If people are coming on to the site after a direct mail drop, but instantly leaving the site, then there is a missed connection from the message in the direct mail piece to the website.

All of this information is powerful and can help to improve the effectiveness of your marketing. However, it must be accurately and consistently acquired. Only with that information, can you maximize the return on investment for your marketing.

In summary

Your external marketing is one more element in elevating your stature as an aesthetic dental practice in your community. Boost your success by defining your message, being consistent, repeating the message five to seven times, placing your message in multiple spots, and tracking the results. Include a strong social media strategy to support your marketing efforts and build relationships with your patients. Track the results and be committed to make the necessary changes to receive the maximum return possible. Do these things and your marketing systems will support your goal of building the aesthetic aspect of your dental practice.

Action steps

1. Individually and as a team, define who you are and what you want your image to express to people in your community and in your dental practice.
2. Develop a budget for marketing. Some 4–6% of your last year's collections are allocated to both internal and external marketing. Taking those allocated monies, design a plan of action for your strategic marketing plan.
3. Connect with a designer or marketing consultant to determine what types of external marketing will support your goals and will be appropriate for you, your practice, and your community.
4. If you choose to create any external marketing pieces or to become involved in any external media, engage professional help, advice, and design. The investment will be worth it.

5. Practice telephone skills. Inbound calls from external marketing are different from inbound calls from personal referral. Make sure you have different telephone skills that are individualized for the various types of calls.
6. Establish monitors or tracking devices that indicate results of any external marketing activity. If desired goals are not being met, take a close look at what is happening and make appropriate changes. Lead the way to success in marketing, just as you do in all systems.

Reference

1. Ferrazzi K. Never Eat Alone. New York, NY: Currency Books, 2005.

7 Communication Skills

Cathy Jameson and Linda Greenwall

> *"Listen before you speak. Understand. Diagnose. Listen with your ears—and your eyes and heart. Find out what the most important behaviors are to the people you're working with. Don't assume you know what matters most to others. Don't presume you have all the answers—or all the questions."*
>
> *Stephen MR Covey, 2006*

Introduction

Great communication equals great production. This hypothesis has been proven through statistical research projects (Jameson, 2000). While it seems to be common sense, proving this statement through validated research gives credence to this principle of good management. If you are interested in building the aesthetic aspect of your dental practice, studying, practicing, and improving communication skills is invaluable. In addition, when a dentist studies transformational leadership (Bennis and Townsend, 2005), which includes the study of communication skills, productivity of the dental practice increases (Jameson, 2010).

Aesthetic dentistry is a personal type of care and connects the dental team and the patient in a special relationship. The communication that is a part of each and every interaction is especially important. The oral cavity is an intimate zone of a human being's body and is a reflection of both personality and confidence.

The smile
Cathy Jameson

The smile – reflection of emotion
The smile – mirror to the soul
The smile – causes a chain reaction
The smile – sometimes straight, sometimes uneven, sometimes easy, sometimes difficult
The smile – sometimes with laughter, sometimes without
The smile – an invitation
The smile – communication at its best
The smile – the first impression
The smile – the subject of painters, musicians, photographers, dental artists
The smile – immortalized by literary compositions
The smile – signature of thespians throughout time
The smile – missed if absent, welcomed if present
The smile – God's gift to humanity as a way of expressing love to one another
The smile – a gift of love you give to yourself and to each other.

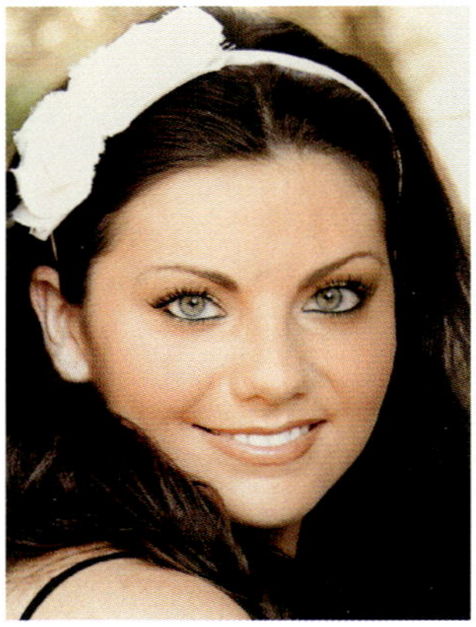

"The first time a patient looked in a mirror with tears in her eyes and reached over to give me a hug, I didn't know what was going on. I had never experienced that before. I had delivered all kinds of dentistry up until that time. But the first time I made an aesthetic change in someone's mouth and saw that their life was dramatically improved, I could have received no fee and would have felt fantastic. This type of dentistry is really rewarding. It motivates me to do it better and better each time – to learn more and more. It is the most fulfilling area of my practice."

Dr Charles Puntillo (interview)

"We have seen aesthetic dentistry truly transform patients' lives. Their emotional well being is every bit as important as their physical well being so why should we ignore the aesthetic aspect of dentistry?"

Cindy Butler (interview), Business Administrator and Treatment Coordinator for Dr Charles Puntillo

Communication is the foundation of excellent relationships and aesthetic or cosmetic dentistry involves a special relationship. Treatment of the oral cavity is an intimate type of care, no matter what the treatment type. However, when you are changing a patient's smile with the goal of enhancing their appearance and, therefore self image too, you are delving deeply into an intimate zone of a person's being.

In your dental practice, no matter what a person's role may be, how they communicate can make all the difference in the world. Communication with a patient can determine whether or not they proceed with treatment, agree to a financial arrangement, or schedule an appointment.

Therefore, it makes sense to study communication to a greater extent. Would you like to accomplish the following as a result of improving your communicative skills?

- improve your personal relationships at work
- acquire a more cohesive team
- reduce burnout and dropout of both you and your team members
- reduce stress for everyone in your dental practice
- increase productivity by a minimum of 10%
- have more patients accept more treatment
- have patients agree to their financial responsibility and reduce disagreements regarding money
- encourage patients to schedule appointments at times that are not only good for them but are also good for you, and to keep those appointments
- have patients come to the dental practice, accept treatment, and stay with the practice over time: no more "falling through the cracks"
- develop the aesthetic/cosmetic aspect of your dental practice.

Hopefully you answered "yes" to all the above statements: "yes," you would like to see improvement in all of these areas and believe that developing better communication could be a part of that improvement.

What is communication?

Communication is an exchange of both information and feelings. A message is sent and a message is received. The key to effective communication is to send messages clearly and succinctly so that your intended message is shared with the recipient. When you receive a message from someone, the only way to determine if you have understood them accurately is to clarify it by listening and speaking. Delivering a message carefully and interpreting a message accurately is important.

Let's look at this more closely. There are four things we do with language: read, write, speak, and listen. In your interactions with your team and patients, all four types of communication bear significance.

(1) Read and (2) write. There are numerous communications that are written and read throughout the ongoing life of your dental practice. Whether you are sending your practice brochure to a potential new patient or sending a newsletter to your existing patient family, how you write and present your ideas can make a difference as to whether a patient comes to you, proceeds with treatment, and stays with you. Be sure to critically review every single written piece of information that is either sent out of your office or is used in your office for inner-office communication.

Everything you do says something about who you are and represents the quality of dental practice you are running. If you aren't an excellent writer or an excellent proofreader, get some professional assistance. A third-party set of eyes may be able to give you a great perspective from a patient's point of view and may be able to pick up those "almost invisible" typos that keep avoiding your eyes.

Remember that the general public doesn't know much about aesthetic/cosmetic dentistry (or any other kind of dentistry for that matter). Your written communication to your patients or to potential patients conveys your interest in your profession, and it enlightens people about what is available in dentistry today. You must accept the responsibility and the opportunity to educate people about what you are doing. Repetition is the key to learning and is also the key to marketing, so put your message out there over and over and do so with excellent written communications.

So much of your written communication presents itself through your website, social networking, and other digital methods. The digital world is an enormous part of dental practices and businesses today. Social networking and social media are here and are drastically impacting how dental practices interact with patients. With digital media, you have a chance to build stronger relationships with present and future patients through continuous and excellent communication.

Internally, the value of the written information that transfers information from the business office to the clinical area and vice versa is another area that requires precision and careful attention. Many miscommunications can be eliminated if the written information (computerized or handwritten) is comprehensive and accurate. Evaluate all of your written communications and ask: "Is our inner-office information being shared in a succinct and thorough manner? Is our written communication clear enough so that people are not constantly asking each other to explain, clarify, or "fill in the blanks"?

(3) Speak. Learn how to communicate your messages effectively. Learn how to say things clearly, professionally, and non-offensively. Agree on the verbal and communicative skills that will enhance your telephone interactions, scheduling, financing, revenue, treatment recommendations, hygiene retention, etc. Spend time, as a team, reviewing the aesthetic procedures you are providing. Discuss the best ways to talk to patients about those procedures in an understandable manner. Use patient-friendly explanations and not dental terminology.

In addition, identify the normal objections you hear in various situations and at various times throughout your day. Practice presenting your ideas and needs or practice protocols. Practice addressing the objections: how to respond to patient enquiries, how to get your message across more clearly, and how to let people know what you expect of them without coming across as aggressive or offensive.

Know that you can say something one way and get a positive response and say something in another way and get a negative response. How you say anything makes a powerful difference.

(4) Listen. In his famous study of motivation, called the Hawthorne Effect, Dr Elton Mayo (1932) says that "one friend, one person who is truly understanding and who takes the trouble to listen to us as we consider our problem, can change our whole outlook on the world." Listening may be the greatest gift we can give to one another.

Listening is essential if you are trying to determine a patient's emotional "hot button" or major motivator. If you have a relationship that is difficult, listening to each other's point of view is critical to resolution. If you have an angry or upset person on your team or in your patient family, listening is the single best way to reduce their heightened emotion so that you can begin an equitable conversation focused on getting the problem solved. It's difficult for a person to really hear what you are saying or to be able to express themselves clearly when emotion is at an intense level. Through listening, the heightened emotion can be reduced and/or calmed. In this more open communication scenario, listening is enhanced.

However, listening is not easy. There are many things that get in the way of good listening: time, busy schedules, interruptions, being unfocused, too much going on at one time, not wanting to listen, being in a hurry to give a solution rather than listening, and egotistically thinking you already know the answer so you don't have to listen. While listening may be considered the most important of all communication skills when establishing and nurturing a relationship, most people have never had a course on the skill of listening.

Dr Mark Hyman of Greensboro, NC, says, "Listening is the hallmark of any long-term relationship. Your patient's goals for their health, circumstances, and priorities are constantly changing. We must listen with every contact we have with the patient, whether that be on the phone, on e-mail or in person. We must be constantly present and focused and communicate our perception of where the patient is at this time in their life."

Listening

Listening is made up of four different and important skills:

- body language
- tone of voice
- passive listening
- active listening.

Body language

Body language accounts for 55% (Mehrabian, 1981) of the perception of the message whether you are sending or receiving a message. Pay attention to what you are saying with your body language. Patients may or may not listen to you or may not think you are listening to them depending on your body language.

Examples of body language expressions that have a constructive influence on communication (Fig 7-1) include the following:

- establish and maintain eye contact
- position yourself on the same level
- be face to face
- touch – in a reassuring and gentle manner (such as on the arm before you lower the chair)
- nod or shake your head in response to the other person's message
- facial expressions – look attentive and responsive
- uncross arms and legs.

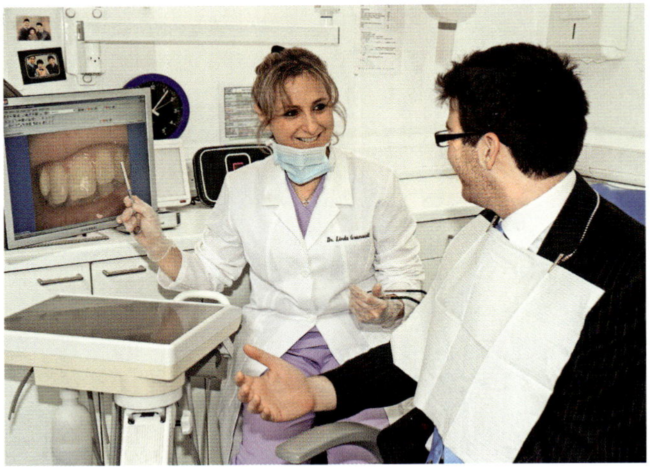

Fig 7-1a Position yourself at the same level as the patient in order to achieve good communication. Be sure to make eye contact with the patient.

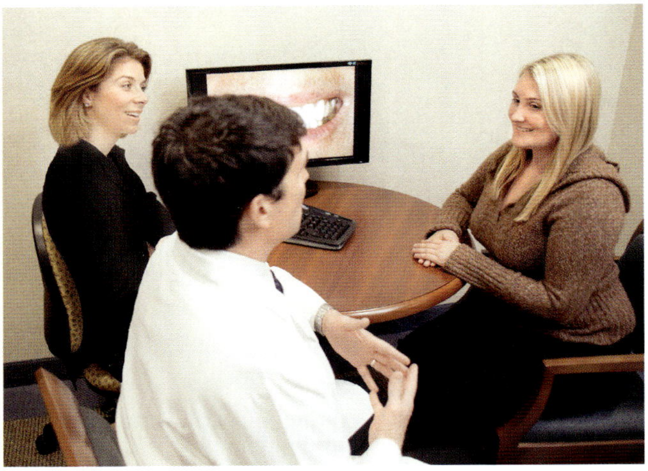

Fig 7-1b Body language is vital to an effective consultation, as demonstrated by Dr Hyman and his treatment coordinator.

Body language is critical in all settings within the dental practice. Every team member will communicate more effectively in their interactions with patients if they pay attention to body language.

When you are speaking or listening to a patient, be aware of their body language and try to make sure you are hearing them accurately, paying total attention, and receiving their message. If patients display negative body language, you might as well stop and go back. Find out what may have been upsetting and deal with that. Otherwise, the patient will not hear another word you are saying. Heightened emotion can stifle a patient's ability to listen to you. These are some of the physical signs displayed when a person is upset, confused and unable to listen:

- emphatically crossing arms and legs
- grasping and clinging to the arms of the chair
- frowning and other negative facial expressions
- angry or frustrated gestures of the hand/body
- slouching posture
- reaching out to touch you, like grabbing your arm or hand
- pulling back from you; distancing themselves
- skin responses – blushing or the opposite, losing all color in the face.

It is said that "actions speak louder than words". There is much truth in that statement. If body language accounts for 55% of a message whether you are sending or receiving that message, it is important to pay attention to this. Body language when connected with a reflective tone of voice impacts your communication as much, if not more, than any words you speak.

Tone of voice accounts for 38% of the perception of the message (Mehrabian, 1981). Be interesting, expressive, and enthusiastic. This doesn't mean you have to be someone you are not. However, all people can develop a tone of voice that encourages others to listen. Try recording yourself (you will not be happy with what you hear, but do this anyway). Record yourself speaking on the telephone and interacting with a patient (you can do this through simulation). Then listen to yourself. Do you interest your own self or do you bore yourself? Vocal training is accessible and worth the effort.

If body language accounts for 55% of a message and tone of voice accounts for 38% of the message, 93% of what you are saying to another person is nonverbal. That, of course, means that 7% of the perception of a message is verbal (Mehrabian, 1981). While the words are critical, no matter how eloquent the vocabulary, without effective presentation, the purpose and impact of the message may be compromised.

Vocal cues

Let's examine the four types of vocal cues: pitch, rate, volume, and quality.

- **Pitch.** Genetics determine the pitch, or the highness and lowness of your voice. The pitch of your voice can be influenced by nervousness, hoarseness, heightened emotion, fatigue, and so on. Relax and breathe.
- **Rate.** The speed at which you speak is considered the "rate". The rate of your speech may be a reflection of your personality. High energy people may speak faster than people who are more relaxed by nature. Your rate may be influenced by where you live, the state of your emotions, your calmness or nervousness. Relax and breathe.
- **Volume.** Loudness or softness of your voice is volume. There may be variances in volume depending on what you are doing, who you are with, and how comfortable you are in a situation. Volume of voice can reflect self-confidence, self-esteem or comfort. Relax and breathe.
- **Quality.** This is the actual sound of your voice. This is the unique sound that becomes your "signature". People can soon recognize you by the sound of your voice. This is the quality. Relax and breathe.

The voice is an instrument and is part of your individuality and your expression of self. If you think you could improve your image, consider vocal lessons. Vocal training is an important part of communicating effectively and can impact the quality of your presentations.

Passive listening

Passive listening means giving the other person verbal cues to go on, to continue, and to give you more information. Passive listening responses are non-stimulating responses that encourage the other person to continue giving you information. You will be listening for insights.

Passive listening can be divided into two types of responses: acknowledgement and door openers.

Examples of acknowledgements are:

- "ok"
- "go on"
- "uh-huh"
- "hmm"
- "really?"

Door openers give a person a specific invitation to continue. Remember, the purpose of passive listening is to encourage the other person to keep talking. You are trying to discover what they mean, what they want or need, or the problem or concern they are bringing to you.

Examples of door openers may be:

- "Tell me about that"
- "Please go on"
- "Can you give me more information about that?"
- "Help me understand that."

You want people to continue sharing their insights with you. When you are listening to a patient seeking care, certainly a person seeking aesthetic treatment, you want to hear them out. You want to know how they feel about their present smile and how they would like to change that smile. When you discover what they want, you can design your own presentation around their individual interests. You can only find out what those interests might be by asking questions and using all of the listening skills. Do not interrupt a person to tell them what you think or to start dictating about treatment recommendations. There will be a time for that. However, if you jump into a presentation before you have determined the patient's emotional "hot button" or major motivator, you may present to the wrong interest and get nowhere. Silence is a communication skill! The most challenging part of passive listening is asking the question and then waiting for the person to respond without interrupting. When you ask a question, be quiet! Let them answer even if a few moments of silence occur.

According to Dr Thomas Gordon (1977), "Silence or passive listening is a potent tool for getting people to talk about what's bothering them, and talking to someone who is willing to listen may be just the encouragement a person needs to keep going."

Active listening

Active listening (Gordon, 1975) means putting into your own words, or paraphrasing, what you think the other person has just said, and reflecting or feeding it back to them so that they can tell you whether you have heard them accurately or not. Kevin Murphy (1987), says, "Listening is the accurate perception of what is being communicated." How many times do we hear the words that another person speaks but totally misinterpret the meaning? Active listening on a daily basis gives you a chance to clarify and to check with the other person to make sure you have not only heard the words they are speaking but you have also clearly and accurately understood the meaning behind the words. This will go a long way to do the following:

- show respect
- establish clear meaning
- capture the intention of a statement or message
- further the relationship
- reduce mistakes
- reduce misunderstandings.

In active listening you pay attention to both the content of the message and the feeling behind the message. Do not think that you can separate emotion out of the equation. Communication is a combination of both information and emotion.

For example:

Patient: "I have always hated my teeth. I don't even like to smile. I don't want other people to see my teeth, so I don't smile. I look unhappy, but I'm not. I just don't smile because I'm embarrassed about my teeth.
Dentist: "You're uncomfortable about the way your teeth look and so you don't smile. But you don't really want people to think you are unfriendly."
Patient: "That's right. People think I'm unfriendly because I look that way. But I'm not. So, I think I need to do something about my teeth."
Dentist: "You've been embarrassed about your teeth for long enough. You want to be able to smile comfortably and confidently, so you are here today to see what can be done to help you get a more attractive smile."
Patient: "Maybe so. Can you do anything for me?"
Dentist: "Once I am very clear about what you want, I will do a comprehensive evaluation of your situation and see what is going on. Then, I will design a plan of treatment that helps you to have the smile you have always wanted. This is what we do here, create beautiful, healthy smiles. I'll show you some examples of other patients who have had a smile makeover and will let you read what they said once they had completed treatment. Together we will determine a plan of action that is right for you. How does that sound?"

By listening, the dentist was able to let the person express their concerns. Actually, through listening, the patient told the dentist what she wanted. So far, the dentist hasn't told her anything. He/she listened and let the patient express their wants, needs, and issues. The patient opened her own door for treatment. You can listen your way to case acceptance.

Eight steps to effective listening

1. Reduce as many distractions and interruptions as possible.
2. Focus your mind on the speaker. Clear away as many internal distractions as possible.
3. Take notes of key issues so that you stay focused and can return to these points when appropriate.
4. Respond to the speaker's total message. Do not pay attention to the words only. Pay attention to the body language, tone of voice, and the emotion.
5. Listen without judgment.
6. Do not be thinking about what you are going to say or how you are going to respond. You will be unable to accurately listen.

7. Keep an open mind when you are listening to another.
8. If you catch yourself not listening, refocus and change your body position to make it more conducive to listening.

When you are speaking to a patient about a smile makeover, listen. You want to know what the patient is seeking and what kind of change of smile is of interest to them. People will never make a decision to proceed with treatment unless they feel that they are listened to, that they are understood, and that they can trust you. You want the patient to tell you what they want. Only then can you provide what they want: a beautiful new smile.

Speaking

Mortimer Adler (1983) says, "The meeting of two minds may consist in their understanding one another while still in disagreement or it may consist in their coming into agreement as a result of their understanding one another." While listening may be the most significant aspect of communication when you are trying to establish and maintain a relationship, certainly how you speak makes a powerful difference, as well.

When you speak, your intention is to get your message across clearly without misunderstanding or inaccuracy. In addition, when you are experiencing a problem yourself, you need to be able to express that concern without hurting the other person or turning a misspoken word into a conflict. Learning to speak clearly and empathetically is one of the essential elements of great communication.

The goals of good speaking are the following (Jameson, 2004):

- To help people *want* to listen to what you have to say.
- To deliver the message in the best possible way.
- To check to see if you were heard (or interpreted) correctly.

As you are building your relationship with a person, you want to make sure that the way you speak and the things you say are conducive to a healthy relationship. In addition, once you have earned the right to present your recommendations to a patient, you want to express your recommendations in the best possible manner. Your goal is to have the patient agree to proceed with treatment, therefore:

- be direct
- be specific
- get to the point
- be positive
- present your recommendations to the other person's motivators
- establish and protect your relationship of trust with the patient.

The flow of communication as part of problem solving

In all communication exchanges, someone sends a message and someone receives it. All messages are interpreted by the receiver based on that person's experiences. Since no one has the same life experiences, any message can be misinterpreted. During the flow of communication, a message is sent (someone says something) and then the other person decodes the message based on their personal understanding. The person receiving the message needs to "check it out." In other words, listen, interpret the message, paraphrase what you think you have just heard, and send this back to the other person to see if you are accurate – or not. This is a great gift you give to yourself and to the other person. How wonderful to truly understand one another and to reduce misunderstandings. Both the speaking skills and the listening skills are a part of this effective problem solving (Adams, 1989).

What does this mean for your dental team? When a person comes to your office seeking care, they are coming to you with a concern or a problem. Often people wrap a solution around a problem before they figure out what is at the root of the situation. Spend time determining what the real problem is and define it in terms of the needs of the people involved. Listen to patients to discover their main interest/desire or their dominant concern/problem. Then build your presentation of recommendations around a solution that meets their "felt" needs. Perhaps the biggest detriment to solving a problem is offering a solution before the actual problem has been determined. Of course, problem solving is not only an ongoing part of your patient relationships; it is a part of your team relationships as well. Problem solving is an important part of strategic planning, goal setting, and dental practice development.

The problem solving technique is outlined below.

- **Define the problem.** Identify the problem in terms of what each party needs. This step of problem solving may take longer than any of the other steps. Take as long as you require. Establish clarity of need before developing solutions.
- **Brainstorm possible solutions.** This is the creative phase of problem solving. Throw out as many ideas as possible to solve the problem. Do not analyze the ideas at this point, simply brainstorm. Write down the ideas that are suggested. Don't give any opinions either affirmatively or negatively. Just set your minds to free-flow and generate possible solutions. Again, do not be critical of anyone for a particular idea, which could shut down the brainstorming process.
- **Discuss each possible solution.** This is the time that you discuss the pros and cons of each idea that was presented during your brainstorming session. Be respectful of each other's ideas. You may not like an idea and you may not agree with it. However, use your positive disagreement skills here. Respect each other's right to their own opinion.
- **Come to a consensus agreement.** Together, determine the solution or solutions that you believe will work best for you.
- **Design a plan of action.** This is when the goal accomplishment steps truly shine. Use the goal accomplishment process and form (Fig 2-5) to design a plan of action as to how you will make the solving of your problem a reality.
- **Put the plan into action.** After all of your efforts to resolve your problem, now is the time to put your action plan into place. Commit to putting it into action and carrying out the responsibilities you have agreed upon.

- **Evaluate.** Determine if the plan of action is working. Revisit the conversation if necessary. Make sure the needs of each party are being met. Both parties need to "win" in order for your problem-solving to be considered successful.

As you study case presentation (in Chapter 10), refer back to this section. You will see that these steps are the basis for an excellent new patient experience and consultation.

In summary

Great communication equals great results and great production. Through effective listening, speaking, and problem solving, communication becomes not only an asset to relationships but also becomes a critical factor in building the productivity of your dental practice. Effectiveness in communication is a lifelong study and one that is worth both time and effort.

Action steps

1. Discuss the definition of communication. Have each person define what communication means to them.
2. As a team, discuss the importance of communication with each other and with patients.
3. Discuss the four types of communication (reading, writing, speaking, and listening), and when and where these are present in your dental practice. Discuss what is going well so that you can continue to do those things. Discuss areas where improvement could be beneficial and what you will do to support that improvement.
4. Read and study the section on listening. Perform practice exercises of each kind of listening.
5. Using a goal sheet (Fig 2-5), write goals related to how you will work to improve communication in your dental practice, including telephone, patient interaction and education, written communication such as website and other marketing, as well as internal written forms, and case presentation. Other areas for discussion can be determined by you.

References

1. Adams L. Be Your Best. New York, NY: Berkley Publishing Group, 1989.
2. Adler M. How to Speak, How to Listen. New York, NY: McMillan Publishing, 1983.
3. Bennis W, Townsend R. Reinventing leadership. New York, NY: Harper Collins, 2005.
4. Covey SMR. The Speed of Trust. New York, NY: Free Press, 2006.
5. Gordon T. Parent Effectiveness Training. New York, NY: Peter H. Wyden, 1975.
6. Gordon T. Leader Effectiveness Training. New York, NY: Peter H. Wyden, 1977.
7. Jameson C. Controlling Stress in the Dental Profession Through Effective Communication. Oklahoma City, OK: JC Educational Services, 2000.
8. Jameson C. Great Communication Equals Great Production. Tulsa, OK: Pennwell Books, 2004.

9. Jameson C. The Impact of Training in Transformational Leadership on the Productivity of a Dental Practice (unpublished doctoral dissertation). Minneapolis, MN: Walden University, 2010.

10. Mayo E. The Hawthorne Effect. Cicero, IL: Western Electric Works, 1932.

11. Mehrabian A. Silent Messages: implicit communication of emotions and attitudes. Belmont, CA: Wadsworth Publishing, 1981.

12. Murphy K. Effective Listening. New York, NY: Bantam Books, 1987.

8 The Business of Bleaching and Tooth Whitening

Linda Greenwall and Cathy Jameson

> *Practicing dentistry is not easy. Practicing aesthetic dentistry is more demanding and involves more complex technologies and a good psychological understanding of the needs, wants, desires, and expectations of our patients, as well as the frustrations and limitations of what we can provide.*
>
> *Dr Ron Goldstein (2002)*

Introduction

Tooth whitening has become one of the most requested aesthetic dental treatments. Many patients do not want extreme changes to their smiles, but want natural enhanced improvements to their existing smile. Tooth whitening treatments improve the appearance of teeth, as lighter teeth appear more youthful and healthy. Many patients who have had whitening then choose to have further aesthetic dentistry. Tooth whitening can be the motivating factor that leads to further aesthetic dentistry.

There are several reasons why teeth discolor and it is essential that the correct diagnosis is made of the cause of the discoloration, so that the appropriate whitening program can be specifically designed for that patient. (For a detailed description of the nature of tooth discoloration, see Greenwall, 2001; Chapter 1)

New patients for whitening

Many new patients who attend the dental practice for the first time request whitening treatment (see Fig 9-3, new patient journey). Tooth whitening is normally the first treatment that is undertaken prior to any other aesthetic or restorative dentistry after any emergency treatment is undertaken (see Appendix 9-5). At the new patient consultation, it is important to ask the patient open-ended questions to fully understand what treatment they are seeking, for example, "How do you feel about the color of your teeth?" Some patients are too shy to ask for whitening. However, when asked, "What are your hopes and aspirations for your smile?" patients often report that "I know my teeth are really yellow, but I do not know what can be done about them."

This can lead to a discussion about whitening. Whitening also has further health benefits such as improved gingival condition, improved oral hygiene and reduced root caries in the elderly (Haywood, 2007), which can be discussed with the patient. Understand at this stage what the patient wants in terms of tooth whitening and the desired shade, whether this is enhanced whitening of their natural shade or an ultra-white "Hollywood white look." Some patients may have unrealistic expectations of the desired outcome and it is essential to understand early on whether these expectations are realistic or unrealistic and unachievable. An outline of the diagnosis process for tooth whitening is shown in Figure 8-1.

Assessment of existing sensitivity

It is also important to ask patients about existing sensitivity as the main side effect of whitening is sensitivity. Up to 50% of patients can experience some type of transient sensitivity during whitening (Leonard et al., 1997). It is important to ask patients about any existing sensitivity or other sensitivity symptoms prior to commencing bleaching treatment (Leonard et al., 2004). Also ask about hot or cold sensitivity, which could mean that there is gingival recession or dentine hypersensitivity present. Asking about sensitivity to heat will elucidate whether the patient has pulpal problems on any teeth. Further questions about pain on biting or cold sensitivity may reveal the presence of a crack on a tooth. Some of these problems such as pulpitis or a crack should be dealt with prior to bleaching the teeth. Figure 8-2 outlines the treatment sequence for managing bleaching sensitivity.

The benefits of tooth whitening:

- improves shade of the teeth by lightening and whitening (Haywood & Heymann, 1989)
- improves the gingival condition
- improves oral hygiene as patients are brushing better and are more interested in their smile
- improves self esteem
- may improve dental caries
- reduces root decay in the elderly (Haywood, 2007)
- gives a more youthful smile (Matis, 2003).

Intraoral assessment for patients requesting whitening

The whitening prescription (Appendix 8-1) has been prepared as a checklist to ensure that all aspects and possible complications are checked and discussed with patients. It is important to check and record the vitality of all darkened teeth. Large restorations should be assessed particularly on the anterior teeth and to ensure that there is sufficient enamel for bleaching. Existing white spots are evaluated and discussed with patients, as white spots get whiter during whitening and this can be alarming to patients.

The following factors should be assessed at the intraoral examination:

- aging enamel
- dehydration lines

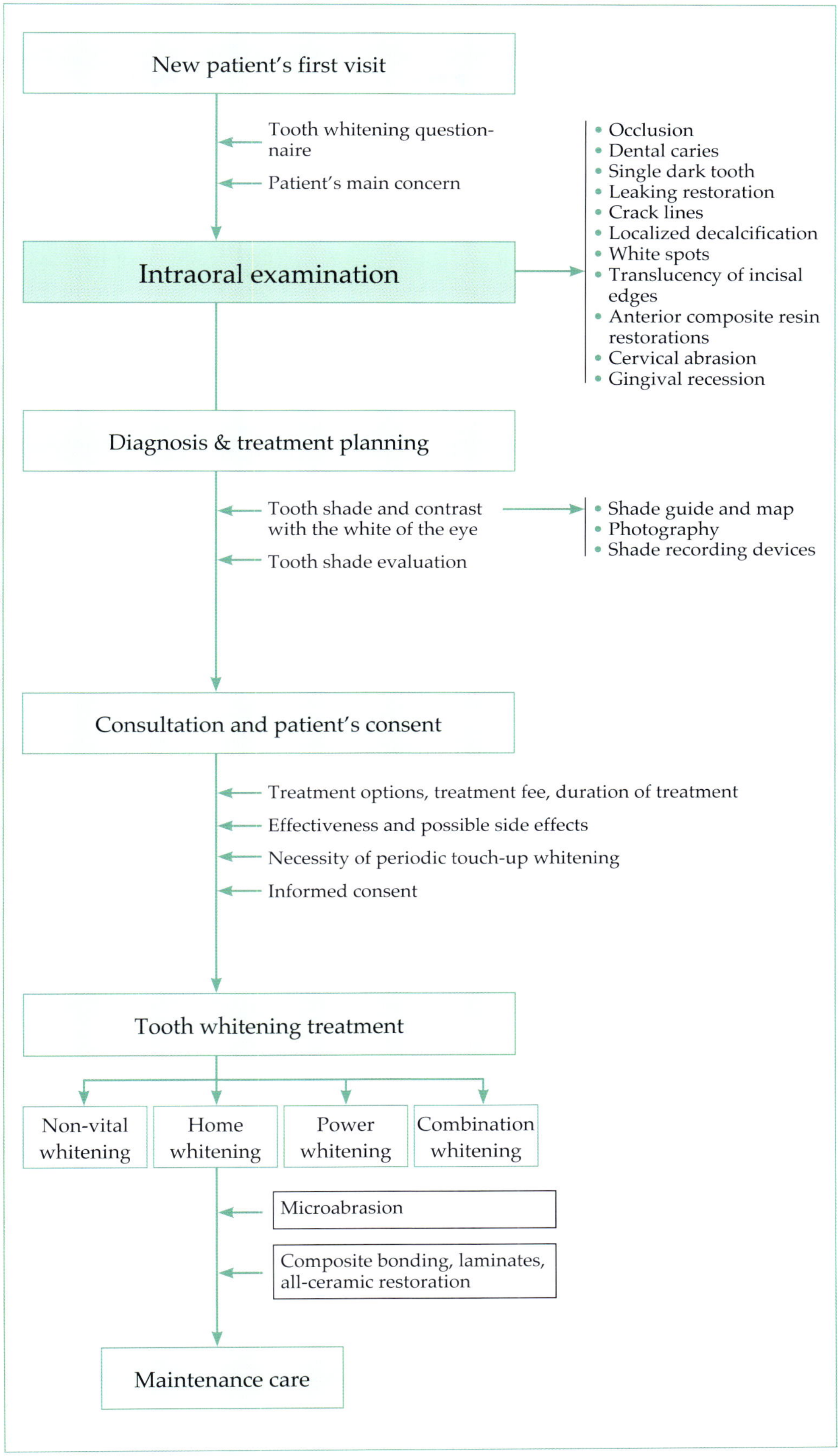

Fig 8-1 New patient whitening journey stages. Diagnosis process for tooth whitening (reproduced from Kwon et al., 2010, with permission from Quintessence Publishing).

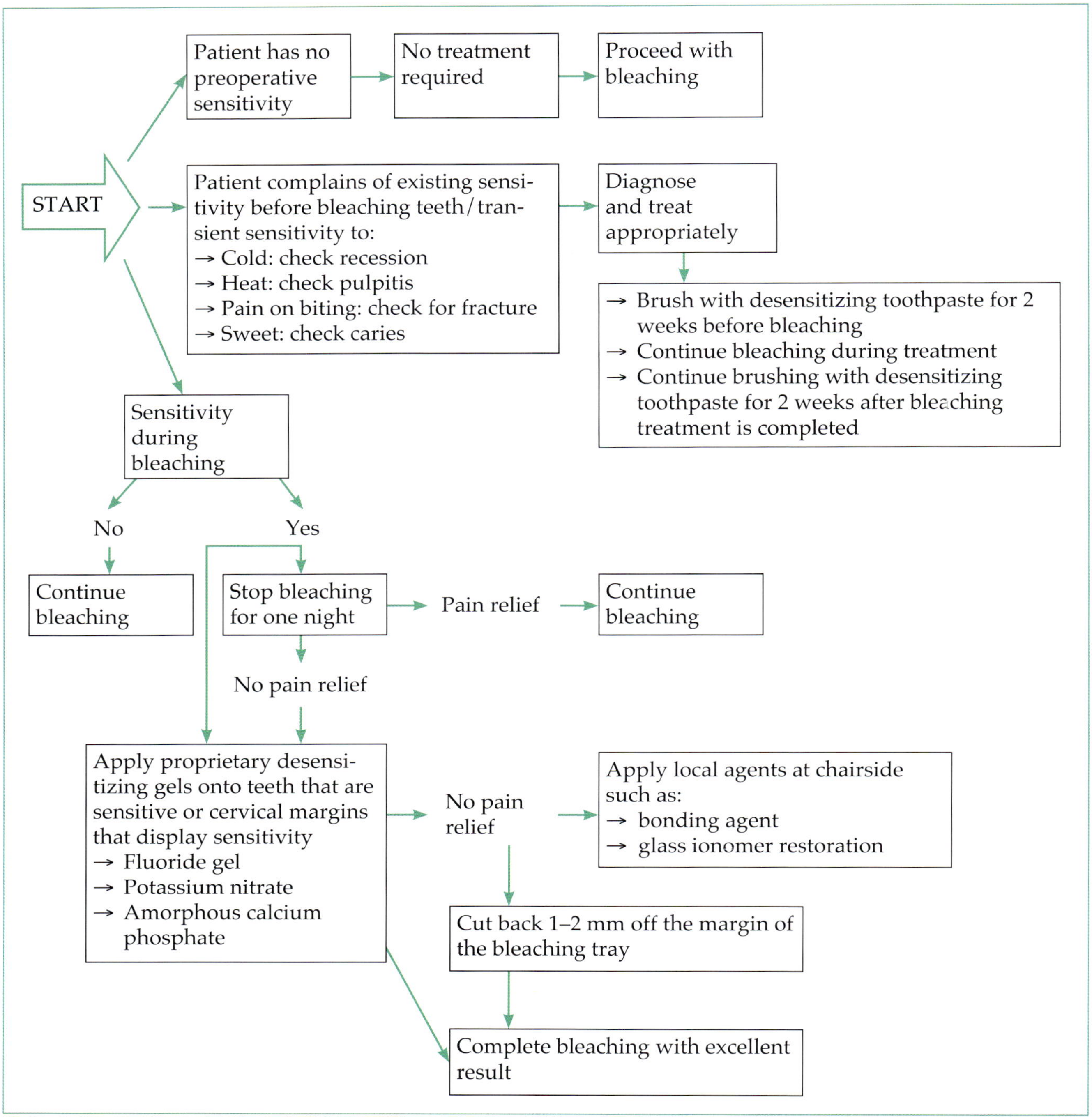

Fig 8-2 Treatment sequence for managing bleaching sensitivity.

- crack lines
- white spots
- internal tooth shading, characterizations
- shading of the teeth, anterior and posterior maxillary and mandibular
- tooth wear
- existing composite restorations

- non-vital teeth
- single yellow vital teeth
- deeper stains or markings
- amalgam staining
- type of discoloration, eg, tetracycline or fluorosis stain
- white markings
- chronological age when damage occurred
- presence of caries or abscesses.

Shade assessment

Assess the patient's baseline shade. Record the shade of the six anterior maxillary teeth as these can all be different. Record the shade of the mandibular teeth. Often there can be a discrepancy between the shade of the maxillary and mandibular teeth. The basic assessment uses the porcelain shade guides (Figs 8-3 and 8-4). Show patients on the shade guide what they may hope to achieve from a realistic point of view. Do not promise something that cannot be achieved in terms of whiteness. Many patients want the whitest shade available and this may not always be possible: further aesthetic dentistry may be necessary. Some patients have all anterior teeth a different shade and this should be individually recorded (Fig 8-5).

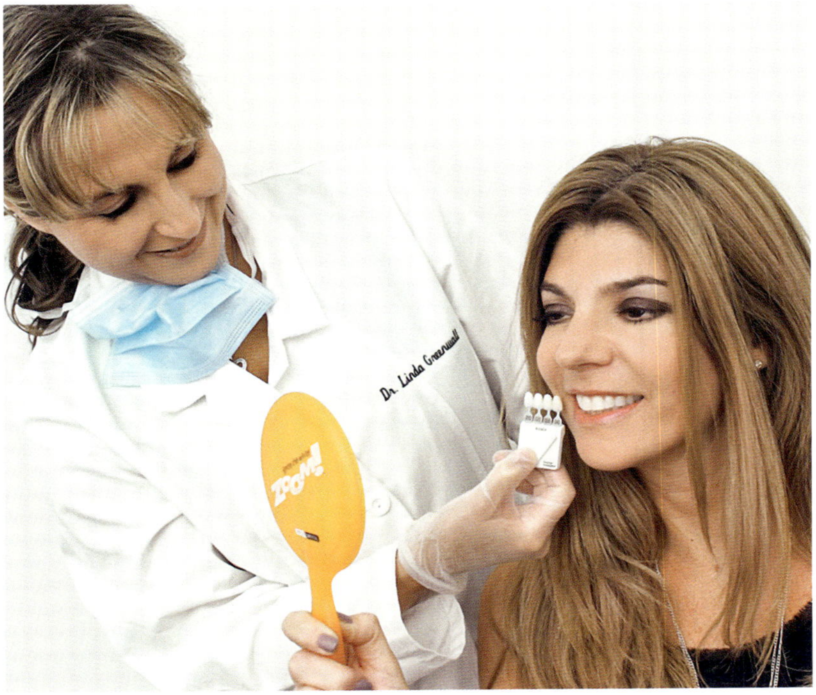

Fig 8-3 Shade assessment. It is essential to involve the patient in the discussion about the shade before, during and after whitening. In this figure the patient is involved in the discussion about the shade of the teeth and uses a mirror to look at the shade guide in comparison to the shade of the teeth.

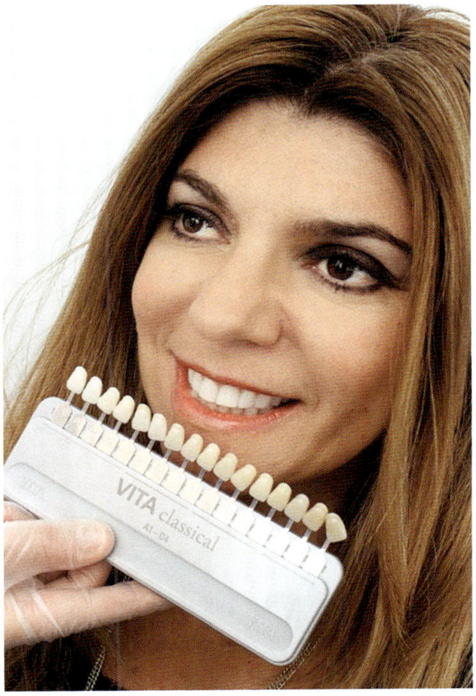

Fig 8-4 The classic Vita shade guide is used to assess the change in color after the whitening treatment. A comparison is made with the shade of the white of the eyes, as after completion of whitening treatment the white of the eyes should match the shade of the teeth.

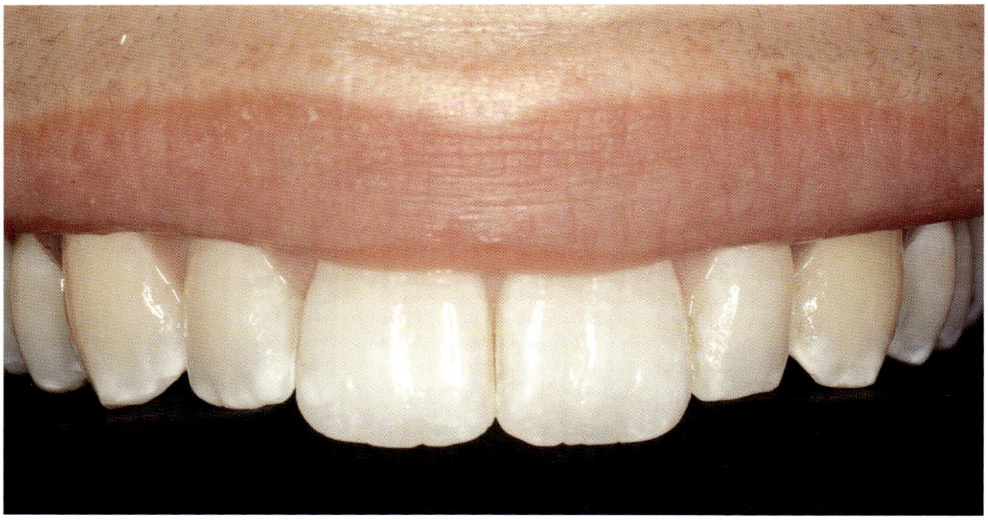

Fig 8-5 This patient's maxillary anterior teeth are different shades. There is a contrast between the shade on the central incisors, the lateral incisors, and the canine teeth. The canine teeth are always darker, and the patient needs to be informed of this. In addition, this patient has numerous white spots in the incisal tips. This should be noted and discussed with the patient, as white spots become whiter and brighter during the initial phases of bleaching. The patient may be alarmed at this if not previously told.

Classification of whitening treatment

Whitening treatments can be classified into three categories, as follows (Kwon et al., 2010).

1. Basic whitening (Fig 8-6)
   - Basic discoloration
   - Home bleaching, 4–6 weeks to achieve B1
   - No restorative dentistry required.
2. Intermediate whitening (Fig 8-7)
   - Combinations of discoloration present, such as non-vital tooth and age yellowing
   - Combination of treatments may need to be undertaken such as non-vital bleaching and home bleaching
   - Some restorative dentistry required afterwards
   - 6–8 weeks to get to B1 and maintain it.
3. Advanced whitening (Fig 8-8)
   - Deep discoloration present, such as tetracycline (Matis et al., 2009) or fluorosis staining
   - Prolonged whitening needed
   - Whitening in combination with advanced restorative dentistry
   - 8–10 weeks to get to B1 owing to complex nature of discoloration
   - Patients who have existing sensitivity may need treatment, and whitening their teeth can be more complex as the sensitivity may need to be managed prior to bleaching, during bleaching, and after bleaching. This would require more time and thus would require more management.

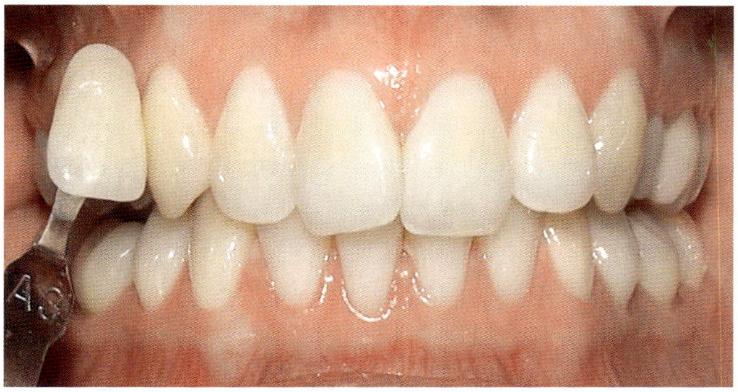

Fig 8-6a Basic bleaching case: appearance of the teeth before bleaching. The patient had healthy teeth that did not require further restorations.

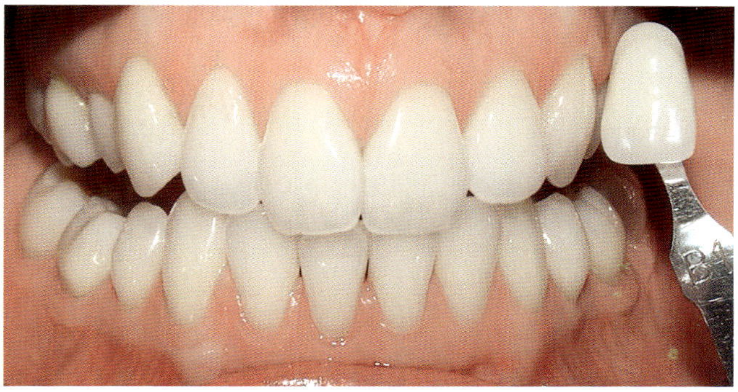

Fig 8-6b Basic bleaching case: results after bleaching. The teeth were lightened to shade B1 and have remained that shade for the last 5 years. The bleaching protocol that was used was that reported by Dr Van Haywood (Haywood & Heymann, 1989).

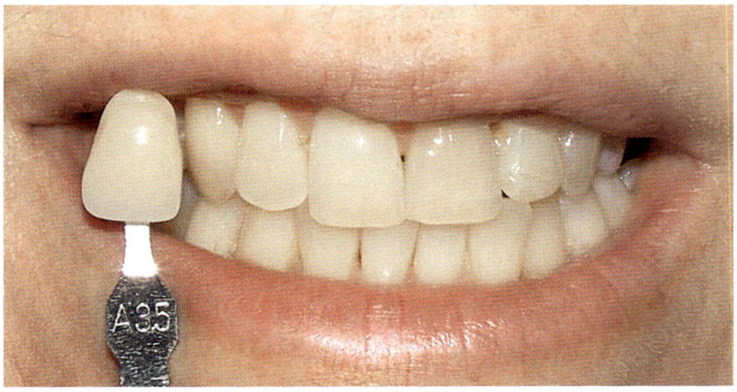

Fig 8-7a Intermediate bleaching case: appearance of the teeth before bleaching. The patient had sustained a fracture to the maxillary left central incisor and the maxillary left lateral tooth. The maxillary left central was root treated and internal bleaching was undertaken. This was followed by home whitening treatment wearing the night guard. A concentration of 10% carbamide peroxide was used in the tray. The maxillary teeth were bleached for 2 weeks, and then the mandibular teeth were bleached for 3 weeks. Although the maxillary left central incisor had experienced trauma, the patient has been told about possible long-term damaging effects of trauma to non-vital teeth.

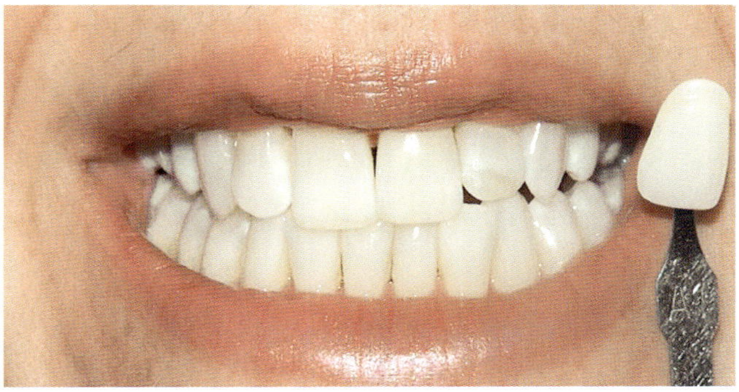

Fig 8-7b Intermediate bleaching case: appearance of the teeth after bleaching. Non-vital bleaching was undertaken for the maxillary left central incisor, and the rest of the teeth were bleached using the home bleaching treatment in the trays.

Treatment planning for patients requesting tooth whitening

The dentist should thoroughly assess and evaluate the patient's aesthetic needs in order to ensure that the most appropriate treatment is provided (Small, 1998). This involves excellent communication with the patient to understand exactly their concerns about their smile. The patient's hopes and aspirations about their smile and their mouth need to be carefully understood. A new consultation involves an interview, an intraoral evaluation, and an examination of the whole mouth. After this thorough assessment (see smile evaluation form [Fig 5-4], new patient questionnaire, and check-

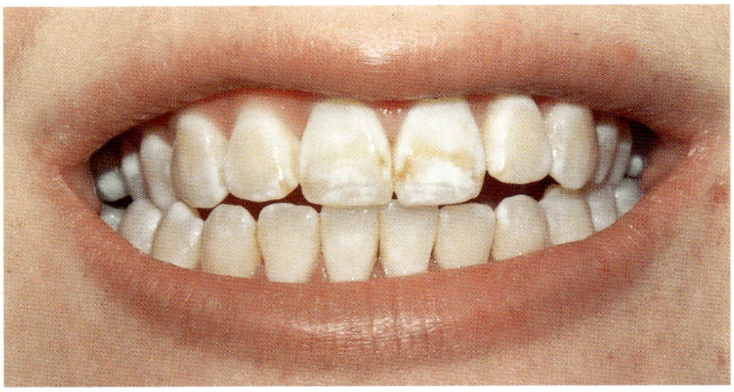

Fig 8-8a Advanced bleaching case: appearance of the teeth before bleaching treatment. This patient suffered from teeth that had a mottled appearance with the presence of brown and white areas across the tooth. The cause was probably due to fluorosis. A specific treatment plan was designed for the patient, where advanced bleaching was undertaken. The teeth were bleached using 10% carbamide peroxide in a bleaching tray for a period of 8 to 10 weeks. The brown stain was removed entirely from the teeth, and then the background of the tooth was lightened. This was followed by two sessions of microabrasion to fade the appearance of the white spots. This was very conservative treatment and the entire enamel surface of the teeth was preserved.

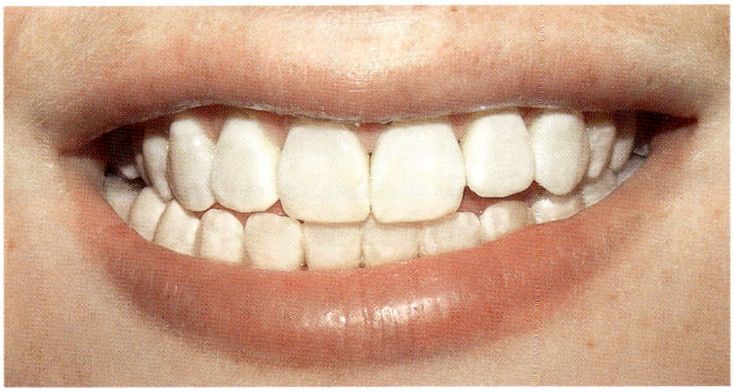

Fig 8-8b Advanced bleaching case: appearance of the teeth after treatment, showing the new lightened shade. After whitening treatment, the patient received two sessions of microabrasion to further fade the white spots.

lists (Chapter 9, Appendixes) – further tests are performed such as vitality testing radiographs, and photographs. Intraoral camera pictures are taken. Once the dentist has all the necessary data, a treatment plan can be designed. The patient is invited back for another appointment for a treatment planning discussion, which is the case presentation (see Chapter 10 for a detailed discussion).

It is important to classify bleaching cases into three categories in order to plan treatment effectively. This also relates to a fee structure, as different bleaching treatments carry a different fee, varying with complexity of treatment and time spent with each patient. So that cases can be well planned, the appropriate appointment sequences should be allocated to the treatment and booked after financial arrangements have been made. Procedure analysis forms (see Chapter 13, Scheduling Aesthetic Dentistry) are completed for all clinical treatment in the dental practice so that systems are well organized. Appendix 8-5 shows a procedure analysis form for home and power bleaching and the associated tray set-ups. At the case presentation and treatment discussion it is important to keep the discussion realistic as to what the patient can expect to happen during whitening. Discuss what will and what will not happen, so the boundaries are kept real to limit the patient's expectations. It is better to underestimate the likely result than overpromise and underdeliver. That way, patients are delighted with the results.

Setting fees for whitening

Fees are based on the classification of the bleaching case and the length of time that it is estimated will be required to complete the case effectively. Darker teeth will take longer to treat than those of a lighter shade and thus will require a different fee. Older teeth will take longer to bleach because of the internal structure of the dentine being highly compacted, and thus the bleach will travel through the teeth more slowly. Older patients will require a different time sequence and allocation for appointments due to the slower nature of the whitening treatment.

Involving the entire team in tooth whitening

It is essential that the entire team is involved in the bleaching (Haywood, 2008). Training and education for the entire team on whitening should be undertaken. Depending on local legislation, each procedure that can be delegated and taught to a dental team member to administer to the patient will save time in the dentist's schedule. The dentist diagnoses the nature of the discoloration and designs the treatment plan for the bleaching treatment and the type of bleaching procedure that is needed.

A dental team that is appropriately trained can be involved in helping with these programs to achieve amazing whitening results. Delegate, according to the laws of your state or country, the whitening treatments to those team members that have been appropriately trained and know the whitening procedure protocols for the dental practice. Completed procedure analysis forms (Appendix 8-5) are part of the dental practice manual and the rooms are prepared for each different whitening appointment following the photographs of the tray set-ups for the treatment room. The appropriately trained hygienist will then manage all the whitening treatment appointments at the dental practice (including home and power bleaching, see Fig 8-16). A dental team member may administer the home bleaching instructions or undertake the chairside whitening procedure.

All team members should be able to take clinical photos according to the recommended guidelines. All team members need to know what advice to give the patient if they are experiencing sensitivity or pain during the whitening treatments. Adjunctive soothing materials may need to be administered.

Continual monitoring is essential throughout the course of whitening treatment to ensure that the patient is motivated to complete the whitening program and to achieve an excellent level of whiteness that is long lasting. Both the dentist and patient should be satisfied with the color achieved. The monitoring appointments should be scheduled in the hygienist's day and the dentist can come through to the hygienist's room to monitor progress.

Again, delegate everything you can, according to the laws and certification requirements of your state or country.

Marketing bleaching treatments

Marketing for whitening can be done externally and internally. Many dental practices do not market their whitening treatments, as patients come in seeking the whitening services. As tooth whitening is such an important service, these aesthetic services are an integral part of the external marketing plan that should be implemented (see Chapter 6). Most dental practices market

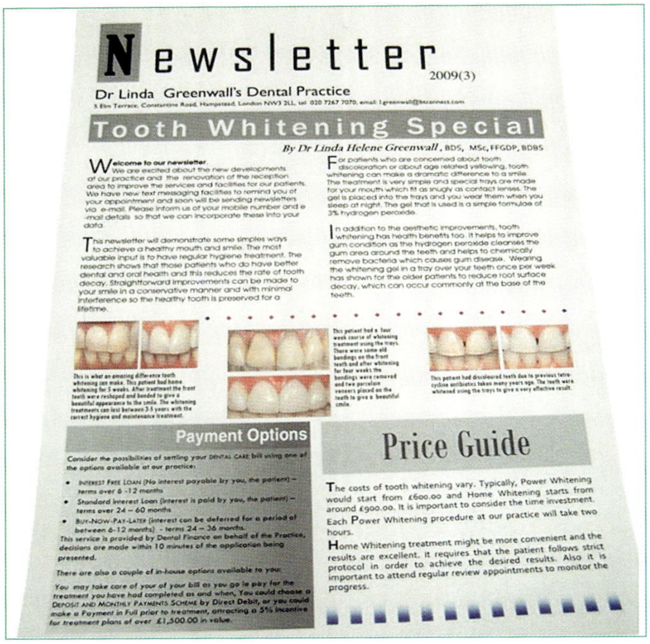

Newsletter 2009(3)

Dr Linda Greenwall's Dental Practice

5 Elm Terrace, Constantine Road, Hampstead, London NW3 2LL, tel 020 7267 7070, email: l.greenwall@btconnect.com

Tooth Whitening Special

By Dr Linda Helene Greenwall, BDS, MSc, FFGDP, BDBS

Welcome to our newsletter. We are excited about the new developments at our practice and the renovation of the reception area to improve the services and facilities for our patients. We have new text messaging facilities to remind you of your appointment and soon will be sending newsletters via e-mail. Please inform us of your mobile number and e-mail details so that we can incorporate these into your data.

This newsletter will demonstrate some simples ways to achieve a healthy mouth and smile. The most valuable input is to have regular hygiene treatment. The research shows that those patients who do have better dental and oral health and this reduces the rate of tooth decay. Straightforward improvements can be made to your smile in a conservative manner and with minimal interference so the healthy tooth is preserved for a lifetime.

For patients who are concerned about tooth discoloration or about age related yellowing, tooth whitening can make a dramatic difference to a smile. The treatment is very simple and special trays are made for your mouth which fit as snugly as contact lenses. The gel is placed into the trays and you wear them when you sleep at night. The gel that is used is a simple formulae of 3% hydrogen peroxide.

In addition to the aesthetic improvements, tooth whitening has health benefits too. It helps to improve gum condition as the hydrogen peroxide cleanses the gum area around the teeth and helps to chemically remove bacteria which causes gum disease. Wearing the whitening gel in a tray over your teeth once per week has shown for the older patients to reduce root surface decay, which can occur commonly at the base of the teeth.

This is what an amazing difference tooth whitening can make. This patient had home whitening for 5 weeks. After treatment the front teeth were reshaped and bonded to give a beautiful appearance to the smile. The whitening treatments can last between 3-5 years with the correct hygiene and maintenance treatment.

This patient had a four week course of whitening treatment using the trays. There were some old bondings on the front teeth and after whitening for four weeks the bondings were removed and two porcelain veneers placed on the teeth to give a beautiful smile.

This patient had discoloured teeth due to previous tetracycline antibiotics taken many years ago. The teeth were whitened using the trays to give a very effective result.

Payment Options

Consider the possibilities of settling your DENTAL CARE bill using one of the options available at our practice:

- INTEREST FREE LOAN (No interest payable by you, the patient) – terms over 6 -12 months
- Standard Interest Loan (Interest is paid by you, the patient) – terms over 24 – 60 months
- BUY-NOW-PAY-LATER (interest can be deferred for a period of between 6-12 months) - terms 24 – 36 months.

This service is provided by Dental Finance on behalf of the Practice, decisions are made within 10 minutes of the application being presented.

There are also a couple of in-house options available to you:

You may take care of your of your bill as you go to pay for the treatment you have had completed as and when, You could choose a DEPOSIT AND MONTHLY PAYMENTS SCHEME by Direct Debit, or you could make a Payment in Full prior to treatment, attracting a 5% incentive for treatment plans of over £1,500.00 in value.

Price Guide

The costs of tooth whitening vary. Typically, Power Whitening would start from £600.00 and Home Whitening starts from around £900.00. It is important to consider the time investment. Each Power Whitening procedure at our practice will take two hours.

Home Whitening treatment might be more convenient and the results are excellent. It requires that the patient follows strict protocol in order to achieve the desired results. Also it is important to attend regular review appointments to monitor the progress.

Fig 8-9 An example of a whitening newsletter sent to all patients.

Fig 8-10 A wedding is often an ideal time to whiten the teeth. Marketing these services to prospective brides may be an excellent idea. The bridal party may all want to have their teeth whitened at this time.

whitening services to their existing patients. Marketing ideas to promote bleaching in the dental practice include:

- Whitening newsletters explaining the procedures available (Fig 8-9).
- Open evenings demonstrating the chairside whitening results.
- Whitening Wednesdays: dedicate an entire day once a month or once a week to whitening. You can offer a special deal on a limited basis and only for the first 25 patients who respond to the newsletter. Time activate the special offer so that patients can respond quickly.
- Whitening special offers: offer no-charge power whitening if patients continue with home whitening.
- Offer combination treatments as a package with home and power whitening undertaken as part of the same course of treatment. This way the power whitening is undertaken to motivate the patient to continue treatment at home.
- Seasonal offers for Summer holiday whitening, or Winter Christmas whitening.
- Special event whitening, eg, a wedding. Special offers may be given for the whole wedding party. The bride and the wedding party often seek treatment prior to this special event (Fig 8-10).

Creating interest in tooth color, lightness, and whiteness

Many patients want to whiten their teeth. Some love their new whitened smiles and they want to continue to whiten their teeth. Other patients may want whiter teeth but never got round to doing the treatment. Some want whiter teeth when asked. When planning aesthetic dentistry for patients it is important to have a discussion about tooth shade and whether the patient has ever thought of whitening their teeth, as it is better to undertake whitening before any further aesthetic treatment is undertaken.

When undertaking a dental examination, an assessment of the patient's existing shade can be undertaken. This can be done by visually evaluating the patient's existing tooth shade against the standard porcelain shade guide. Take photographs of the patient's teeth with the shade tab present. Put the shade tab into the smile shot and record the actual shade of existing teeth for the patient. The patient may ask why this is being done and this may create interest in what the actual shade of the teeth is at present. Patients may ask to see the whole shade guide and ask how their present shade compares with the rest of the shades on the shade guide and in the general population. This can lead to a further discussion on tooth whitening options. Always record the present shade using the porcelain shade tab opposite the left maxillary canine. That way the eye runs from left to right and onto the shade tab to assess the present shade. This helps to standardize the process of shade documentation for each case.

The hygienist can also take out the shade guide and have a discussion about shades and tooth whitening during the hygiene appointment. Show patients the comparison of the lighter shades on the shade guide and hold these up to the patient's teeth while the patient holds a hand mirror, so that the patient can see the comparison of the lighter shades with their existing shades.

Put the photos on the screen when the patient walks into the room so the patient can see what their smile looks like in a photograph. By assessing and recording the shade on an annual basis, patients can be involved in the discussion about tooth shade and whitening options. When discussing tooth whitening or shade lightening, we always underestimate the possible results so patients are not disappointed with the final result.

The dental team should have white teeth!

If needed or desired, the entire team should also have their teeth whitened to demonstrate their beautiful smiles. It is also essential that the entire team have good smiles. If a team member does not have a beautiful smile, this can be created by the dentist. Then the staff member will be an excellent walking advertisement for the dental practice. Often staff members are stopped in the street by strangers who may admire their beautiful smiles. Team members should always carry business cards with them as they are frequently asked about their smiles. Team members should give patients their business cards to help answer any questions that they may have concerning their whitening treatments.

Whitening maintenance programs

Most patients are delighted with their new, whiter smiles. Some patients want to continue to whiten their teeth continually. This is not necessary. The tooth whitening programs should be of a specific length and until the white shade of B1 or beyond is achieved or until the patient is happy with the shade. The program is completed. Further evaluation and monitoring of the shade can take place during the hygiene appointment. Patients can be advised on how to maintain their white smiles, and effective home care methods and advice can be given on whitening toothpaste. It is not advised that patients buy over-the-counter products to use as maintenance treatments, as these may be open to abuse and overuse.

Maintenance whitening treatments are normally undertaken a few years later (Leonard, 1998). The hygienist will dispense the whitening gel after obtaining the dentist's consent, and advise the patients how to use the gels and the length of time over which this should be undertaken. It is good to review the patient after this maintenance treatment.

Summary

It is important to involve the entire team in the whitening programs of the dental practice. Following these guidelines will lead to successful whitening treatment. Success strategies will help to build and organize your entire dental practice as you prepare to undertake more whitening procedures.

Action steps

1. Prepare and ensure an excellent new patient journey.
2. Treatment plan the case effectively.
3. Classify the type of whitening treatment to be undertaken.
4. Set fees for the whitening treatments according to the classification. Itemize all the services relating to bleaching to ensure that all aspects are treatment planned and costed accordingly. Prepare a sheet for all the bleaching materials that are given out to patients to keep track of how many and which materials are used.
5. Train and educate the entire team on all the bleaching protocols and photography. Prepare excellent advice sheets on all aspects of bleaching for your patients.
6. Learn how to manage sensitivity during bleaching treatments. Each team member should know his/her role and responsibility in dealing with sensitivity experienced as a result of bleaching.
7. Prepare excellent advice sheets on sensitivity management for patients at home and explain that they may experience sensitivity during whitening treatment.
8. Complete procedure analysis sheets for all the bleaching procedures that are offered in the dental practice.
9. Take photos of tray set-ups for each procedure to help train assistants and hygienists who will be involved in bleaching.
10. Ensure good monitoring and supervision of the bleaching treatments and good aftercare.
11. Ask patients to complete testimonials (with their permission) once they have completed the bleaching treatments. These can be used for marketing purposes and be shown on the website.
12. Prepare a photo book of before-and-after whitening cases so that you can record your excellent results to demonstrate to other patients.

References

1. Goldstein RE. Esthetics in Dentistry. Ontario, Canada: Decker Publishing, 2002.
2. Greenwall LH. Bleaching Techniques in Restorative Dentistry: An Illustrated Guide. London, UK: Informa Healthcare, 2001.
3. Greenwall LH. The Business of Bleaching. Smile-on e-learning program, 2006.
4. Haywood VB. Whitening and caries control in the elderly. Aesthetic Dent Today 2007;1:4.
5. Haywood VB. The bottom line on bleaching. Inside Dent 2008;4:82–89. Available at: http://www.vanhaywood.com/articles/pdf/2008Bottom%20Line%20on%20Bleaching.pdf.
6. Haywood VB, Heymann HO. Nightguard vital bleaching. Quintessence Int 1989;20:173–176.
7. Kwon SR, Ko SK, Greenwall LH. Tooth Whitening in Esthetic Dentistry. London: Quintessence Publishing, 2010.
8. Leonard RH. Efficacy, longevity, side effects and patient perceptions of nightguard vital bleaching. Compend Contin Educ Dent 1998;9:766–781.
9. Leonard RH Jr, Haywood VB, Phillips C. Risk factors for developing tooth sensitivity and gingival irritation associated with night guard vital bleaching. Quintessence Int 1997;28:527–534.
10. Leonard RH, Smith LR, Garland GE, Caplan DJ. Desensitizing agent efficacy during whitening in an at-risk population. J Esthet Restorative Dent 2004;16:49–56.
11. Matis BA. Tray whitening. What the evidence shows. Compend Contin Educ Dent 2003;24(4A):254–262.
12. Matis BA, Cochran MA, Eckert G. Review of the effectiveness of various tooth whitening systems. Operative Dent 2009;34:230–235.
13. Small B. The application and integration of at-home bleaching into private dental practice. Compend Contin Educ Dent 1998;9:799–807.

Further reading

American Dental Association website. Available at: www.americandentalassociation.com

British Dental Bleaching Society website. Available at: www.bdbs.co.uk

Greenwall LH. Bleaching Techniques in Restorative Dentistry, 1st edition. London: Martin Dunitz, 2001.

Haywood VB. Tooth Whitening: Indications and Outcomes of Nightguard Vital Bleaching. Chicago, IL: Quintessence Publishing, 2007.

Linda Greenwall's website. Available at: www.lindagreenwall.co.uk

Van Haywood's website. Available at: www.vanhaywood.com

Whitening prescription form.

Appendix 8-1

Examination, diagnosis & prescription sheet for whitening		
Patient details Title	Surname	First names
Address		

Date of birth		Male/female		Tel no. home	
Tel no. mobile				Tel no. work	
Hopes & aspirations for tooth whitening					
Medical history (medication taken)					
Diagnosis of discoloration					
Type of discoloration			Basic	Intermediate	Severe
Current shade			Expected shade		
White spots			Fluorosis		
Brown spots			Tetracycline		
Dehydration line			Dark crack lines		
Other					
Lasting sensitivity	Yes	No	Treatment for sensitivity	Yes	No

Radiographs & photographs							
Radiographs taken date				Radiographs checked date			
Periapicals		Bite wings		Full mouth series		OPG	
Photographs taken date: Extraoral				Photographs taken date: Intraoral			
Vitality testing							
Intra-oral examination							

Recession																
Treatment required																
Existing restoration																
	8	7	6	5	4	3	2	1	1	2	3	4	5	6	7	8
Existing restoration																
Treatment required																
Recession																

Significant gingival condition:	Yes	No	
Patient will need further restorative treatment as follows:			

Dentist's signature		Date			
Whitening prescription					
Please provide whitening for the above patient.					
Type of whitening procedure:	Basic		Intermediate		Advanced
Medical history checked date		Medication review date			
Patient has existing:	Patient's attention has been drawn to the following issues:				
Fillings (anterior composite)		Gingival condition		Gum recession	
Crowns		White spots		Lichen planus	
Implant crowns		Brown spots		Existing sensitivity	
Veneers		Existing fillings		Dehydration line	
		Crowns		Fluorosis, tetracycline line	
Home whitening		Power whitening			
Products provided for whitening procedure:					
Product name					
Product name					
Concentration					
De-sensitizing products prescribed					
Disclaimer discussed				Date:	
Patient's consent to treatment:					
Patient's signature:				Date:	
Parent's consent given for under 16 year olds:				Date:	
Parent or guardian's signature:				Date:	
Completion of treatment:					
How many appointments		Review appt. date:			
Final appointment date:					
Final photographs taken date:		Final shade achieved:			
Patient referred back to (dentist's name): for treatment diagnosed prior to whitening.					
Date of referral: Signature of referrer:					

Appendix 8-2

Whitening examination record sheet (© Linda Greenwall).

Patient whitening record sheet		
Name		
Date bleaching started	Age	
Patient's main complaint		
Discoloration type	Preoperative shade	Shade guide used
Patient's desired color		
Informed consent: The patient is informed that there are no guarantees as to the amount of lightening that can be achieved with whitening treatment. Further dental treatment may be required to whiten the teeth. These options may include microabrasion, bonding, porcelain laminate veneers, crowns, or combinations of the above. The patient is instructed to discontinue the whitening treatment should any problems occur.		
Patient's signature:	Date:	
Whitening method		
Non-vital tooth: tooth number	Root canal treatment present	
Patency of apical seal	Radiograph checked	
Bleaching method: walking bleach	Inside/outside technique	
Bleaching material used	Concentration	
Power bleach	Maxillary teeth	Mandibular teeth
Bleaching material	Concentration	
Radiographs checked		
Home bleach	Maxillary teeth	Mandibular teeth
Presence of anterior composites	Patient informed they may need to be replaced	
Bleaching material used	Concentration	

Whitening audit					
	Appointment date	Arch	Bleach used	Amount dispensed	Problems
1					
2					
3					
4					
5					
6					
7					
8					
9					
10					

Postoperative assessment	
Shade preoperative	Shade postoperative
Recommended re-bleaching	Problems encountered
Maintenance	Further aesthetic treatment

Appendix 8-3

Patient instructions for managing sensitivity during home bleaching (© Linda Greenwall).

How to manage sensitivity during whitening treatment

Sensitivity of teeth is the most common side effect of whitening treatment. This usually occurs around the necks of the teeth. Patients can experience some degree of sensitivity which ranges from mild awareness to a throb on a specific tooth. Up to 50% of patients suffer with some sensitivity.

If you are experiencing sensitivity during your whitening treatment, these are the different treatments that you should follow.

1. We will provide you with a desensitizing material called Soothe to place in your bleaching trays. This should be placed in the trays in exactly the same way that the bleaching material is placed. You should alternate each night, one night with the Soothe and the following night with the bleaching material, or you can apply it onto the tray for 1 hour per night. This should be continued until the sensitivity disappears.
2. We will provide you with some preformed trays which are called Ultra-eze trays. You should wear these trays for one night only. These should relieve your sensitivity.
3. We will provide you with GC Tooth Mousse. This can either be put in your bleaching trays or you can rub it into an individual tooth where it is sensitive.
4. You can also use a desensitizing toothpaste such as Sensodyne. You can brush with the desensitizing toothpaste during the whitening treatment. Place a small amount of the toothpaste on your finger and rub it into the sensitive area. You should repeat this each night until the sensitivity disappears.
5. You can stop the whitening for one night if the sensitivity is too severe. Do not stop for more than two nights otherwise the effect of the whitening will slow down. Sometimes the gums may also feel a little sensitive. If you notice the gums are feeling sore, you need to refrain from bleaching for one day or reduce the concentration of the whitening gel.

Appendix 8-4 Protocol for home whitening.

Whitening Protocol

1st appointment

1. Confirm patient has a signed treatment plan for the whitening procedure planned for them.
2. Take upper and lower alginate impressions and complete laboratory sheets. Always state to the lab the date you require the trays back. Any special requests should be placed under the section that reads comments. Sterilize impressions and wrap them well.
3. Complete patient's clinical notes and arrange a follow-up appointment.
4. Write up impressions in lab book.

2nd appointment

1. Prepare paperwork before appointment. A bleaching pack (Fig 8-11) should contain:
   - ☐ Bleaching log form
   - ☐ What to Expect leaflet
   - ☐ Two consent forms
   - ☐ Quick help sheet
   - ☐ Calendar
   - ☐ Brochure.
2. Go through paperwork with patient and ask them to sign two consent forms. Discuss the What to Expect leaflet with the patient.

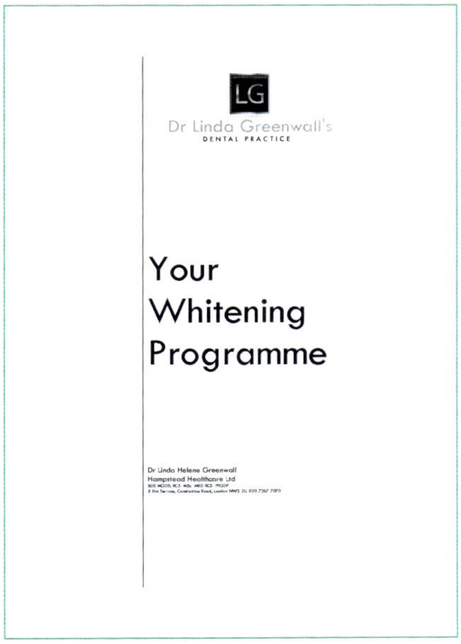

Fig 8-11a An example of the whitening booklet that all patients receive who are undertaking home whitening treatment.

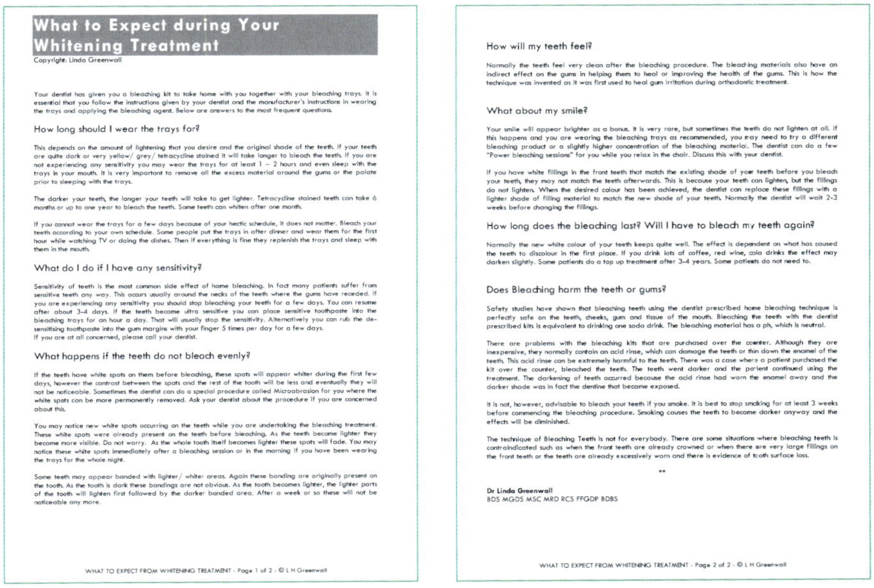

What to Expect during Your Whitening Treatment

Copyright: Linda Greenwall

Your dentist has given you a bleaching kit to take home with you together with your bleaching trays. It is essential that you follow the instructions given by your dentist and the manufacturer's instructions in wearing the trays and applying the bleaching agent. Below are answers to the most frequent questions.

How long should I wear the trays for?

This depends on the amount of lightening that you desire and the original shade of the teeth. If your teeth are quite dark or very yellow/ grey/ tetracycline stained it will take longer to bleach the teeth. If you are not experiencing any sensitivity you may wear the trays for at least 1 – 2 hours and even sleep with the trays in your mouth. It is very important to remove all the excess material around the gums or the palate prior to sleeping with the trays.

The darker your teeth, the longer your teeth will take to get lighter. Tetracycline stained teeth can take 6 months or up to one year to bleach the teeth. Some teeth can whiten after one month.

If you cannot wear the trays for a few days because of your hectic schedule, it does not matter. Bleach your teeth according to your own schedule. Some people put the trays in after dinner and wear them for the first hour while watching TV or doing the dishes. Then if everything is fine they replenish the trays and sleep with them in the mouth.

What do I do if I have any sensitivity?

Sensitivity of teeth is the most common side effect of home bleaching. In fact many patients suffer from sensitive teeth any way. This occurs usually around the necks of the teeth where the gums have receded. If you are experiencing any sensitivity you should stop bleaching your teeth for a few days. You can resume after about 3-4 days. If the teeth become ultra sensitive you can place sensitive toothpaste into the bleaching trays for an hour a day. That will usually stop the sensitivity. Alternatively you can rub the desensitising toothpaste into the gum margins with your finger 5 times per day for a few days.
If you are at all concerned, please call your dentist.

What happens if the teeth do not bleach evenly?

If the teeth have white spots on them before bleaching, these spots will appear whiter during the first few days, however the contrast between the spots and the rest of the tooth will be less and eventually they will not be noticeable. Sometimes the dentist can do a special procedure called Microabrasion for you where the white spots can be more permanently removed. Ask your dentist about the procedure if you are concerned about this.

You may notice new white spots occurring on the teeth while you are undertaking the bleaching treatment. These white spots were already present on the teeth before bleaching. As the teeth become lighter they become more visible. Do not worry. As the whole tooth itself becomes lighter these spots will fade. You may notice these white spots immediately after a bleaching session or in the morning if you have been wearing the trays for the whole night.

Some teeth may appear banded with lighter/ whiter areas. Again these banding are originally present on the tooth. As the tooth is dark these bandings are not obvious. As the tooth becomes lighter, the lighter parts of the tooth will lighten first followed by the darker banded area. After a week or so these will not be noticeable any more.

WHAT TO EXPECT FROM WHITENING TREATMENT - Page 1 of 2 - © L H Greenwall

How will my teeth feel?

Normally the teeth feel very clean after the bleaching procedure. The bleaching materials also have an indirect effect on the gums in helping them to heal or improving the health of the gums. This is how the technique was invented as it was first used to heal gum irritation during orthodontic treatment.

What about my smile?

Your smile will appear brighter as a bonus. It is very rare, but sometimes the teeth do not lighten at all. If this happens and you are wearing the bleaching trays as recommended, you may need to try a different bleaching product or a slightly higher concentration of the bleaching material. The dentist can do a few "Power bleaching sessions" for you while you relax in the chair. Discuss this with your dentist.

If you have white fillings in the front teeth that match the existing shade of your teeth before you bleach your teeth, they may not match the teeth afterwards. This is because your teeth can lighten, but the fillings do not lighten. When the desired colour has been achieved, the dentist can replace these fillings with a lighter shade of filling material to match the new shade of your teeth. Normally the dentist will wait 2-3 weeks before changing the fillings.

How long does the bleaching last? Will I have to bleach my teeth again?

Normally the new white colour of your teeth keeps quite well. The effect is dependent on what has caused the teeth to discolour in the first place. If you drink lots of coffee, red wine, cola drinks the effect may darken slightly. Some patients do a top up treatment after 3-4 years. Some patients do not need to.

Does Bleaching harm the teeth or gums?

Safety studies have shown that bleaching teeth using the dentist prescribed home bleaching technique is perfectly safe on the teeth, cheeks, gum and tissue of the mouth. Bleaching the teeth with the dentist prescribed kits is equivalent to drinking one soda drink. The bleaching material has a ph, which is neutral.

There are problems with the bleaching kits that are purchased over the counter. Although they are inexpensive, they normally contain an acid rinse, which can damage the teeth or thin down the enamel of the teeth. This acid rinse can be extremely harmful to the teeth. There was a case where a patient purchased the kit over the counter, bleached the teeth. The teeth went darker and the patient continued using the treatment. The darkening of teeth occurred because the acid rinse had worn the enamel away and the darker shade was in fact the dentine that became exposed.

It is not, however, advisable to bleach your teeth if you smoke. It is best to stop smoking for at least 3 weeks before commencing the bleaching procedure. Smoking causes the teeth to become darker anyway and the effects will be diminished.

The technique of Bleaching Teeth is not for everybody. There are some situations where bleaching teeth is contraindicated such as when the front teeth are already crowned or when there are very large fillings on the front teeth or the teeth are already excessively worn and there is evidence of tooth surface loss.

**

Dr Linda Greenwall
BDS MGDS MSC MRD RCS FFGDP BDBS

WHAT TO EXPECT FROM WHITENING TREATMENT - Page 2 of 2 - © L H Greenwall

Fig 8-11b A What to Expect leaflet is included in the bleaching pack.

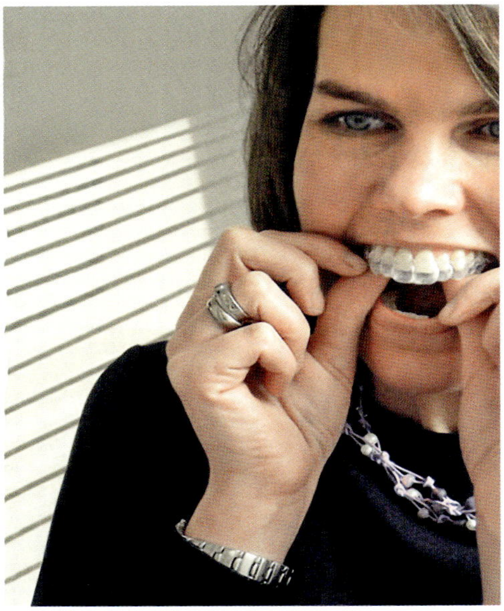

Fig 8-12 Patient applying the bleaching tray at home and checking the fit of the tray in the bathroom mirror, after receiving instructions on how to apply the gel into the tray. Patients need to be shown exactly how much gel to insert in the bleaching tray so that they can comply with the home care instructions.

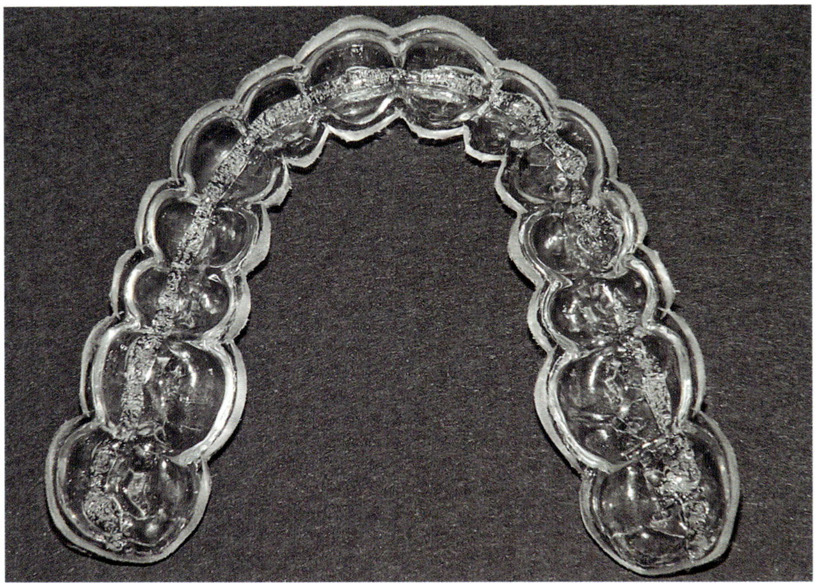

Fig 8-13 The bleaching tray. This photograph demonstrates the amount of bleaching gel that should be placed into the tray for overnight application. A small amount of the gel is placed directly into the buccal outer section of the tray in order for the bleaching gel to travel to the outside and inside surface, and coat the teeth with sufficient bleaching gel to obtain a good whitening effect. The tray should be in close contact with the teeth.

3. Take a present shade of the patient's upper and lower teeth and write it in the patient's clinical notes. Give the patient a mirror and show them the present shade and, using the shade guide, show them the shade you hope to achieve. Always underestimate the result.
4. Take photographs of patient's teeth using cheek retractors. Ask patient to close upper and lower teeth together whilst taking the picture.
   - Frontal view with blue sheet
   - Patient's smile
   - Retractor smile at 2/3 stop with shade tab
   - Two photos, one of just the teeth and the other with the present shade in. You can ask the patient to hold the chosen guide against one of the lateral teeth. (Camera should be set on 2/3 stop for an in-focus picture.)
5. Show patient the bleaching tray you are going to give them and try it into the patient's mouth to check that it fits correctly. A good fitting tray should extend over all of the teeth and there should not be too much of the tray on the gingivae.
6. Take a tube of the material you have chosen to use and show the patient how to place it into the tray and the amount required (Figs 8-12 and 8-13). You should mark with a pen in the tray any crowned teeth so that patient does not apply material to these areas.

7. Place the tray with the material into the patient's mouth and show how to wipe off any excess material with a cotton wool roll.
8. Once the patient is comfortable with the tray placement explain how they should clean away the material from their tray and teeth.
9. Give the patient a bleaching log sheet and ask them to write down how long they wear their trays for and note if they have any sensitivity.
10. Give the patient their bleaching pack. Explain to patient that if they have any sensitivity they should place proprietary tooth desensitizing gel in the tray for one night until sensitivity subsides. They can also brush with Sensodyne toothpaste.
11. Organize a review appointment for 2 to 3 weeks.

3rd appointment: review upper bleach

1. Collect log sheet – ask about sensitivity.
2. Review patient shade.
3. See whether patient needs more material.
4. Motivate and encourage the patient.
5. If shade B1/A1 can stop now (or if the patient is happy).
6. Give lower tray – take photos.
7. Arrange appointment for 3 weeks.

4th appointment

1. Review lower bleaching.
2. Check shade of lower teeth.
3. Ask for log sheet.
4. Discuss shade with patient.
5. Take photos.
6. Treatment of sensitivity.
   - Explain that 70% of people get sensitivity during home whitening.
   - It is transient and not long-lasting, and patients will not be left with permanent sensitivity.
   - Patients can either:
     - use proprietary desensitizing material in the tray
     - use UltraEz in the tray
     - brush with Sensodyne toothpaste
     - skip a night
     - document the sensitivity so it can be reviewed at the next appointment.

Appendix 8-5

Procedure analysis forms for home and power whitening, with tray set up.

Procedure: Fitting bleaching trays

Time: 30 min

- Greet and seat patient, check medical history.
- Check soft tissues, soft/hard deposits.
- Remove any stain, hard deposits if needed.
- Go through the consent form with the patient: need to sign both copies.
- Go through What to Expect leaflet and Patient Log (see paperwork folder below).
- Show the patient their trays, demonstrate how to apply the gel.
- Explain procedure if patient has sensitivity.
- Go through Quick Reference Bleaching Instruction sheet (see paperwork folder below).
- Dentist must check that the trays fit.
- Take a shade, and photos (shade guide and retractors).
- Complete documentation, and schedule review appointment for 2–3 weeks.

To set up (Fig 8-14)

- Patients notes, current radiographs.
- Patient bib, glasses.
- Gloves, mask, and shield.
- Mouthwash, salivary ejector, wide bore suction.
- Tray with mirror, probe (perio and straight), tweezers.

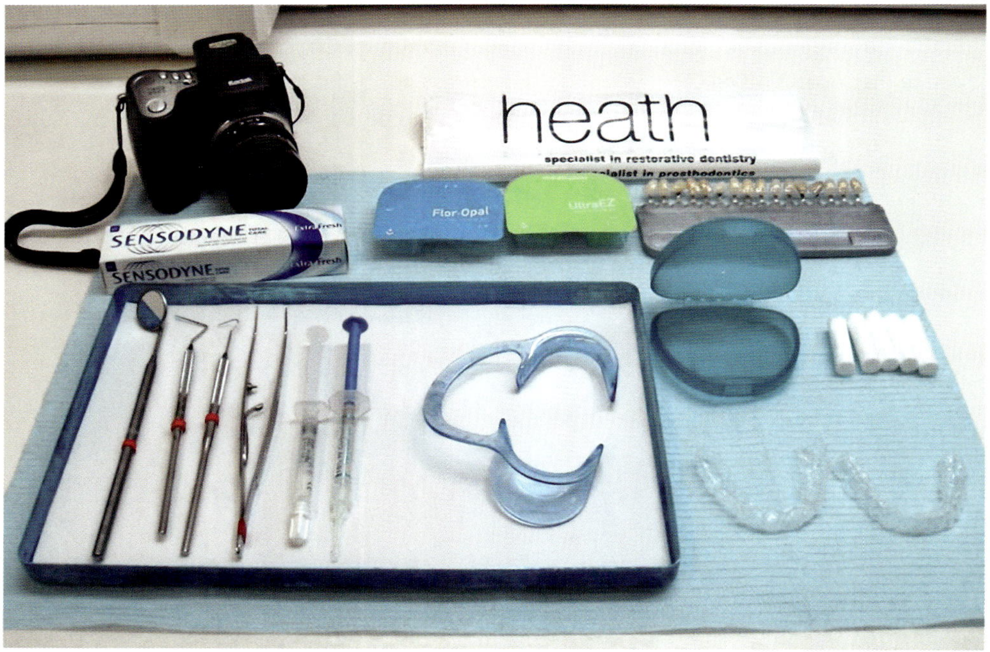

Fig 8-14 Items required for set-up when fitting bleaching trays (Appendix 8-5).

- Patient's trays.
- Paperwork folder.
- Syringes of whitening gel.
- Soothe, Sensodyne, single-use fluoride trays.
- Case for trays.
- Cotton wool rolls.
- Shade guide.
- Heath Health Care bag.
- Camera (and blue background).

Whitening take-home bag

- Trays (and the case).
- Bleaching gel (as prescribed by dentist).
- Soothe.
- Cotton wool rolls.
- Sensodyne whitening.
- Single-use disposable fluoride trays.

Home bleaching paperwork folder (see Fig 8-11)

- Home bleaching instructions and consent form x 2 (one for patient's notes and one for the patient).
- What to Expect leaflet.
- Quick Reference Bleaching Instruction sheet.
- Patient Log.
- Dentist's business card x 2.
- Bleaching brochures, and newsletter.

Procedure: Bleaching review

Time: 15 min

- Greet and seat the patient, check medical history.
- Check if patient has any sensitivity – Patient Log.
- Check shade, before and present.
- Photos (need retractors).
- Issue more gel if required.
- Complete documentation, make next review appointment.

To set up (Fig 8-15)

- Patient's notes, current radiographs.
- Patient bib, glasses.
- Gloves, mask, and shield.
- Mouthwash, salivary ejector, wide bore suction.
- Basic cons tray.
- Shade guide.
- Cheek retractors.
- Camera (and blue background).
- Extra bleaching gel if required.

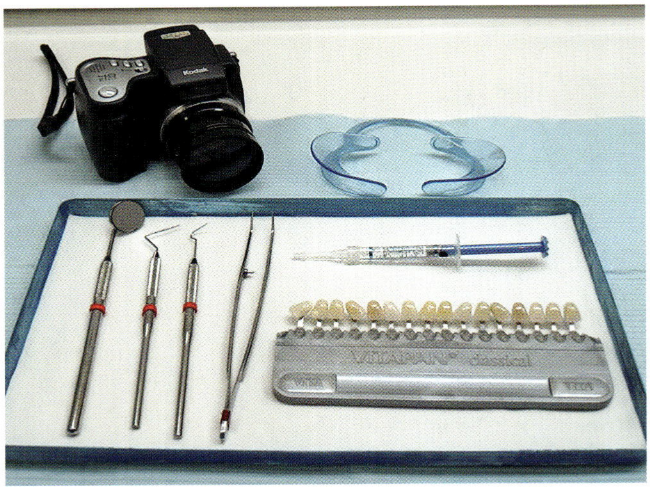

Fig 8-15 Items required for set-up of bleaching review (Appendix 8-5).

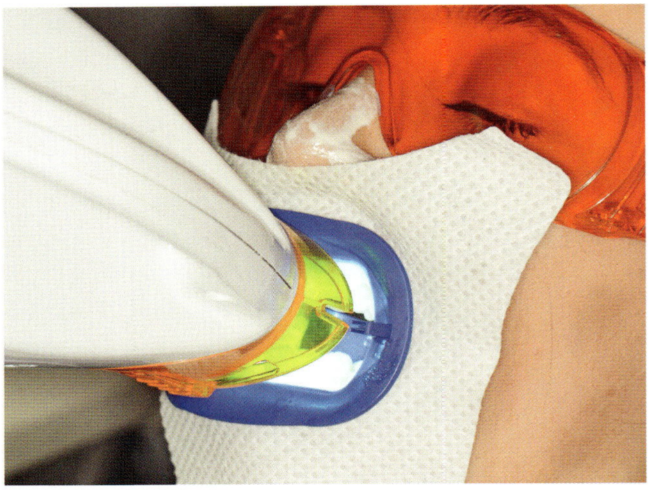

Fig 8-16 The power bleaching procedure in progress.

Procedure: Power bleaching (Fig 8-16)

Time: 2 hours

- Greet and seat patient, check medical history.
- Check the consent form is signed.
- Explain the procedure to the patient.
- Take a shade.
- Take preoperative photos (with a blue background).
- Apply face cream, Vaseline to the lips
- Place retractors in patient's mouth, long cotton wool rolls, and napkin.
- Apply liquid dam, tack to cotton wool.
- Apply gauze to protect soft tissues including cheeks.
- Apply bleaching gel to the teeth.
- Position the Zoom 2 light, make sure it is correctly lined up.
- Light is on for 15-min intervals.
- Remove gel and rehydrate teeth with water and cotton wool rolls.
- Repeat procedure two more times.
- Following third cycle, remove liquid dam and cotton wool rolls.
- Ask patient to rinse (plain water).
- Apply fluoride gel to teeth.
- Take postoperative photos.
- Postoperative instructions, trays, and material supplied to patient if continuing with home bleach.
- Complete documentation.
- Ask patient if they have any questions, run through what treatment has been carried out today, and what to expect at their next visit.
- Schedule next appointment.
- Decontaminate surgery and set up for next patient.

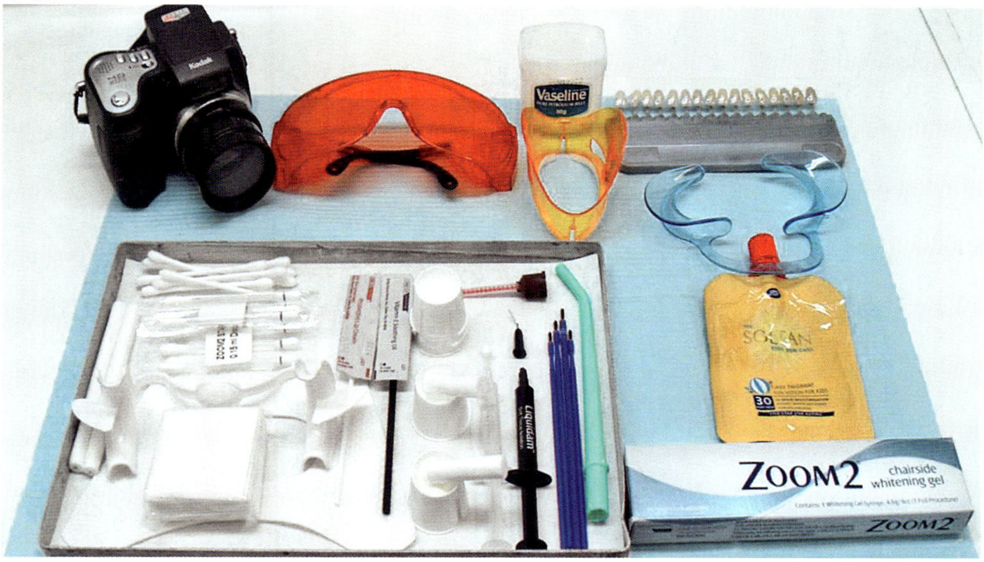

Fig 8-17 Tray set up and additional items required for power bleaching treatment using Philips Discus products (Appendix 8-5).

To set up, and instruments for power bleaching procedure (Fig 8-17)

- Patients notes, current radiographs (ensure the radiographs are up on computer monitor).
- Patient bib, glasses.
- Gloves, mask, and shield.
- Mouthwash (colorless), salivary ejector, wide bore suction and surgical suction tip.
- Basic examination tray (mirror, probe, and tweezer).
- Camera, shade guide, retractors.
- Cotton wool rolls (long and short), gauze, napkin, retractor, Q-tips.
- Face cream, Vaseline, dappens dishes, cotton rolls.
- Suction tips, applicator brushes.
- Liquid dam.
- Power bleaching material and light.
- Soothers (fluoride gel, potassium nitrate, and amorphous calcium phosphate).

9 Treatment Planning and Diagnosis of Aesthetic Dentistry

Linda Greenwall and Cathy Jameson

> *The goal of treatment is to establish a biological compatible dentition that is aesthetically acceptable to the patient.* — *Galip Gurel (2003)*

What does the patient want?

Treatment planning of aesthetic dentistry can be a complex issue. It is essential from the outset that the dentist fully understands what the patient wants to achieve when seeking aesthetic dentistry (Fig 9-1). While some patients may only want a minimal change to improve their smiles, others may request further advanced and extensive treatment. While the aesthetic look may be a personal choice, it is the dentist and team members who need to ask the correct, relevant and open-ended questions so that they fully comprehend what the patient is trying to achieve. As with all dentistry, it is important to understand the patient's main motivation first. This is the subjective opinion.

Many of the initial questions can be handled with the use of a questionnaire (Appendix 9-1). This may be sent or emailed to the patient to complete prior to the initial consultation.

When it comes to tooth whitening, many patients request only a natural enhancement of their existing shade. They may be concerned that the teeth become too white too quickly. However, as the whitening process progresses they invariably request to continue lightening to the lightest shade on the shade guide. It is essential for the dentist to guide the patient through the process of tooth whitening and to continue to motivate and encourage the patient to continue whitening until the desired shade is achieved.

There are many options for aesthetic dental treatment, and patients need to be informed of the choices available, the side effects, advantages, and dis-

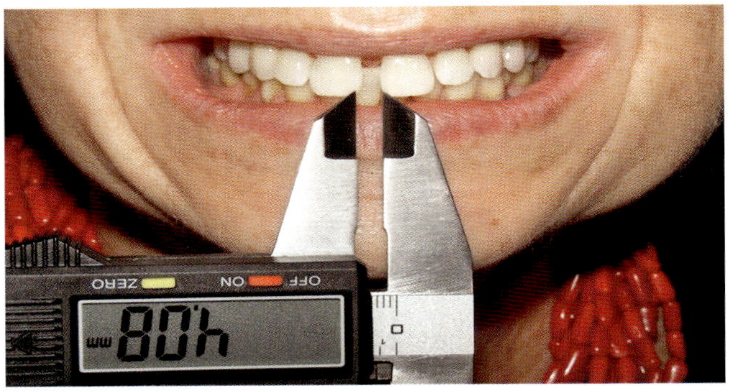

Fig 9-1 Some patients love having a midline diastema. Others would like the space closed. It is important to understand the patient's requirements. This patient first undertook whitening treatment and then was motivated to look at treatment options for closing the midline diastema.

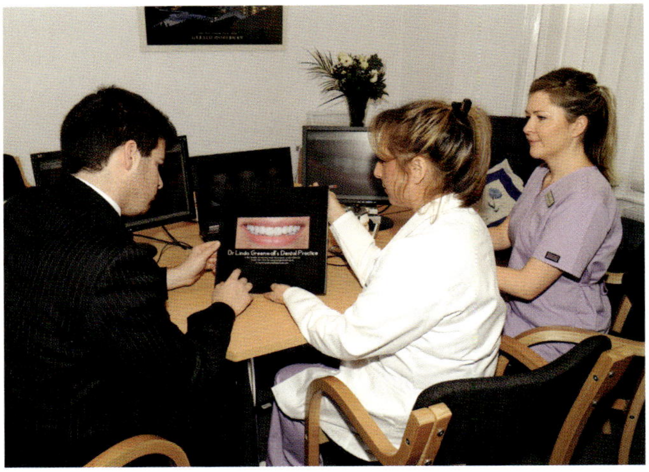

Fig 9-2 The initial patient interview is very important.

advantages of the different treatment options in order to make an informed decision about the treatment. Patients need to be aware of the full implications of treatment and also what can and what cannot be achieved. The patient's expectations need to be assessed as to whether these are realistic or unrealistic.

Treatment planning is an extremely important aspect of the aesthetic dental practice. The planning of treatment can be ongoing and dynamic, and may change as a patient gets older, breaks a tooth, suffers from added stress, changes their diet, or does not comply with recommendations.

There are four key stages of the treatment planning and diagnosis phase:

1. assessment
2. planning
3. implementation
4. evaluation.

1. Assessment: the initial interview and information/ data gathering

Conducting an excellent initial interview with the patient is essential to understand their requirements (Fig 9-2). Enough time should be given to allow the patient to talk about any concerns that they may have. It may be difficult for some patients to express themselves to adequately describe what they hope to achieve with a new smile. It is best not to undertake this interview in the dental surgery but rather in a separate room or area away from the clinical area. The consultation room is a non-threatening environment for the patient where they can feel comfortable and relaxed. They should be able to express their hopes and aspirations or any concerns that they may have about their teeth. Some patients have built up many issues about the state and appearance of their teeth, and are embarrassed to talk freely about their dental problems. By using active listening you can allow the patient to relax and discuss these concerns. Often when questioning patients about their hopes and aspirations they may break down and cry, as they have never been asked this question before. They need to gather their thoughts and need time to do so.

A checklist for the dental team for the preparation of the interview is shown below.

- Has the patient completed the paperwork: medical questionnaire or health history form, smile evaluation (Appendix 9-2), other dental information?
- Is the room prepared?
- Are the notes made up with all the required sheets?
- Are the computer records completed with all the necessary information?
- Medical history completed?
- Advance payment for new patient consultation.
- Hygiene appointment coordinated after new patient consultation.

The patient should feel comfortable that they can express any issues about their teeth that they would like addressed. It is important that the dentist actively listens at this stage. It may take time to get the full picture of what is concerning the patient. Sometimes it may be difficult for them to express their concerns. When the patient says that they don't like their teeth, find out why. There is a big difference between not liking the color of the teeth and not liking the appearance of the teeth. These two factors should clearly be separated early on in the interview in order to understand their requirements. When questioning patients it is also important to ascertain the patient's expectation of the dentist, the dentistry, and the service requirements of the patient in the dental practice.

New patient interview questionnaire checklist:

- What does the patient want? "How can I help you?"
- What is the main complaint?
- What do they want from me? "What are your expectations of me?"
- How do you feel about your smile?
- What do you like most about your smile?
- What do you like least?
- What about the color?
- If you could change anything, what would you do?

Appendix 9-1 is a detailed example of a new patient questionnaire.

Educating the patient: developing perceived need

It is the dental team's responsibility to continue to educate the patient at every contact appointment. That way the patient can learn about the situation in their mouth and how improvements can be made. Educating the patient helps them to understand that although they do not experience pain in the tooth, there is decay present that needs to be removed or a periapical area underneath an old crown that will need attention. When undertaking the initial interview, ask open-ended questions to get the patient to explain their concerns. Often they may not have any specific concerns but their hopes and aspirations will reveal what they are looking for or hoping to achieve. This can help to understand what dentistry is necessary and essential, and what is optional or elective. Often the case may be complex and require a longer treatment time and an interdisciplinary approach (see Appendix 9-5), which will need to be carefully explained to the patient (Winter, 2007).

Developing your skills

The successful aesthetic dentist should acquire the following skills.

Clinical:

- Continual dedication to improving clinical skills and that are specific for aesthetic dentistry.
- Pursuit of excellence in clinical skills.
- Attention to detail.
- Knowledge of the literature and the evidence for successful outcomes.
- Sound scientific knowledge of the clinical aspects of aesthetic dentistry.
- Dedication to continually acquiring the necessary skills.
- Willingness to go the extra mile for patients.
- The 10,000 hour rule (Gladwell, 2009).
- Artistic talents to create beautiful smiles.
- Manual dexterity to undertake complex procedures.

Professional:

- Honesty.
- Listening and understanding skills to determine what the patients want.
- Sincerity.

Personal:

- Striving for excellence.
- Well-organized.
- Clear goals and vision in place.

Managerial and other qualities:

- Be of the highest integrity (Goldstein, 2010).
- Strong ethics.
- Never be afraid to speak up when something is wrong.
- Be outstanding.
- Organizational skills to have the practice protocols geared up for aesthetic dentistry cases.
- Wisdom to know what will work and what not to do.
- Artistic talent to create beautiful smiles.
- Manual dexterity to undertake complex procedures.
- Creativity.
- Enthusiasm.
- Drive and determination.
- Passion for aesthetic dentistry.
- Dedication.
- Striving for excellence.
- Professionalism.

The new patient journey (Fig 9-3)

a. The patient makes contact with the practice via website, email, or telephone.
b. Telephone contact is made by the practice coordinator with the patient, calls handled well so the patient is enthused to book an appointment.
c. The patient makes an appointment.
d. The patient attends the New Patient Appointment, which includes patient interview, clinical assessment, full mouth radiographs, intraoral photography, digital photographs, and standard views recommended by the American Academy of Cosmetic Dentistry (AACD).
e. The patient returns for treatment planning discussion or consultation appointment.
f. The financial agreement is determined and signed.
g. Commencement of treatment begins – sometimes in phases.
h. Completion of treatment.
i. The patient is enrolled in hygiene maintenance program.
j. Review, monitor, follow up, and maintain for a lifetime.

The existing patient journey (Fig 9-4)

a. The existing patient is a patient of record.
b. The patient is involved in a hygiene maintenance program.
c. The patient has emergency dental situations requiring attention.
d. The patient expresses an interest in having an emergency situation taken care of and also requires aesthetic treatment.
e. The patient rebooked for a full and thorough reassessment, as the situation may change.
f. Full assessment carried out, which may include full mouth radiographs, periodontal indices, intraoral camera views of each tooth, and new photography.
g. The patient returns for treatment planning discussion, which includes all options for treatment and the most suitable for the patient, with priorities given to disease eradication.
h. The patient signs consent form and financial responsibility form.
i. An appointment for appropriate length of time is scheduled.
j. Treatment commences.

2. Planning

The treatment planning essentials can be thought of as "four legs of a table" supporting a successful dental practice (Fig 9-5).

- The administration: Everything along the way to get to this point – the patient journey, and the financial agreement.
- The aesthetic dentistry service: The clinical dentistry. Plan from the disease eradication process after emergency situations are taken care of. Ensure that the mouth is healthy and stable prior to undertaking any advanced aesthetic treatment. The patient may need provisionals for a time until the mouth is more stable.
- The marketing: What does the patient need to get to this point? How did the patient find out about the dental practice? Who referred them? It is

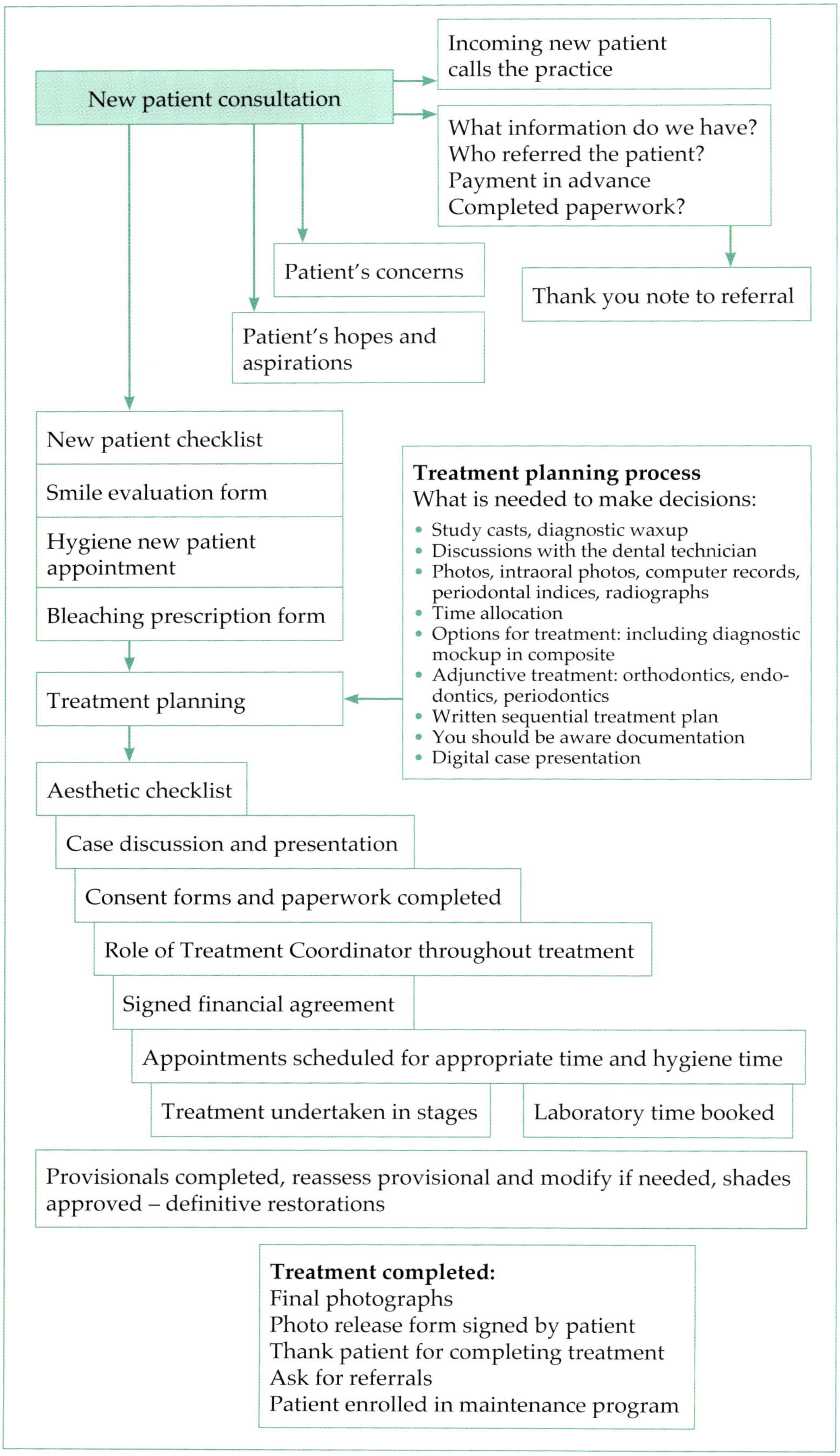

Fig 9-3 New patient journey.

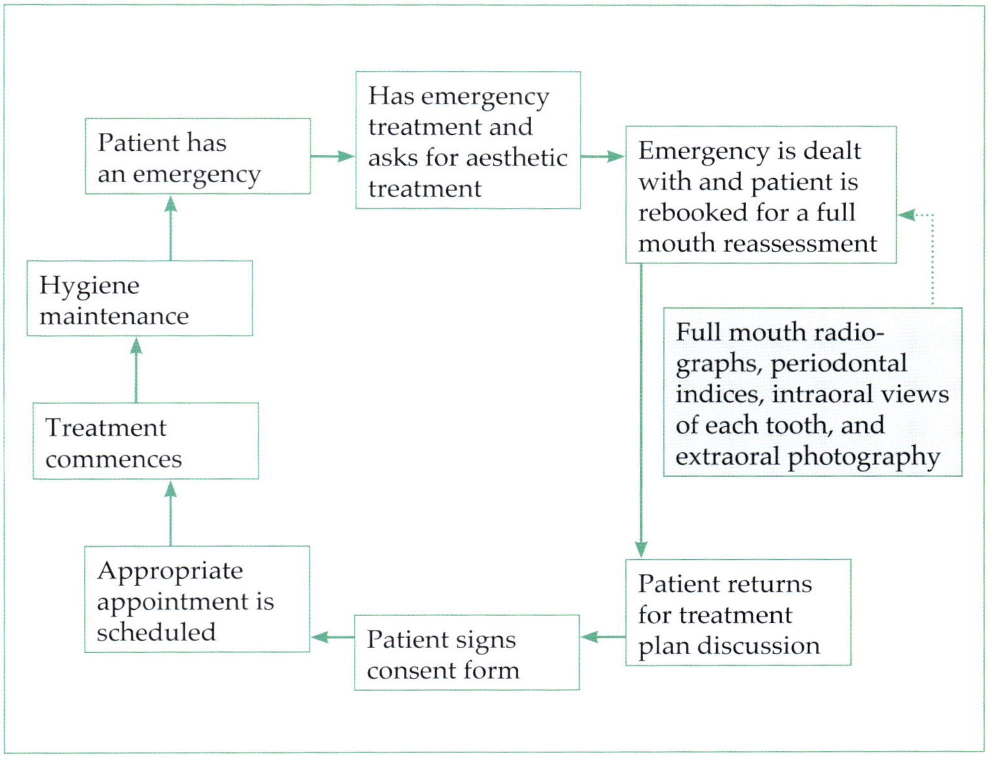

Fig 9-4 Existing patient journey.

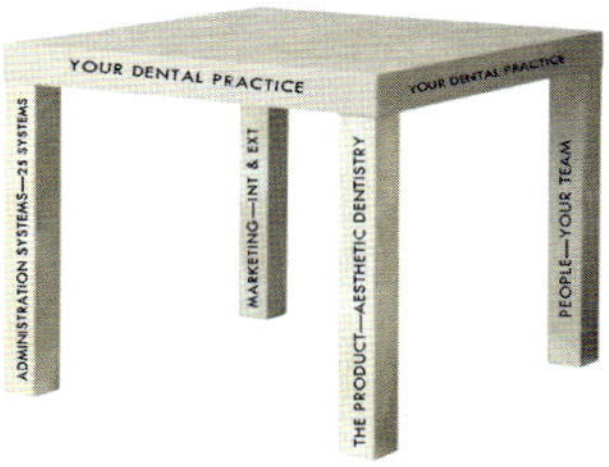

Fig 9-5 Four legs of the table. Each needs to be a good and stable support for the aesthetic dental practice (modified from Ackerman et al., 2010, with permission).

helpful for patients to see examples of treatment that other patients have undertaken to help the patient understand the types of treatment that are available. Before-and-after photos are useful for patients to see (Fig 9-6). These can be placed with the patients' permission on the dental practice website, in before-and-after treatment albums, and in advertisements for the dental practice.
- The team: The team who will be involved in the treatment procedure: preparation, sterilization, meeting, greeting, and coordination.

During the planning phase, all the information is collated and reviewed concerning the new patient interview, data collected from the intraoral examination, as well as the diagnostic records, radiographs, and photographs.

The formulation of your diagnosis should include the following components (Winter, 2007):
- Development and prioritization of a problem list.
- Identification of the etiology.
- Development of treatment goals, which includes options for each problem.
- Visualization of the final biologic and aesthetic outcome.

Table 9-1 shows a list of the "dos and don'ts" for planning treatment.

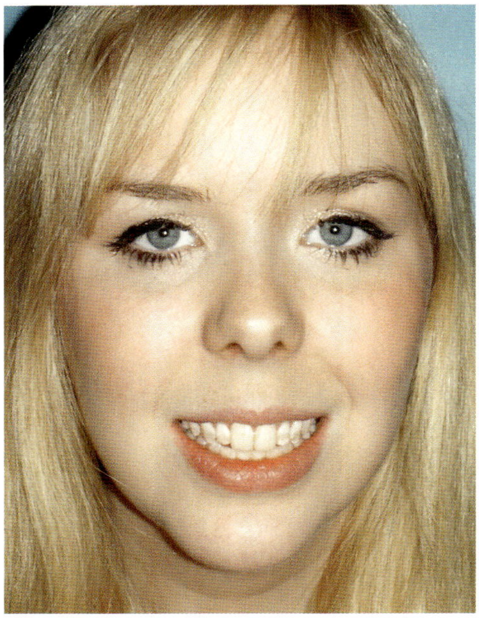

Fig 9-6a The appearance of the teeth before whitening.

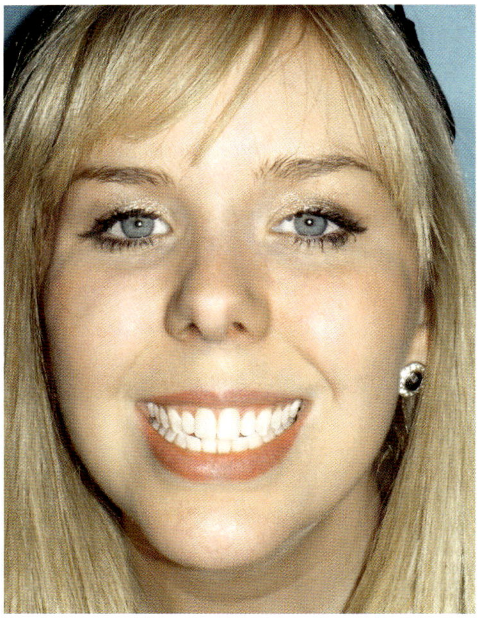

Fig 9-6b The appearance of the teeth after whitening. The existing resin composite bondings were removed and the teeth were whitened using 10% carbamide peroxide gel in the home trays. As this patient had fluorosis mottling, the treatment involved extended bleaching for a period of 8–11 weeks followed by two sessions of microabrasion to remove the white spots that still remained after prolonged bleaching.

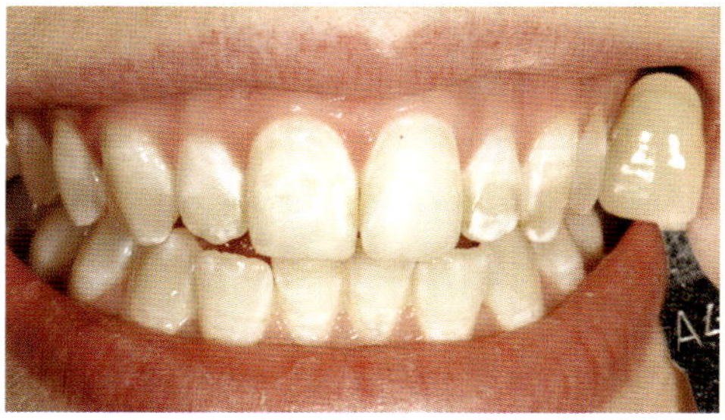

Fig 9-6c The appearance of the teeth before bleaching. The patient has severe fluorosis staining and mottling on the teeth. This is considered to be an advanced bleaching case as whitening the teeth will take longer to undertake. The existing resin composite bondings on the central incisors were removed and the teeth were whitened using 10% carbamide peroxide gel in the home trays for a period of 8–10 weeks.

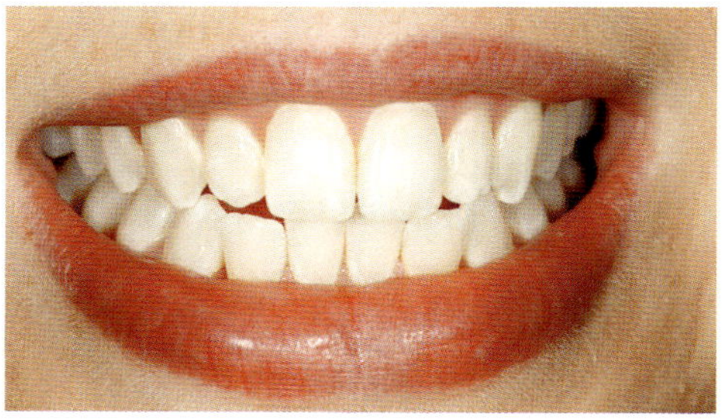

Fig 9-6d The appearance of the teeth after completion of treatment. Note the disappearance of the brown, yellow, and orange staining from the teeth. This disappeared after the prolonged bleaching treatment with 10% carbamide peroxide. The white marks and banding were faded by administering the microabrasion technique. Microabrasion paste (Opalustre from Ultradent/Optident [UK]) was used, containing 5% hydrochloric acid, and pumice and silica carbide particles.

Table 9-1 "Dos and don'ts" for planning treatment

Do	Don't

• Ensure that adequate uninterrupted time is allocated for planning the case (normally at least 1 hour per week, or 1 hour at the middle of the week and 1 hour at the end of the week).
• Set aside enough time to be able to sit quietly and plan, in a step-by-step manner. You may need at least 1 hour to plan the case, as it may be complex.
• Allow time to consider all the treatment options for the patient.
  • Get further advice from additional specialists such as endodontic evaluation and detailed periodontal report.
• Schedule treatment-planning time/appointment into the appointment schedule. This can be the same time each week or may need to have more time devoted to it as case load increases.
  • Ensure the patient fully understands what is involved in the treatment.
	• Treat a patient in a hurry. **Warning:** do not treat a patient in a rush without first treating the emergency situation. Ensure that the patient knows the financial responsibility first and agrees to pay the fee. Reschedule another appointment after the emergency situation is taken care of.
	• Rush or pressurize a patient into treatment.
	• Make assumptions (Goldstein, 1999):
	  • eg, if the patient has rejected the proposed treatment in the past they may not necessarily do so again.
	  • as the patient's circumstances may have changed. Previously the patient may have requested that the tooth be patched, but has finally realized the need for a crown.
	  • based on what you think the patient can afford.

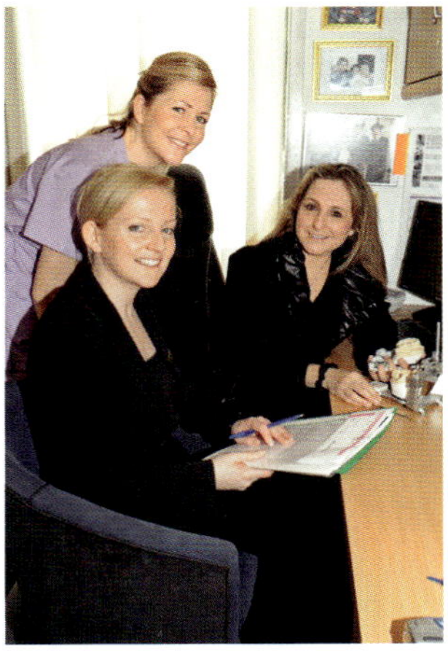

Fig 9-7 Treatment planning session with treatment coordinator and dental assistant.

Taking time to plan

Treatment planning should have special time allocated, and this time should be uninterrupted. The dentist needs to have all the documentation (such as treatment planning forms, either computerized or written forms) and data present in order to make treatment-planning decisions. The additional data required includes radiographs, photos, study casts, preoperative casts, diagnostic waxups and stents, CT scans, intraoral camera views, and clinical data such as periodontal indices. The treatment coordinator can ensure that all this is gathered and ready for the planning session, and should sit in at this session (Fig 9-7). With all the information gathered where the treatment planning will take place, decisions can be made in a clear and concise manner. In order to get in the habit and to focus on the task at hand, a treatment planning checklist can be used (Appendix 9-3).

Radiographic evaluation

To start the treatment planning process, first look at the radiographs. This will give a general view of the situation. Scan the bone levels to look at the overall health of the mouth, and the support structure for the periodontium. Look at the general health of the teeth. Then focus on individual teeth to look for tooth decay. Look at all the apices of the teeth for widening of the apical area or any periapical lesions, endodontic sclerosis, incomplete root canal treatment, perforations, internal/external resorption, and problems associated with posts (Wise, 1995). With the digital radiography, it is easy to use the magnification process in order to obtain a clearer picture. Look at the integrity of individual restorations or existing crowns or fixed partial dentures. Look for any root fractures that may be present.

- Assess endodontic lesions at the apices of all teeth.
- Assess any questionable areas for further testing.
- Focus on individual teeth. Start in a systematic manner from the maxillary right side and focus on each tooth.

- Check the radiographs for existing decay, and decay under restorations.
- Check existing restorations and indirect restorations such as crowns and fixed partial dentures.
- Check bone levels around implants.
- Further information.

CT scan evaluation (Appendix 9-4)

- Scan the bone levels in the area that you wish to place implants.
- Scan the rest of the teeth for endodontic lesions.
- Look at the state of the periodontium through the rest of the scan.

Intraoral photo evaluation

- Assess the photos with the radiographs to verify which teeth will be receiving treatment.
- Which teeth need urgent treatment?
- View the intraoral shots of the smile from different angles.

Assessment of the photographs

It is best to view all the photographs of the face first, then the smile from central and left and right lateral views. This is when the dark premolars that have existing large amalgams are visible. The patient may have noticed this before, and this is visible on the photos. Does the patient have a midline diastema that they want to close? Look at (Fig 9-8):

- tooth size discrepancy
- tooth shape discrepancy
- gingival height
- gingival color
- gingival zeniths
- arch shape
- occlusion
- lip line
- smile line.

Assess what needs to be improved and what options are available for the patient.

Assessment of the diagnostic waxup

- Can it achieve the look that the patient wants?
- Are the central incisors symmetrical?
- Do the teeth achieve the desired aesthetic effect on the waxup?
- Will there be sufficient space?
- Does it give a good overall appearance of the whole arch?
- Will the closing of the diastema improve the overall shape of the teeth?

Assessment of the duplicate casts and stents

- Are they satisfactory?
- Will there be any problems using them?

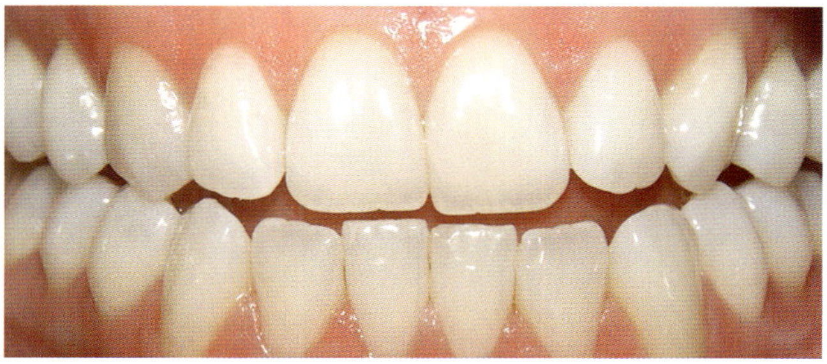

Fig 9-8a The ideal proportions of teeth for smile design teeth and zenith lines. This patient has a beautiful natural dentition. Although the smile does not follow many of the recommended guidelines, she has a beautiful natural smile.

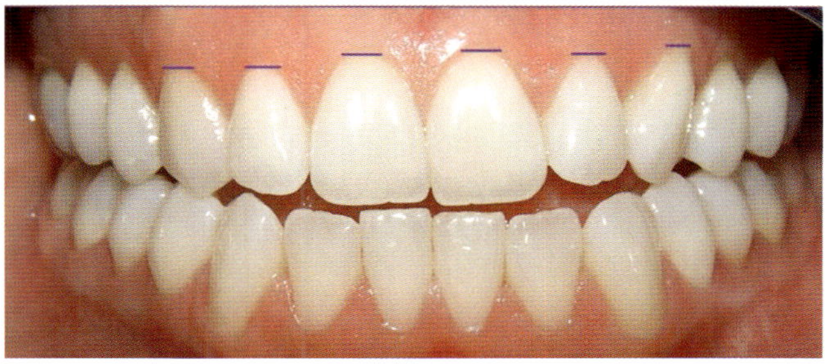

Fig 9-8b Assessing gingival heights and zenith lines. This patient has a difference in the heights of the right and left canines. There has been recession on the maxillary left canine of 2 mm. The midlines are coinciding, but the alignment of the central incisors in not straight. The lengths of the central incisors are different. However, the smile is generally aesthetically pleasing and no changes beyond whitening were recommended.

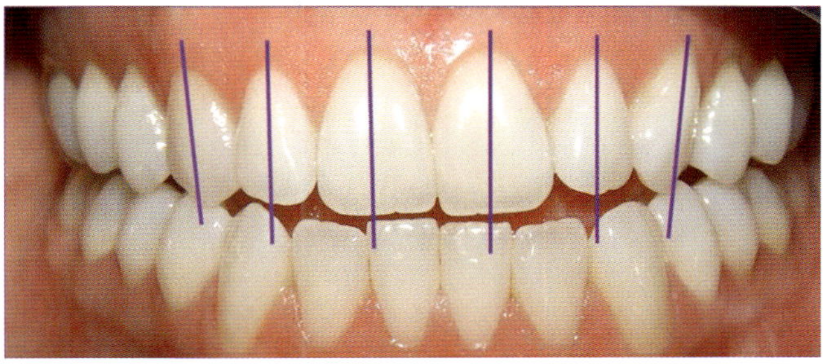

Fig 9-8c Assessing the ideal positions of the teeth for smile design: angle of inclination of the teeth.

- Is there sufficient space for minimal preparation or will further tooth reduction be required?
- Adjunctive treatment?
- Does the patient need periodontal treatment?
- Will the patient need crown lengthening?
- Root canal or re-root canal treatment?
- Are there any hopeless teeth?
- Will the patient need extraction of the tooth and an implant placed?
- Provisionalization: what is needed?
  - temporary fixed partial denture
  - adhesive fixed partial denture
  - immediate provisional implant restoration.

Writing down the treatment plan – notation

- What is the patient's main motivation or concern?
- Does this need to be managed first?
- What are the patient's hopes and aspirations?
- Can I design a plan according to the patient's wishes?
- Classify and clarify whether this is a basic, intermediate, or advanced case? What does that imply?

- What is needed to get to this treatment phase?
- What should be done first to eliminate the dental disease?
- Tooth-by-tooth assessment on an individual basis?
- Tooth-by-tooth assessment from the occlusal planes?
- Occlusal vertical dimension. Does the bite need to be opened up or is it satisfactory at present? Are there any over-erupted teeth that need reduction?
- What is the prognosis for each tooth – is it good/guarded/hopeless?
- What types of restorations are needed for each tooth?
- Which surfaces and materials are to be used?

Length of each appointment and time intervals

- How much treatment is to be provided at each appointment?
- Appointment length.
- Can more than one tooth be treated in the same sextant for better treatment ease and local anesthetic and to reduce number of appointments for the patient?
- It is better for the patient, dentist, and team to have longer appointments to do more necessary dentistry for the patient during that visit, than multiple short appointments.
- The order in which treatment is to proceed.
- The length of time necessary for each appointment.
- The time between appointments.
- The phase and stage of treatment.

Further options to be discussed

- Treatment priority:
  - urgent: immediate treatment
  - necessary: should be done
  - elective
  - ideal treatment.
- Maintenance program and intervals of review.

Outcome at the end of the treatment planning stage

- A treatment plan which may be staged.
- Before-and-after photos of a similar case.
- A digital case presentation incorporating a summary of all the relevant data is prepared on power point.
- A copy of the digital case presentation is given to the patient on USB stick.
- The patient has a copy of the treatment planning booklet.

The treatment planning booklet (Fig 9-9)

- The details of the treatment without the fees so that the patient first focuses on the clinical dentistry that is being presented.
- The photos of the patient.
- A clinical charting system that the patient can understand.

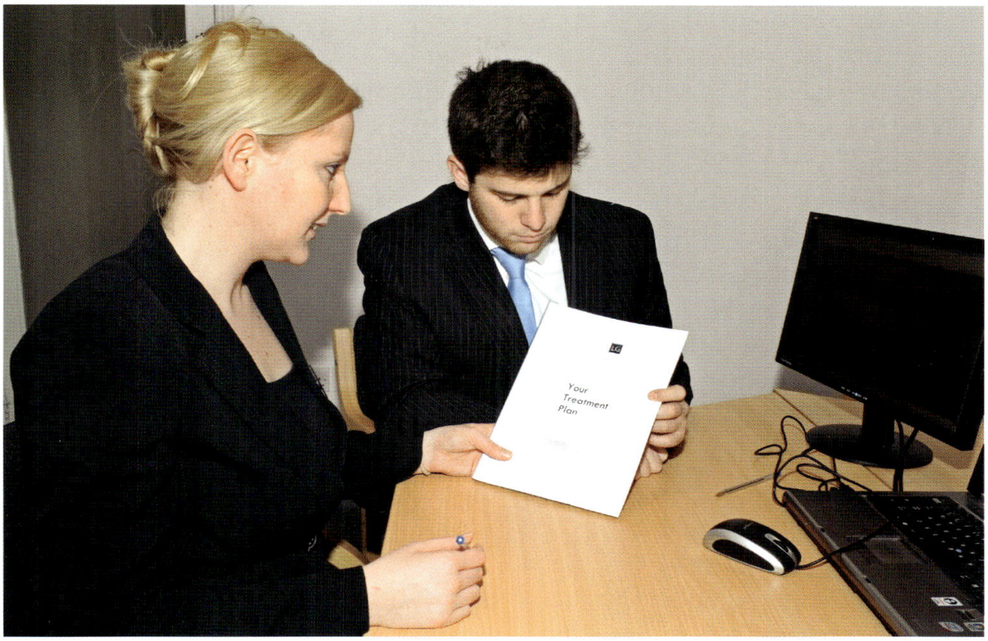

Fig 9-9 The treatment coordinator giving the patient their treatment planning booklet.

- Implant staging sheet for the patient to understand the process of implant treatment.
- The treatment broken down into phases.
- Photos of a similar before-and-after case.
- Terms and conditions.
- Financial responsibility form to be signed.
- Practice newsletter, calendar and other marketing information on the back page.
- What to Expect leaflet.
- Patient's charter form.

Success strategies in aesthetic dentistry

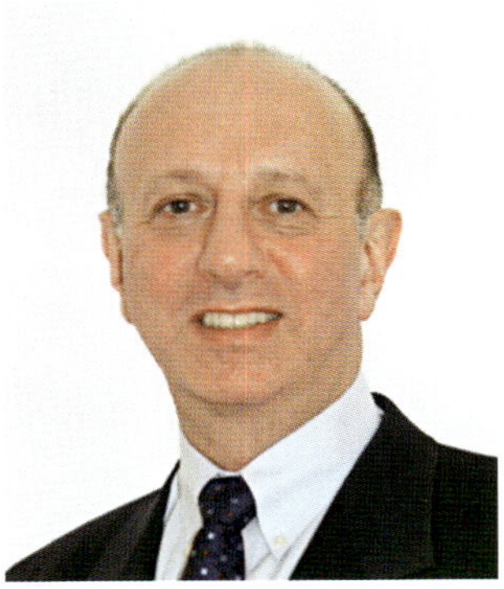

Dr Michael Wise,
Specialist in Restorative Dentistry and Oral Surgery, London

Always:

1. Carry out a full dental examination and record the findings. Do not just carry out an esthetic assessment.
2. Plan treatment carefully and ensure that sufficient time is allocated for this.
3. Explain the risks, advantages, and disadvantages of treatment and the alternative options for treatment, ensuring that the patient understands them.
4. Obtain consent.
5. Ensure that you do not become a single treatment dentist, eg, always providing veneers, or always providing implants.
6. Do not promise the impossible. Ensure that your technician is capable of providing the results that you and your patient are striving for.

3. The planning process: implementation

Trends in clinical aesthetic dentistry

There have been many trends in aesthetic dentistry over the last few decades. Some have been dentist-driven, some patient-driven, and some media-driven through the television and fashion industry. There are several problems that have arisen with some of these trends, which need to be considered when planning aesthetic dental treatment for patients.

Realistic or unrealistic expectations

Some patients are pursuing unrealistic expectations as to what can be achieved with a new smile or smile makeover. It is essential to know what is not possible. It is important for the dentist to understand what the patient is trying to achieve in the certain look that they want. Sometimes it is better not to undertake treatment for patients with unrealistic expectations as the treatment or dentist can never live up to these expectations and this can be a source of conflict.

The need for perfection

Although many patients may seek the perfect smile, perfect smiles can look artificial. There is a constant quest for perfection of the body, the face and the teeth. The problem with seeking perfection is that perfection in life does not exist. There is always some feature that is not perfect, which adds to the natural beauty of the smile and the face. Smiles can be designed along certain smile design principles that follow certain guidelines. However, certain factors may not always allow for perfection and thus the patients may be disappointed with the result. It is essential to assess the patient's occlusion, occlusal pattern, and whether these can be accommodated in the quest for perfection (Miller, 1999).

The whitest shade possible

White teeth are a beauty feature but some patients want the whitest shade possible, which can also look unnatural. This extreme whiteness may either look opaque or blue and either case is not appealing to everybody. However, it is the patient who wants this look even though the dentist does not like the extreme whiteness, and aesthetic dentistry is elective so the patient will need to approve the shade of the porcelain. Changes in shade or porcelain cannot be made after cementation.

Whole mouth correction for a single problem

There has become the need for correction of the whole mouth when a small problem exists on one single anterior tooth. Other options may need to be considered such as orthodontics, which can correct the position of the tooth. There are new options for more aesthetic orthodontics, which include lingual placement of brackets and clear aligners, which are more acceptable for patients.

Mass destruction of healthy teeth and enamel to create "the look"

Destruction of enamel leads to many further problems, which include sensitivity and pain. The patient is committed to a lifetime of repeat aesthetic dentistry as dentistry has a finite lifespan.

> *"Because of the growing sophistication of today's global public who are educated to understand the power of an attractive smile, an increasing number of patients seek aesthetic dental treatments. With this opportunity to improve a patient's oral health and aesthetics also comes a responsibility to do no harm."*
>
> *Dr Cherilyn Sheets (interview)*

The patient in Figure 9-10 wanted to improve her smile without mass destruction of healthy teeth. First a diagnostic waxup was undertaken, followed by a resin composite mockup to show the closure of the diastemata between the central and lateral incisors. Photos were taken of the patient with the mockup in place to show how the look could be created.

The patient took the resin composite mockup home to see if she liked the look. She then returned to have the treatment. Treatment involved whitening using trays, direct bonding to both central incisors to close the central black triangle, reshaping of the distal parts of the central incisors so that the teeth would not look too wide, and then no-preparation resin composite veneers placed directly over the maxillary left and right lateral incisors and canines. Figures 9-10h–j show the final result that was achieved for the patient. This case highlights the importance of careful treatment planning.

The persistent quest for beauty (Dunn, 1996)

This can be psychological and there are some patients who suffer from dysmorphophobia. Dysmorphophobia is an unnatural focus on the body as unattractive. These patients may never be happy or satisfied with the treatment that is provided, not due to the treatment or the result itself, but because of their psychological condition (Feinman & Harris, 1984). Dentists need to be aware of this condition and may need to make the diagnosis or refer to a psychologist/psychiatrist for a further opinion prior to contemplating any clinical treatment, as it may be a mistake to carry out any treatment at all on these patients.

The Hollywood/celebrity smile

There is a trend towards requesting the Hollywood cosmetic smile. The media and movie industry dictate the design of certain smiles for celebrities. While some patients want to emulate this look, it may not be to the dentist's liking. Aesthetic dentistry is based on personal taste, and the choice is very personal. A certain look in a patient's smile makeover that looks fake may be what they want to achieve. This smile design is not for everybody – many others want natural smiles.

The trend towards natural enhancement

There has now been a backlash against the Hollywood smile, which has been fabricated towards the naturally enhanced smile with minimal or no destruction of healthy enamel. Patients want to keep their existing teeth and whiten a few shades lighter to enhance the natural beauty of their own natural teeth. Most of the time, this improvement can be achieved with home

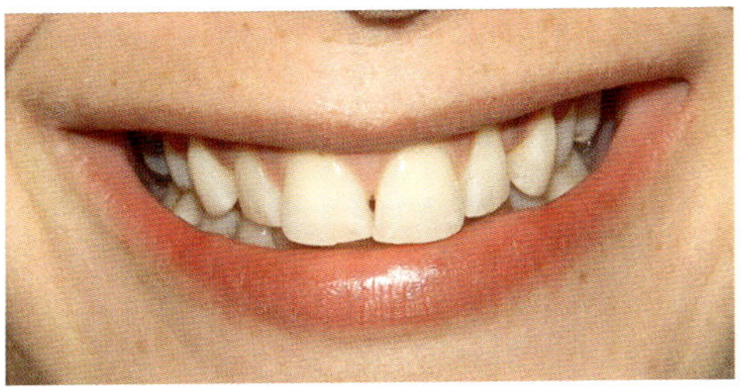

Fig 9-10a The patient before treatment and whitening. Conservative treatment was planned involving bleaching, tooth contouring to reduce the size of central incisors, direct bonding, and indirect laboratory fabricated resin composite veneers.

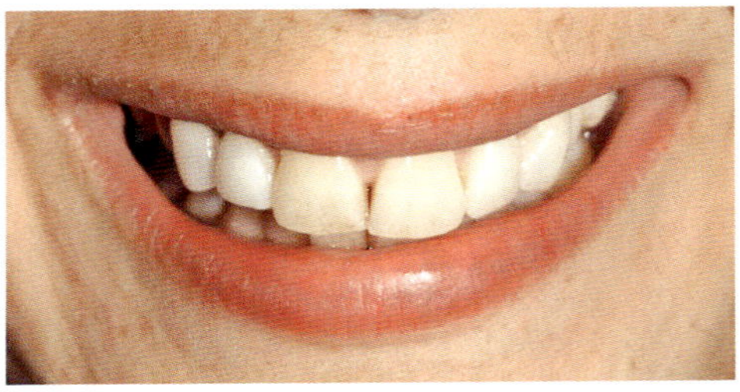

Fig 9-10b Patient with resin composite mockups to check the shape of the teeth with the diastema closed.

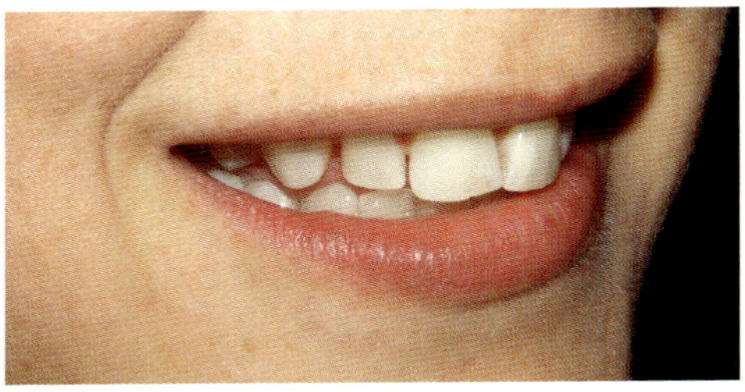

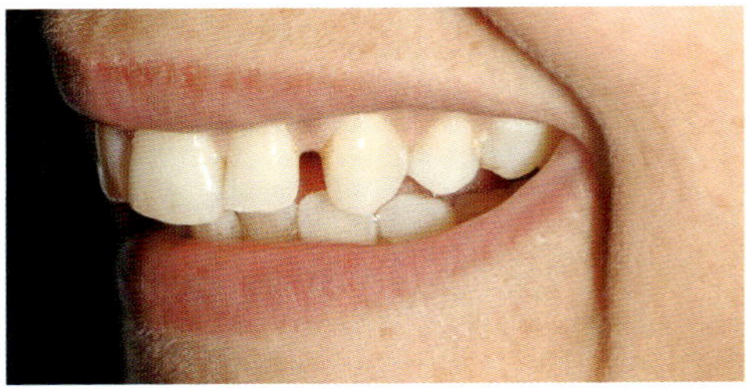

Figs 9-10c and 9-10d Lateral views showing diastemata before treatment.

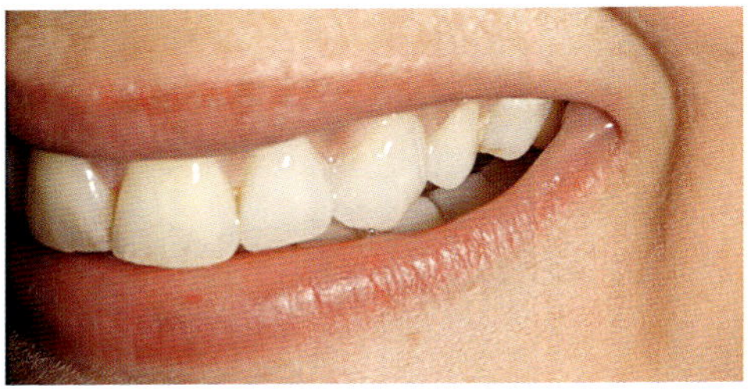

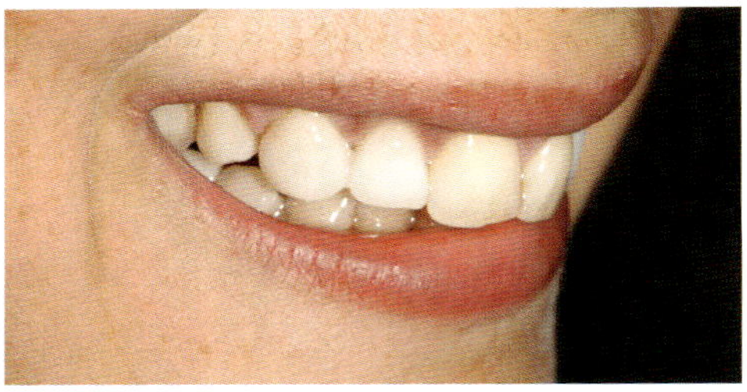

Figs 9-10e and 9-10f Lateral views of the patient with the mockups in place for the patient to assess.

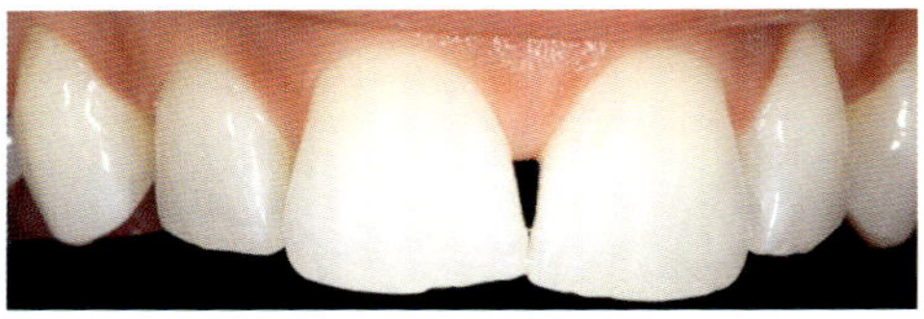

Fig 9-10g The smile after whitening but before bonding.

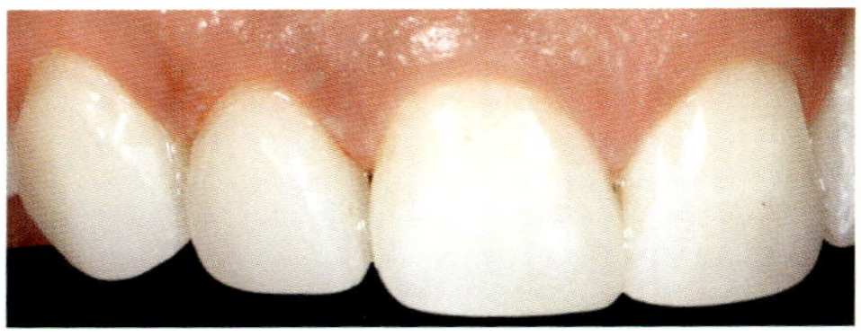

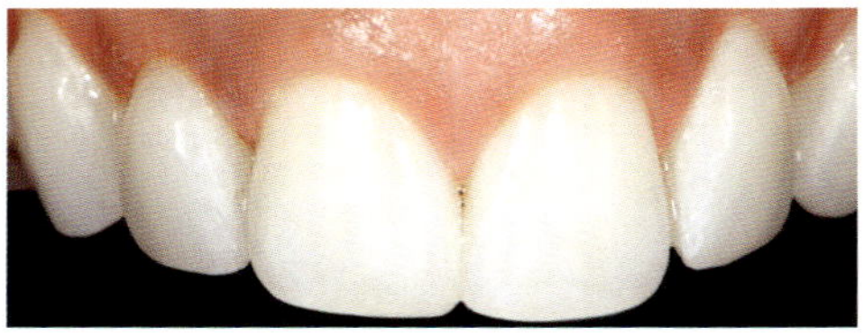

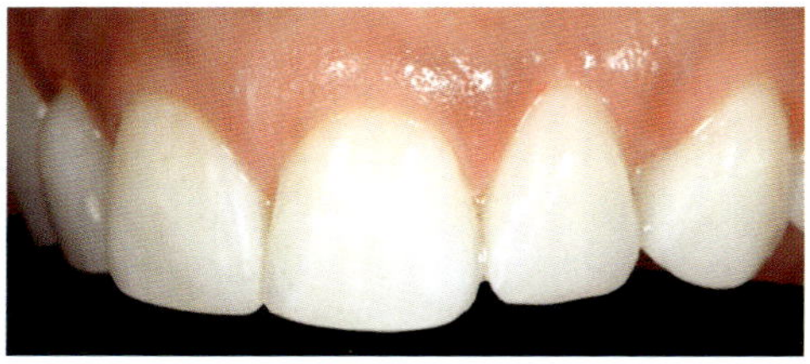

Figs 9-10h to 9-10j The final outcome.

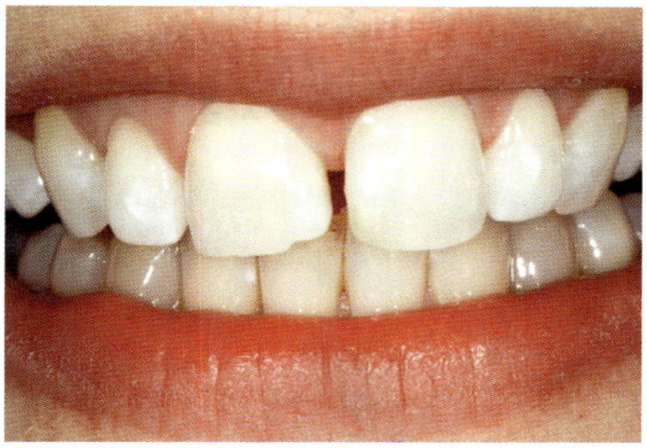

Fig 9-11a This patient did not like the appearance of her teeth. Specifically, she wanted to close the midline diastema and whiten her teeth. The treatment that was undertaken was whitening first, followed by Invisalign treatment, and then final resin composite bonding on the central incisors, in order to achieve harmony and symmetry for the smile.

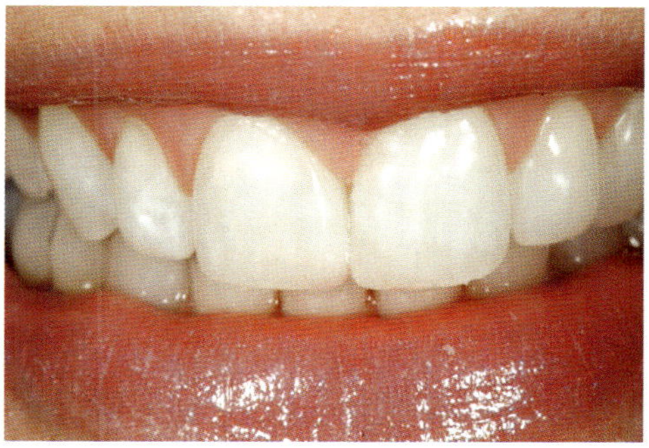

Fig 9-11b The appearance of the teeth after completion of the Invisalign treatment, whitening and bonding. The closure of the midline diastema took approximately 9 months to complete.

bleaching and resin composite bonding. The patient in Figure 9-11 underwent whitening first. This was followed by Invisalign treatment to close the midline diastema. After completion of the Invisalign treatment the central incisors were bonded (Fig 9-11b) to improve the shape and symmetry of the anterior teeth. This treatment plan follows the trend toward minimal natural enhancement. The patient's enamel is preserved with an improvement of the smile in a natural way.

The minimalist trend

The trend has swung towards enhancing the natural look and keeping the existing enamel. This is the trend towards only bleaching the teeth to give a lighter, whiter shade of a patient's existing teeth. This may be followed by direct or indirect resin composite bonding of the teeth, which is seen as a less invasive option without heavy destruction of enamel. The minimalist trend may lead to compromising the final look as teeth are mainly kept in the natural state. As long as the patient understands that and is not disappointed, it is fine to go ahead with treatment. This look can be achieved with bleaching, direct bonding, and cosmetic contouring (Fig 9-12).

No-preparation veneers

Although no removal of healthy enamel and only minimal enamel preparation may be advocated, postoperative problems may still arise. These may not be suitable for patients whose natural teeth are very dark. It may be better to bleach these teeth prior to undertaking any veneer treatment. Bleaching may improve the situation, so that veneers may not be necessary. Teeth that have been bleached using the night guard vital bleaching method have

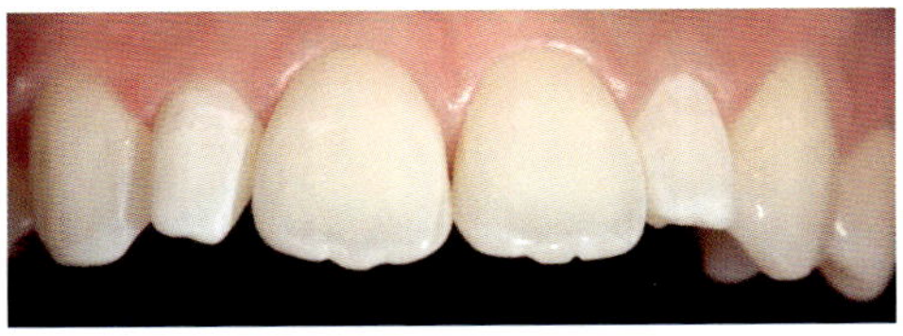

Fig 9-12a The teeth before bonding for the peg-shaped lateral teeth. At this stage the peg-shaped lateral teeth have been etched ready to commence the bonding treatment. Simple conservative options should be discussed with patients first to preserve as much healthy enamel as possible.

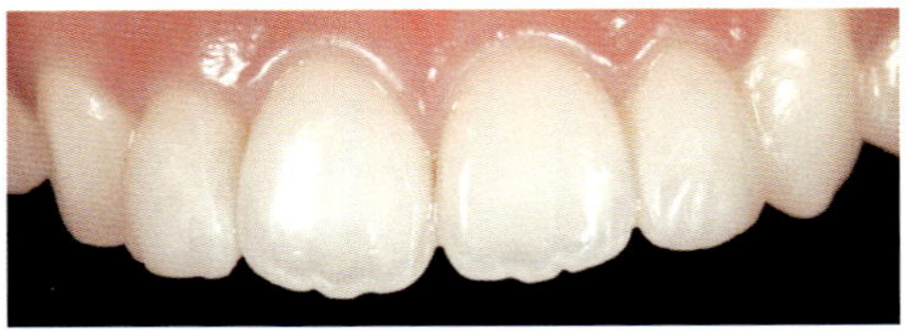

Fig 9-12b The result after direct resin composite bonding to improve the shapes of the peg-shaped lateral teeth.

a reduced enamel bond strength, which needs to be considered as veneer treatment should be delayed for 2 to 4 weeks, depending on how long the home bleaching procedure was administered. This treatment option may be provided if a waxup has demonstrated that to achieve the desired look, it may not be necessary to prepare the underlying teeth. Many patients like the option of leaving their own healthy teeth underneath and placing the veneers directly over the unprepared natural teeth, as it is considered as a less invasive option.

Bleachorexic or bleachaholic?

Some patients become obsessed with the whiteness of the shade of their teeth that they have achieved through whitening or bleaching their teeth. They continue to bleach their teeth daily for fear of the shade reverting back to the previous yellow shade. For them the shade of the teeth is not white enough and they continue to purchase bleaching materials from the dentist and over the counter or on the internet. There is a certain shade of lightness that can be achieved and then no further whitening is possible. It is best for these patients to undertake the proper protocol for a bleaching progam, and then to reach an end point for bleaching when both the dentist and patient are happy with the white shade. Then treatment should be terminated. It is not necessary to continually whiten on a daily basis.

The clip-on smile

This is a trend in which the patient can have clip-on teeth made which they can wear when they go out or for different occasions, similar to people having different color contact lenses, while still keeping their natural teeth underneath. This has not taken off and is merely a gimmick. It is not considered as a recommended solution for treatment in aesthetic dentistry.

The daughter test (Burke & Kelleher, 2009)

There is concern expressed at the extensive amount of elective aesthetic dentistry. Burke and Kelleher (2009) have come up with a test called the Daughter Test to help dentists consider if the treatment proposed is in the patient's best interest. Dentists should ask themselves a question first about the proposed treatment.

Would you undertake the treatment that you, the dentist, are proposing on your own daughter or member of your family? If in your heart of hearts the answer is no, then you need to reconsider the treatment plan for that patient. There is an ethical and moral obligation to provide the patient with all options for treatment. It is essential to always try the minimalist approach first (Burke & Kelleher, 2009). Dentists should be providing treatment plans with the least possible dentistry required to get the look that the patient wants to achieve. Preservation of healthy enamel for a lifetime is essential. Direct resin composite bonding is an excellent option and often should be considered as the first alternative to treatment as it can be easily removed, added to, and rebonded and resurfaced.

Success strategies in aesthetic dentistry

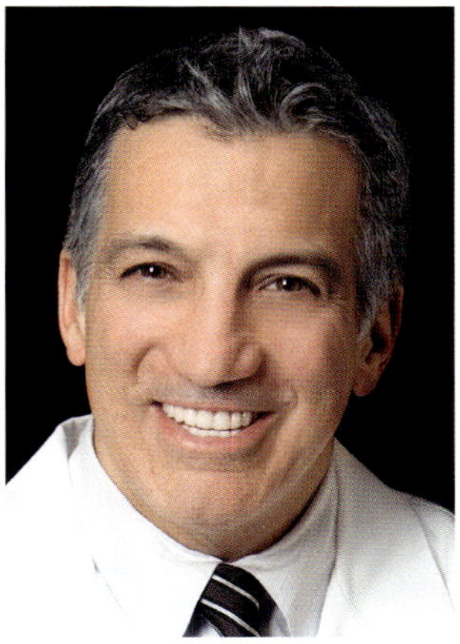

Dr Gerry Curatola, Aesthetic Dentist, New York, NY

1. Listen to the patient! Doctors are used to telling patients what they need – but not in aesthetic dentistry. Here the patient must tell you, and you MUST listen. I have had patients with a large diastema that love it, and I have had others bothered by seemingly small cosmetic problems that would not have been a concern to me. Again, LISTEN to the patient.
2. Walk the talk! You can't promote aesthetic dentistry if you or members of your dental team do not have beautiful teeth or aren't recipients of aesthetic dental treatment.
3. Create a clinic environment that is aesthetically oriented. At Rejuvenation Dentistry, we create a "thematic experiential environment" around "rejuvenation" with furnishings, amenities, materials, music, lighting, and so on. It has a profound and supportive effect on a patient's commitment to treatment. You can't be successful if your environment looks like "Little Shop of Horrors".
4. Make it possible for patients to attain. Aesthetic dentistry should not just be for the rich and famous. I have school teachers, bus drivers and even fishermen who want a nicer smile and my staff are well trained to help them meet the financial commitment when they understand the treatment and are ready to commit to what they need.
5. Build "ambassadors" of your dental practice. By creating a life-changing experience in a pleasant "patient centered" environment, patients will be eager to speak praises to their friends and family. Nothing beats the success of the good old "word of mouth."

The treatment planning checklist

The key to a successful outcome is to use a logical step-by-step process to fully understand potential treatment options before you begin, and to develop interdisciplinary relationships to provide planning or procedural support when needed (Appendix 9-5).

Urgent/emergency treatment

Disease control: periodontics, restorative decay removal, functional management. Are there broken teeth that need temporary fillings?

Stabilizing the mouth

Check the bone levels together with the periodontal indices. Does the patient need further periodontal treatment prior to the treatment? Will the patient be able to keep their teeth for a lifetime?

Look at all the root apices in the full mouth series, then look at the three-dimensional CT (computed tomography) scan as further lesions will become visible and this may help to clarify areas that may be questionable on the periapical radiograph. Assess the status of the roots. Are there any widened apices or endodontic lesions? What is the status of the existing root canal treatment? Is it acceptable on the radiograph? Are there problems?

Occlusion

The existing occlusal relation, its stability, the occlusal plane, vertical dimension, existing restorations, wear, deflective contacts, and parafunctional habits all require attention. Does the occlusion need adjustment?

Provisional restorations

Provisional crowns.

Definitive treatment

The definitive treatment can only begin to be completed once the mouth is stable and there is evidence that the patient can maintain periodontal health and excellent home care. The initial periodontal cleanings should be completed. At this stage there should be healing of the infection under root canals, the implants should be integrated, and there should be no further caries present in the mouth. It may be essential to take new radiographs to assess the healing of the caries lesion. Is there evidence and data that show that the mouth is stable?

The patient should be happy with the appearance and color of the provisional restorations.

Definitive try in of porcelain restorations: Is the occlusion stable? Are there enough contact points on the articulating paper in the correct locations? Is it holding shim stock in the correct locations? On both sides? Are they equal the sides?

Photos taken

The anterior teeth:

- central incisors: correct length, shapes, symmetry of both centrals, no visible black triangles, good incisal length and transitions, line angles are well defined
- lateral incisors: good shapes and contact points
- canines: good color and buccal emergence profile.

Color

Check the color:

- is light enough
- is translucent in the correct areas
- characterization of neck, body and tip
- blends in with the natural teeth.

The lip lines and smile lines are good.

The contact points are acceptable: floss checked on all points. Interproximal contacts?

Use of interproximal brushes checked and allocated.

4. Evaluation: completion of the case

- Review occlusion.
- Embrasure spaces: floss and brushes and interspace brushes.
- Patient's smile.
- Check that they know how to maintain good dental health.
- Hygiene appointments scheduled to dovetail.
- Exit interview: ask the patient to complete a testimonial form.
- Consent for photos should be sought in order to use these cases for patient education and internal and external marketing on website and within the dental practice.

The evaluation phase is the final stage of the treatment-planning journey. Once the treatment has been completed it is essential that an evaluation takes place where the dentist evaluates whether the treatment objectives that were planned at the treatment planning phase have been fulfilled. Any issues or problems should be discussed with the patient, along with any possible further long-term treatment. It is also important to ensure that the patient knows exactly how to maintain and clean the new and existing restorations and be able to maintain excellent oral hygiene.

The patient should be enrolled in a maintenance program with the hygienist and monitoring at monthly, and then at 3-monthly intervals to ensure that a successful outcome can be achieved. Continuous monitoring is essential for a successful outcome. This monitoring and evaluation phase is just as critical as any other component of the treatment planning process. It is always ongoing and includes the evaluation for any future needs (Winter, 2007).

Appendix 9-6 shows a checklist for the complete aesthetic case. Implant treatment can be tracked using Appendix 9-7.

Action steps

1. Block out time in your schedule to treatment plan every week. If this is insufficient then book time every second day.
2. Ensure that you have sufficient unhurried quality time for this process. Take more time than you think you need as there are many

patients who will need comprehensive treatment planning and time to assess radiographs and CT scans.

3. Ensure that the team member (treatment coordinator) has all the data present to make decisions about the clinical treatment required.
4. Prepare a space in your office where treatment planning happens regularly so that all data can be stored ready for treatment planning.
5. Prepare a treatment planning sheet on which all information can be recorded and documented.
6. Ensure that all clinical aspects are documented on the treatment plan in order to ensure proper time allocation on appointment sequencing.
7. Ensure that you have excellent knowledge of your computer software and its treatment planning function, and use this to insert radiographs and photographs into the treatment plan letter to patients.
8. Complex treatment planning requires more time: identify those patients who need complex planning.
9. Prepare and categorize standard paragraphs that be used for complex treatment plans and can be adapted for treatment planning reports.

Success strategies in aesthetic dentistry

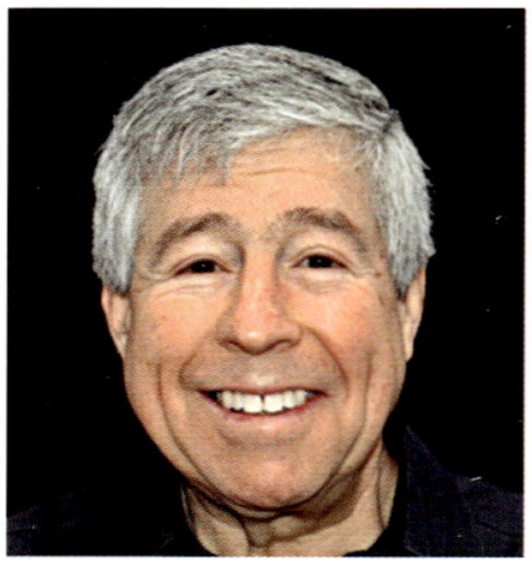

Dr Mervyn Druian, Cosmetic Dentist, London

1. Everyone in the dental practice must have good self-esteem – necessary for case presentation.
2. The dental practice must have the gift of empathy.
3. The dental practice must have knowledge, care, skill, and judgment to look after people coming for care.
4. Be available to new patients 24/7/365.
5. Get a mentor for the dental practice. Not only to continue being a cutting-edge practice, but for everyone to be great human beings.

Success strategies in aesthetic dentistry

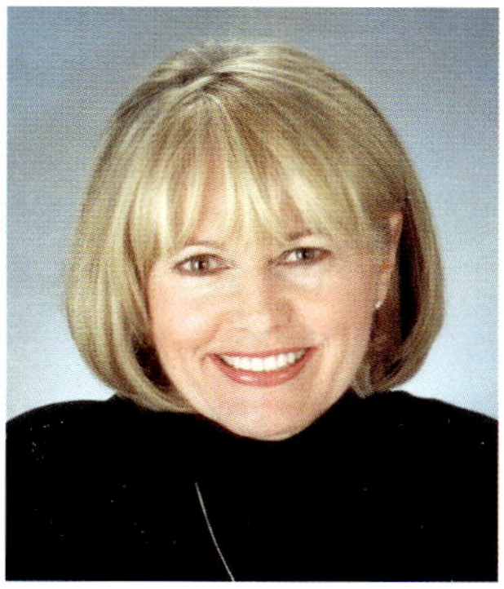

Dr Cherilyn Sheets, Prosthodontist, Newport Beach, CA

1. Excellence as a constant in everything.
2. Treat patients and staff as family.
3. Invest in yourself and staff in continuing education.
4. Invest constantly in your business in appropriate new technology and upgraded equipment.
5. Constantly reinvent yourself in positive ways so that you never lose your passion.
6. Be a dental philanthropist. Help others.

Success strategies in aesthetic dentistry

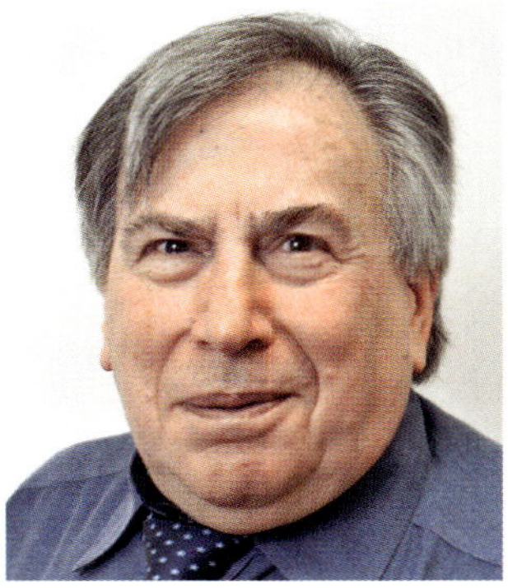

Dr David Klaff, Prosthodontist and Aesthetic Dentist, London

1. Treatment based on a totally honest policy in describing clinical skills and education.
2. Treatment based on a "First Do No Harm" approach.
3. Treatment based on a clear policy of informed consent.
4. Treatment based on a proven scientific approach.
5. Expertise of multi-disciplinary specialists where needed.

Success strategies in aesthetic dentistry

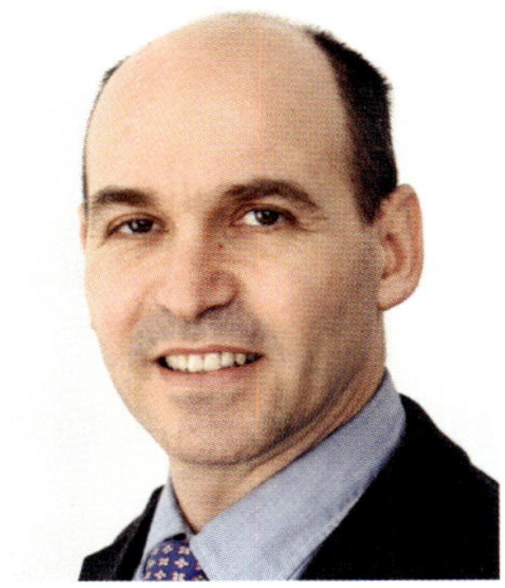

Dr Basil Mizrahi, Prosthodontist, London

1. "Visualize before you finalise." Make sure you get on the same wavelength as your patient as early as possible in treatment and continue to work towards this throughout treatment. Before commencing treatment, allow ample time for discussion and use visual aids such as pictures, waxups, mockups, and later temporaries to make sure the final result is not a surprise. Aesthetics is subjective. If you try to convince the patient that the final result you have given them is correct, that's an excuse. If you educate them before and during treatment as to what to expect, that's an explanation.
2. Take into account the personality, demands, and expectations of the patient when quoting your fees. One size does not fit all. Once treatment has started, it's too late to change your fees.

3. Don't carry out any treatment on a patient that you wouldn't carry out on your own child.
4. Your cosmetic results are only as good as the underlying foundation. Failure to adhere to good biologic principles will reduce the longevity of the restorations. There are no short cuts to technical excellence.
5. Multidisciplinary problems need multidisciplinary treatment. Keep up to date and well informed so you can offer/discuss with your patients the optimal treatment available, even if you are not able to provide all the treatment yourself.

Success strategies in aesthetic dentistry

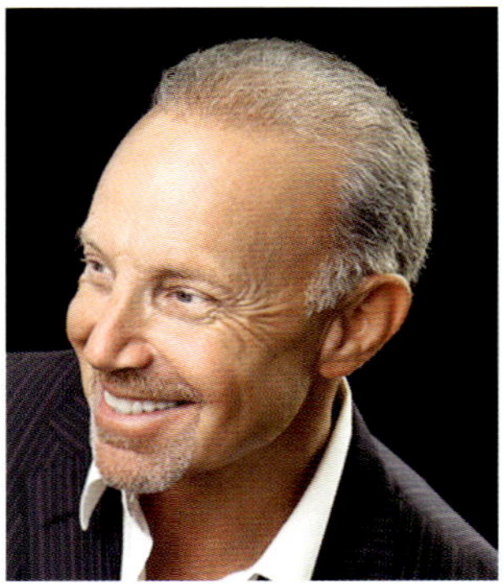

Dr Larry Rifkin, Cosmetic Dentist and Prosthodontist, Beverley Hills, CA

1. Practice and live with passion for what you do and the people around you. Your energy will impact your staff and patients.
2. Enjoy the journey as much as the results. Your patients will appreciate the experience and love coming to you for care and refer others.
3. The aesthetic practice demands a foundation in art as well as science. Take classes in art and expand your vision and ability to design smiles that are natural and believable.
4. Develop a team approach to comprehensive care that includes your essential dental technologist as well as all the dental specialists.
5. Incorporate meaningful technologies that are the tools to enhance your knowledge, performance, and precision.

Success strategies in aesthetic dentistry

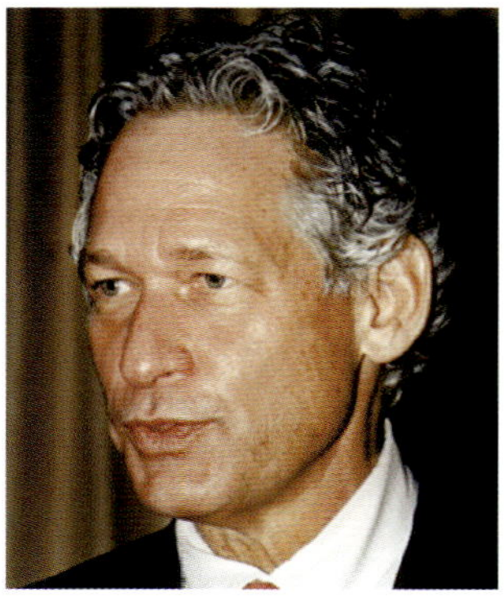

Dr Oded Bahat, Implant Surgeon and Periodontist, Beverley Hills, CA

1. The final solution should be optimal for the patient and not tailored to the dentist's ability.
2. A comprehensive treatment plan including long-term and short-term prognosis of the entire dentition and individual units should be precise and accurate.
3. View the final goal of the reconstruction and illustrate it to the patient through aesthetic stents, 3D models, and simulation etc.
4. Consider different prosthetic solutions to a given situation.
5. Delineate multiple surgical approaches which will allow the dentist to achieve the final goal.
6. Review alternative modalities of treatment to resolve any complications.
7. Know when not to treat.

References

1. Ackerman RA, De Bruyn P, Ackerman S. A Sprat to Catch a Mackerel. Key Principles to Build Your Business. Johannesburg: Jonathan Ball Publishers, 2010.
2. Burke FJ, Kelleher MG. The "daughter test" in elective esthetic dentistry. J Esthet Restor Dent 2009;21:143–146.
3. Dunn WJ, Murchison DF, Broome JC. Esthetics: patients' perceptions of dental attractiveness. J Prosthodont 1996;5:166–171.
4. Eaton K, Nathan K. The MGDS examination: a systemic approach. 3. Part 2 of the examination: diagnosis, treatment planning, execution of treatment, maintenance and appraisal, writing-up log diaries. Primary Dental Care 1998;5:113–118.
5. Feinman C, Harris M. The diagnosis and management of psychogenic facial pain disorders. Clin Otolaryngol Allied Sci 1984;9:199–201.
6. Gladwell M. Outliers: The Story of Success. Ed 1. London: Penguin Books, 2009.
7. Goldstein R. Considerations for smile-generated long-range treatment planning. Thoughts and opinions of a master in aesthetic dentistry. J Esthetic Dent 1999:11:1:49–53.
8. Goldstein RE. Personal communication, 2010.
9. Goldstein RE, Haywood VB. Esthetics in Dentistry: Volume 2: Esthetic problems of individual teeth, malocclusion and special populations. Hamilton, Ontario: BC Decker, 2002.
10. Greenwall LH. Bleaching Techniques in Restorative Dentistry. Ed 1. London: Martin Dunitz Taylor and Francis Publishing, 2001.
11. Gurel G. The Science and Art of Porcelain Laminate Veneers. Berlin: Quintessence Publishing, 2003.
12. Miller L. Masters of Esthetic Dentistry. The symbiosis of esthetics and occlusion. Thoughts and opinions of a Master of Esthetic Dentistry. J Esthet Restor Dent 1999;5:155–165.
13. Winter RR. Interdisciplinary treatment planning. Why is this not a standard of care? J Esthet Restor Dent 2007;19:284–288.
14. Wise MD. Failure in the Restored Dentition. Ed 1. London: Quintessence Publishing, 1995.

Further reading

Ahmad I. Digital and Conventional Dental Photography. Ed 1. Chicago, IL: Quintessence Publishing, 2004.

Butler Brown T. 50 Success Classics: winning wisdom for work and life from landmark books. London: Nicolas Brearly Publishing, 2004.

Davidson J. Essential Management Checklists. Ed 1. London: Kogan Page, 1986.

Dorfman B, Lombardi P. Billion Dollar Smile. A complete guide to your extreme smile makeover. Nashville, TN: Rutledge Hill Press, 2006.

Fradeani M. Esthetic Rehabilitation in Fixed Prosthodontics; A systematic approach to prosthetic treatment. Volume One: Esthetic Analysis. Chicago, IL: Quintessence Publishing, 2004.

Gawande A. Checklist Manifesto: How to get things right. London: Profile Books, 2010.

Goldstein RE. Change Your Smile. Chicago, IL: Quintessence Publishing, 2010.

Greenwall LH. Bleaching Techniques in Restorative Dentistry. Ed 1. London: Martin Taylor and Francis Publishing, 2001.

Koch R. The 80:20 Principle. The Secret of Achieving More with Less. London: Nicolas Brealey Publishing, 1998.

Robbins A. Awaken the Giant Within. How to take immediate control of your mental, emotional, physical and financial destiny. Ed 1. New York, NY: Fireside Books; Simon and Schuster, 1991.

Terry DA, Leinfelder KF, Geller W. Aesthetic and Restorative Dentistry: Material Selection and Technique. Stillwater, MN: Everest Publishing, 2009.

New patient questionnaire.

Appendix 9-1

New Patient Pre-Examination Questionnaire Copyright: Linda Greenwall				
Patient's Name: Date:				
Complains of:				
What can I do for you?				
Hopes and aspirations for dentistry:				
What would you like from me?				
What would you like done?				
Hopes to keep teeth:				
Special dislikes/worries about treatment:				
Previous dental history:	Last dental visit:			
	Regular attendee:			
	What was done:			
Past experience: ie, Why did you leave your last dentist:				
Smoker:	Yes/No	How long?	Ex-smoker	
Pain: Nature of pain:				
Sensitivity from:	Hot	Cold	Sweet	Pressure
Gingivae:	Bleeding gums:			
Calculus formation:	Other gum problems:			
Previous hygiene treatment: Interval				
Disclosing	Brushing	Flossing	Diet Sheets	
Smile: Look at lip line and smile line:				
What do you like most about your smile?				
What do you like least about your smile?				
If you could change anything about your smile what would you want to do?				
Teeth:				
Root canal treatment				
Previous orthodontic treatment				
Teeth missing:	Teeth replaced:	Bridges:		
Fillings:	Migrating teeth/Loose teeth:	Crowns/Caps:		
Food impaction:				
Wisdom teeth:				
TMJ:	Clicking	Bruxing	Clenching	
Past experiences with:	LA	GA		
Anything else:				

Appendix 9-2 Smile analysis sheet to assist with treatment planning.

Smile Analysis Sheet to Assist with Treatment Planning Copyright: Linda Greenwall							
Date:				Date of birth:			
Name:							
Patient's concerns and main complaint:							
Assessment of the face:				**Assessment of the teeth:**			
Proportions:				**Occlusion:**			
Forehead:	Midface:	Mandible:		Skeletal pattern:	Class 1		
Facial musculature:					Class 2 division 1		
Vertical dimensions:					Class 2 division 2		
in proportion to face:	Over closed:				Class 3		
Loss of occlusal vertical dimension:				Occlusal alignment:			
Tooth visibility:				Interferences: ICP = RCP			
Lip line:	High	Low	Other	ICP-RCP slide type:	Vertical	Horizontal	
Smile line:				First point of contact:			
Type of smile: upper lip curvature				**Lateral guidance:**	Working side contacts		
Negative space: lateral negative space					Non-working side contacts:		
	Present:	Absent:		**Canine guidance:**			
Smile symmetry:				Group function:			
Gingival morphology:				Dental midline:			
Amount of attached gingivae:				Presence of diastemas:			
Gingival health:				Golden proportion:			
Gingival disease				Tooth arrangement:			
Color of gingivae:				Axial alignment:			
Recession:				Arch type:			
Type of gingivae:				Square:	Narrow:	Rounded:	Tapered:
	Thick:	Thin:	Collagenatous:	**Existing maxillary anterior tooth length:**			
Planning:					Centrals:	Laterals:	
Diagnostic waxup needed:				**Tooth width:**			
	Yes:	No:	Mounted study casts:		Centrals:	Laterals:	
Bleaching alone will solve aesthetic requirements?:				Contact points:	High:	Low:	
Further treatment required:				Tooth wear:			
				Tooth shade:			

ICP, intercuspal position; RCP, retruded contact position

Appendix 9-3

Example of a treatment planning checklist from Dr Greenwall's dental practice.

To be checked and ready:	To be completed and checked by:
Treatment plan and financial agreement written up and signed by Dr Greenwall and additional specialist Periodontist/implant surgeon report	Day before appointment
Photos, intraoral photos and radiographs to be printed for notes and saved in P drive/dental eye	Day before appointment
Make sure reception and surgery is covered – appointment will take as long as necessary	When booking appointment and during morning meeting
Make sure treatment plan coordinator is available, and there is adequate time for the appointment	When booking appointment and during morning meeting
Consulting room ready: pens, highlighter, calculator, patient notes, treatment plan pack, before-and-after photo books, credit card machine	On day of appointment, no later than 30 min before appointment so that any problems can be rectified in time
Make sure all three screens are working and patient radiographs, photos, and PowerPoint are ready on the laptop	On day of appointment, no later than 30 min before appointment so that any problems can be rectified in time
Follow-up – ensure appointment is booked, consent is signed, and financial agreement is documented clearly	During appointment

Appendix 9-4 Checklist for assessing CT scans (© Linda Greenwall).

Vertical plane	Horizontal plane	Cross sectional cuts
Bone Teeth Maxillary sinus	Bone Teeth Maxillary sinus	Bone Teeth Maxillary sinus

Maxilla: anatomy	Mandible: anatomy
Sinus: • shape • size • pnematization • grey areas: mucosal thickening • pathology that is visible • does it need an ENT consultation?	Anterior mandible: • bone density • bone angulation • resorption patterns • borders
Maxillary bone: • bone density • bone angulation • resorption patterns • borders Interior	Posterior mandible: • bone density • bone angulation • resorption patterns • borders
Anterior maxilla: Ridge contour • vertical height • horizontal height • labial concavities Posterior maxilla: • vertical height • horizontal width	Nerve position: • mental foramen • mandibular canal • anterior branch of mental nerve visible
Incisive canal: • width • shape • interference	Bone/ridge width Lingual concavities in the anterior mandible
Teeth: • pathology • periapical lesions • periodontal problems • fractures	Teeth: • pathology • periapical lesions • periodontal problems • fractures

Treatment planning checklist: clinical aspects. Adapted and modified from Eaton and Nathan (1998) and Greenwall (2001) with kind permission.

Appendix 9-5

Stage 1

Initial assessment

- What does the patient want?
- What are the hopes and aspirations?
- Is the patient in pain?
- What is the main complaint?
- What is the patient's wish list?

Emergency treatment: elimination of pain

- Dressings
- Emergency relief of pain
- Emergency root canal therapy
- Extractions
- Control of infections.

Study models

- Initial study models
- Diagnostic waxup
- Articulated study models
- Indices and stents and models.

Treatment planning management

- Discuss possible treatment options
- Treatment implications.

Paperwork

- Consent forms
- Financial arrangements.

Stage 2

Elimination of active disease and achievement of oral stability: disease control

Periodontal:

- Assessment with indices
- Oral hygiene instruction
- Scaling and prophylaxis
- Root surface debridement (root planning and curettage)
- Surgery
- Other treatment.

Caries control:

- Chemical application:
  - use of fluorides: topical applications, mouthwash
  - amorphous calcium phosphate
- Dietary counseling and diet sheet.

Bleaching treatments:

- Assessment of the initial shade and desired shade
- Home or power bleaching
- Classify case type as basic, intermediate, or advanced bleaching treatment
- Monitor progress for patient
- Reassess shade achieved.

Provisional restorations and simple restorations:

- Intracoronal restorations: glass ionomers, resin composites
- Extracoronal restorations: provisional direct bonding, crowns, bridges, prostheses
- Root canal treatment
- Extractions: routine, surgical
- Occlusal analysis and adjustment
- Orthodontics
- Referral for advice/treatment
- Other treatment: consider bleaching after elimination of active disease.

Stage 3

Definitive and restorations: once oral stability has been achieved

- Monitor periodontium
- Monitor caries (non-active lesions)
- Record indices as applicable
- Assess long-term implications with patient (costs, ability to maintain)
- Periodontal: monitoring, crown lengthening, other
- Bleaching
- Definitive restorations:
  - veneers/laminates
  - crowns
  - bridges
  - prosthesis
- Orthodontics
- Implant fixture placement
- Oral surgery
- Other (including post-treatment photographs).

Stage 4

Maintenance and monitoring at monthly intervals

- Record indices
- Check radiographs
- Review preventive advice: dietary assessment, oral hygiene instruction, fluoride applications
- Oral prophylaxis
- Repeat aspects of Stage 2 and Stage 3 if applicable (such as implant abutment connection and implant prosthesis).

Stage 5

Administration

- Written treatment plan with financial responsibilities sent to patient
- Financial arrangements for patient
- Estimated laboratory bill
- Patient's written acceptance of treatment plan
- Total time estimated
- Appointments scheduled accordingly
- Total fees planned and earned
- Terms and conditions.

Appendix 9-6 Aesthetic case checklist.

Patient's name.. Date.........................	
1. Case requirements and treatment planning	
Study casts	
Working casts, diagnostic waxups	
Stents buccal, lingual	
Custom trays, temporary trays, bleaching trays	
Photos	
Intraoral camera shots	
Cosmetic imaging	
Digital radiographs	
2. Case presentation with all data present	
3. Consent forms signed and photo release form signed	
4. Financial arrangements signed and organized	
5. Laboratory booked for the case	
Dates and turn-around times confirmed	
Photos emailed/sent to the lab for reference	
6. Treatment sequence and appointments scheduled	
7. Hygiene scheduled	
8. Number of appointments	
9. Bleaching treatment maxillary and mandibular teeth first	
10. Shade evaluation	
11. Hygiene check	
12. Prep appointment	
13. Review appointment, date scheduled 3–5 days later	
Adjust temporaries	
Length and lip support	
Photos taken	
Casts of temporaries	
Review gingival healing and patient cleaning	
14. Cementation appointment	
Overall shade checked with water glycerin	
Cement shade	
Patient approval: signed sheet	
Postoperative photos taken/checked	
Postoperative written instructions given	

15. Hygiene and home care	
Additional products	
Tooth mousse	
MI paste floss	
Interproximal brushes	
16. Written warranty: if patients come every 3 months for hygiene maintenance, replace the veneers free of charge during 1 year	
Testimonial sheet given	
17. Postoperative appointment	
Final contouring	
Flossing	
Occlusion	
Patient's satisfaction	
Length on lip support	
18. Take to the consultation room and show the photos	
19. Ask for referrals for similar cases	
20. Send a thank you card	
21. Send final photos sent together with two business cards	
22. Send a gift	

Appendix 9-7 Implant treatment tracking form.

Implant treatment tracking form

Patient Name: ....
Date of Birth: ....
Telephone no:
(home) .... (work) .... (mobile) ....

Diagnostics

	Date booked/ taken	Date sent	Where sent	Date received back/read and checked
CT scan				
Full mouth series				
OPG				
Study casts Stent needed				

Treatment plans

	Date completed Done	Date sent
Dr Greenwall		
Implant surgeon		
Periodontist		

Consultations

	Date booked
Dr Greenwall	
Implant surgeon	

Financial arrangements

Financial arrangement made	Date deposit paid or full amount

Components

Components ordered	Date ordered	Date received

Hygiene

Appointments required	Date booked

Anesthetist

Appointments required	Dates booked

Medical history forms

	Date sent	Date received back
Medical history sheet		
Sedation consent		
Consent to treatment		

10 Effective Case Presentation

Cathy Jameson and Linda Greenwall

> *Educate, motivate, activate.* — Dr John Jameson (2009)

The fulcrum of your dental practice

The fulcrum of your dental practice is your comprehensive diagnosis, complete and carefully documented treatment planning, and excellent case presentations. In Chapter 9, you were introduced to comprehensive treatment planning and the outline for case presentation was given. In this chapter, we will go into the details of establishing and implementing the "system" of case presentation. There will be some repetition. That's great. Remember: repetition is the key to learning.

Introducing new and existing patients to aesthetic possibilities is only the first step in building the aesthetic aspect of your dental practice. It's an important step, but it is only the beginning.

Getting from the initial appointment to the place where a person agrees to treatment is a long and important journey – the patient journey.

Case presentation is an essential system within the dental practice. There are six major steps in your case presentation system. Each step is significant. Every person on your team has the opportunity to make or break a relationship with the patient or to help or hinder a person from making a decision to go ahead with treatment. Do not underestimate the value of each interaction.

The goal of presenting your recommendations is to gain acceptance of the recommendations you are making.

▶ *"During your initial appointment and during your consultation, you have a chance to educate, motivate, and activate a patient to move ahead. These are two of the most important appointments in your schedule. Offer patients the very best, make the financing of the treatment comfortable, and get out of the way so that patients have a chance to say 'yes' to the very best. Don't do your presentations without careful preparation. Plan the case, prepare your presentation, and then present to the best of your ability. This is some of your most productive time. If a patient walks out your door saying they have to 'think about it,' everyone loses."*

Dr John Jameson (2009)

Listen your way to case acceptance

Most people, when asked, would like to change something about their smile. The operative word here is "ask." Open the door for conversations about smile enhancement by asking questions and listening without judgment. You may not always agree with the other person, but out of respect for them, listen without imposing your own values and opinions on others. You may think a person's smile is just fine the way it is. However, the patient may hate their smile. Listen without judgment.

Recall that there are four things we do with language: read, write, speak, and listen. Each of these four skills penetrates every one of your days. However, in order to establish and maintain an excellent relationship with patients, the skill of listening may be the most powerful (see Chapter 7).

Most people have not had specific courses on the skill of listening even though they agree that it is a vital part of communication.

▶ *"I have learned that the most critical aspect of any case presentation is creating a sense of urgency. But, I cannot create a sense of urgency for a patient without knowing their main motivation. I learn this by listening. If I have listened carefully, performed an excellent comprehensive evaluation, and studied the data, we can design a treatment plan that offers an optimal way for the patient to accomplish their goals. Listening is the key."*

Dr Mark Hyman (interview)

As people become more aware of aesthetic opportunities through the media and other sources, you may find that people will ask you questions that they have not asked in the past. Your patient's questions may expose interest in aesthetics. Some people have such negative feelings about their smile that they are too embarrassed to bring up any questions. Therefore, when you learn to ask open-ended questions, when you use photography appropriately, and when you show respect for people's personal opinion of their smile, doors may begin to fly open.

There are six steps of the case acceptance system:

1. Build the relationship
2. Establish the need
3. Educate and motivate
4. Ask for the commitment
5. Financial arrangements
6. Schedule the appointment.

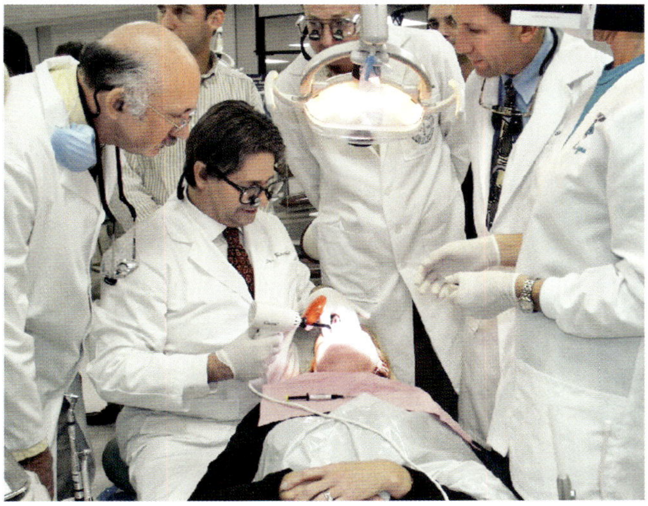

Fig 10-1 Dr Larry Rosenthal provides quality, comprehensive care during the Aesthetic Advantage Continuum.

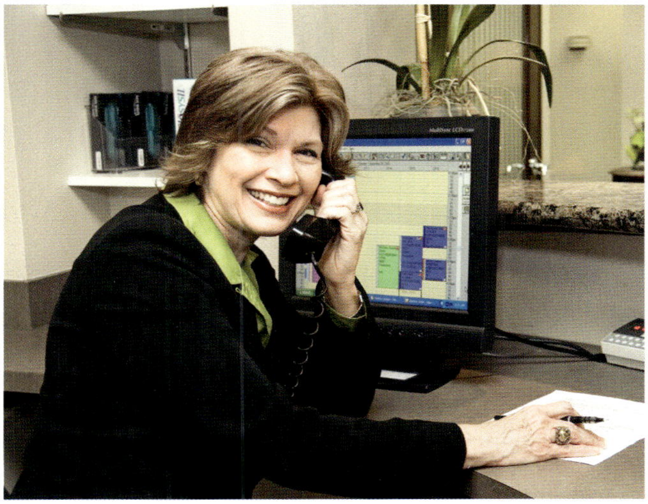

Fig 10-2 The telephone: the window of your dental practice.

Step 1: Build the relationship

Without a healthy, trusting relationship, no one will purchase your product or service. This relationship must have a strong foundation of both trust and confidence: confidence in you and your team, in the service you provide, and in the results you will obtain. In addition, patients must be able to count on you to stand behind your treatment.

▶ *"No one walks out my door unless I am completely satisfied with the result. As a team, we care about these people. Plus, these people are our ambassadors. We want them to walk out of our door ready to tell others about us and to be able to show a beautiful smile to other people who may be interested. We will do whatever we need to do to make sure that both the patient and we, as a team, are not just satisfied, but in fact, thrilled with the result of treatment."*

Dr Larry Rosenthal (interview; Fig 10-1)

Initial contact

In most dental practices, a patient's first contact is on the telephone (see Chapter 5 on Internal Marketing). Certainly, if you have been doing any external marketing, patients may know something about you. If they come to you as a personal referral, they have some knowledge of you and may have even seen the results of your treatment on friends, family members, or colleagues. However, *as vital as these introductory events may be to your dental practice, nothing you have done up to the point of the initial phone call matters if the answering of the phone is not terrific.*

The telephone is your most important marketing tool. A person calling your dental practice makes a subconscious decision about the dental treatment they will receive by the way they are treated on the telephone. The telephone must be answered with professionalism, grace, and enthusiasm. How can you expect a patient to be enthusiastic if the people on your team are not enthusiastic, including the person answering your phone? They are your window to the world. Your patients will reflect your energy and the energy of your team. They need to be really good (Fig 10-2).

Telephone etiquette

On the initial telephone call, listening is as important as speaking. Certainly, during this call there are things you will want to discuss with the patient. However, nothing is more important than building that relationship with the patient and you do this by asking questions and listening. Through effective listening you can determine their wants and needs. *Here is the key to case acceptance: determining a patient's wants and needs and focusing on these during your presentation*. The gathering of this critical information begins on that initial call.

An inbound caller will give you about 30 seconds to "sell them" on the benefits of coming to your dental practice. The person answering your phone must never seem too busy to make an outstanding first impression. You never know – the caller may be that person who is seeking you as the dentist who will remodel their smile.

Below we will expand on the section on telephone skills from Chapter 5. The photographs that accompany this section on case acceptance were taken in the practice of Dr Ken Hamlett in Dallas, Texas.

The phone should be answered in the same manner by all people. For example, "Good morning, Dr Hamlett's office. This is Pam. How may I help you?" Let the person know they have reached the right number. Give them a name so that the relationship has a beginning. And present your purpose, which is to help them.

Once you have asked how you can help them, listen. What is it that they are seeking? Use active listening to make sure you are hearing them accurately. If and when someone poses questions about aesthetics, answer those questions briefly and in layman's language. Do not go into elaborate detail. Encourage a person to go on, to continue, and to give you more information.

The goal of this initial call is to schedule an appointment for either a comprehensive oral evaluation or for a complimentary cosmetic consultation. Track not only the number of people who schedule a new patient appointment, but also track the number of people who call and ask about your dental practice but never schedule. This data may give you an indication that your telephone skills could benefit from further development.

When a patient calls your office, they are interested in what you can do for them. *Gather information about every inbound caller.* Your main goal of this initial call is to find out the primary interest of the inbound caller and to "sell" the person on your dentist and your dental practice to schedule an appointment.

Write brief, thirty-second scripts about the aesthetic options you offer in your dental practice. Then, practice these scripts. Certainly, people will put their own personality into the conversations. Team members will answer the telephone properly and productively if they have practiced the scripts with the correct verbal skills. If there are normal questions raised regarding money, insurance, time, and so on, determine how you are going to respond to these objections. Practice these verbal skills. Then use them!

For example:

Mr Smith: "I saw a television program about people who have their smile changed. They discussed veneers on the show. Does your practice do that kind of dentistry?"

Business administrator: "We do. Thank you for asking. Are you interested in changing your smile?"

Mr Smith: "Well. Maybe. I have terrible teeth and I didn't really know that I could do anything to change them. So, I am wondering if there is something that would work for me."

Business administrator: "Sounds like you are uncomfortable with your smile as it is at the present time and would like to find out if we could do something that would make your teeth and smile more professional."

Mr Smith: "Yes. I just thought I would see what's available."

Business administrator: "I am so glad you called us, Mr Smith. We do provide many different types of aesthetic treatments in our practice. We do our best to make sure people are happy with their smiles, which is exactly what we would do for you. Our dentist is excellent and very experienced. Let's schedule a time when you and the dentist can evaluate your situation and then he can inform you of the options and possibilities that are right for you. Would that be acceptable?"

The important factor in any initial call is to find out what the patient wants before you dive into an "oration" about anything. Ask questions and listen first. Reflect back to the person who is speaking what you think they are saying, making sure that you are hearing them accurately.

During the initial call, gather all the necessary information regarding the patient so that contact can continue and so that the clinical team can be introduced to the new patient before their arrival (Fig 10-3). Send a welcome pack (Fig 10-4), including the smile evaluation form (Fig 10-5; see Chapter 5 for further details).

Once again, the goal of the initial phone call is to start building the relationship of trust and confidence and to schedule the first appointment. Everything you do has as its ultimate goal to encourage the person to accept your treatment recommendations. If people do not say "yes" to treatment, no one wins. Tom Hopkins (2001) says, "The closing starts at the beginning of the transaction, when you first make contact with your prospect (potential patient)" (Hopkins, 2001).

You have gathered information and sent the welcome pack. Now it is time for the patient to arrive at your dental practice.

PATIENT COMMUNICATION SLIP

Date: ______________ New Patient ❑ Patient of Record ❑ Adult ❑ Child ❑ Age ______

Name: ______________________________ ______________________
(Pronounced)

Referred By: ______________ Family Member ❑ Friend ❑ Parent/Guardian of Child: ______

Address: ____
(Street) (City) (State) (Zip)

Daytime Phone: ______________ Home Phone: ______________

Work Phone: ______________ Cell Phone: ______________

Email Address: ______________________________

Purpose of Call

Emergency ____ How long? ______________

Describe how it feels: ______________

____

____

____

Where is the problem located? ______________

Swelling? ______________

Sensitive to hot/cold? ______________

Other: ______________

Premedication necessary? ______________

New Patient Evaluation ____ Last seen by a dentist? ____

Date of last FMS: ______ Doctor: ______________

New patient evaluation scenario explained: ______________

1. Hard & soft tissue evaluation: ______________
2. Necessary radiographs: ______________
3. No cleaning: ______________
4. Statement of philosophy: ______________
5. Questions & Answers: ______________
6. Statement of payment expectations: ______________
7. New Patient Information Sent: ______________

Insurance Information

Subscriber Name: ______________ Date of Birth: ________ Soc Sec Number: ______________

Employer: ______________________________

Insurance Carrier: ______________________________

Policy Number: ______________________________

©Jameson

Fig 10-3 Jameson Management's patient communication slip.

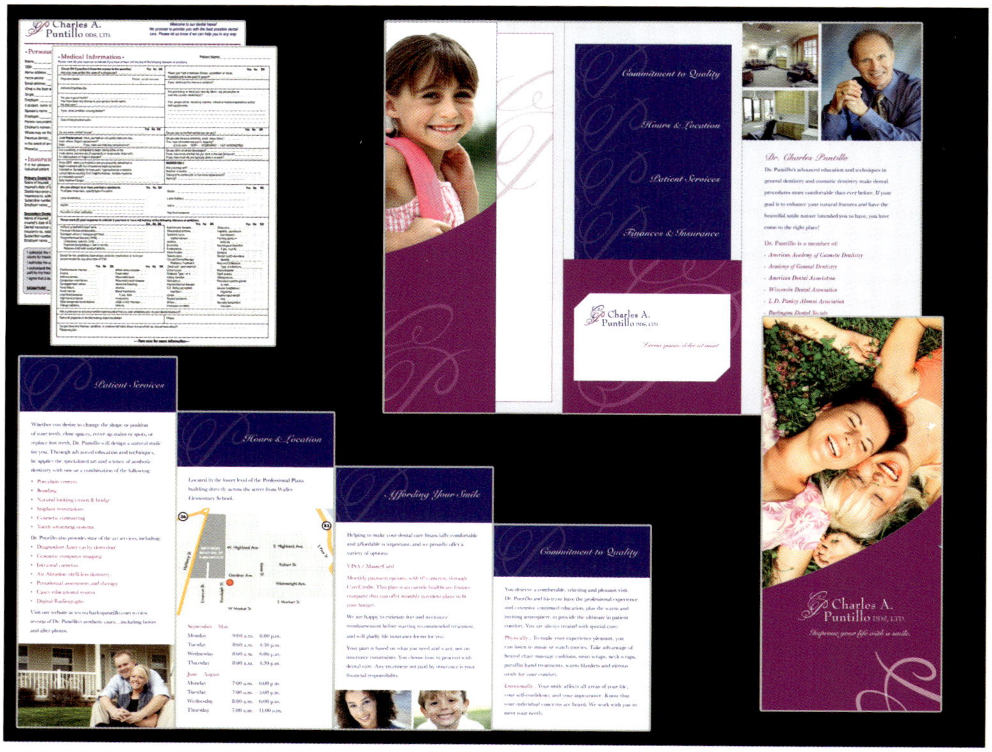

Fig 10-4 Dr Charles Puntillo's welcome pack.

Charles A. Puntillo DDS, LTD.

190 Gardner Avenue • Suite 6
Burlington, Wisconsin 53105
(262) 763-8360 Phone
dds@charlespuntillo.com
www.charlespuntillo.com

Smile Evaluation

"Improving lives by designing healthy, beautiful smiles with care and passion."

If you could improve your self-image and boost your confidence by having the smile that you want, would you?

Do you like the appearance of your teeth? ☐ Yes ☐ No
Please explain:______________________________

Are your teeth all in alignment (straight)? ☐ Yes ☐ No
Please explain:______________________________

Do you have spaces between your teeth? ☐ Yes ☐ No
Please explain:______________________________

Are you happy with the color of your teeth? ☐ Yes ☐ No
Please explain:______________________________

Are your teeth chipped? ☐ Yes ☐ No
Please explain:______________________________

Are your teeth wearing on the biting surface? ☐ Yes ☐ No
Please explain:______________________________

Are you happy with the shape of your teeth? ☐ Yes ☐ No
Please explain:______________________________

Do you have missing teeth that you would like to replace? ☐ Yes ☐ No
Please explain:______________________________

Do you have old, silver fillings that you would like replaced with tooth-colored fillings? ☐ Yes ☐ No
Please explain:______________________________

If you could change anything about your smile, what would you change?
____
____
____

Name:______________ ***Phone:***______________ ***Email:***______________

Address:______________ ***City/State:***______________ ***Zip:***______________

Best day to contact you? ☐ Monday ☐ Tuesday ☐ Wednesday ☐ Thursday ☐ Friday
Best time to call you? ☐ AM ☐ PM

Fig 10-5 Dr Charles Puntillo's smile evaluation form.

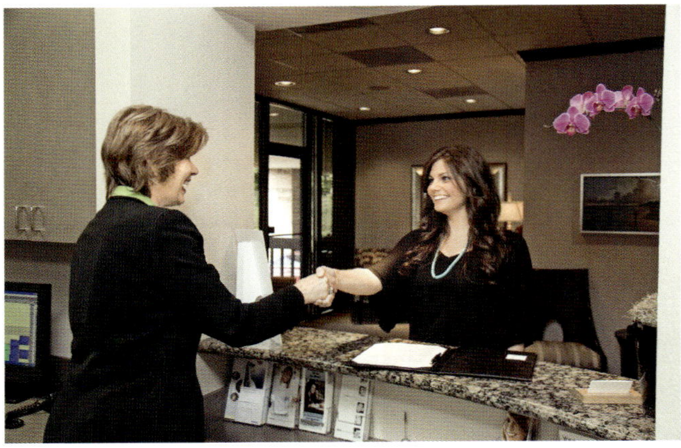

Fig 10-6 Greeting the new patient.

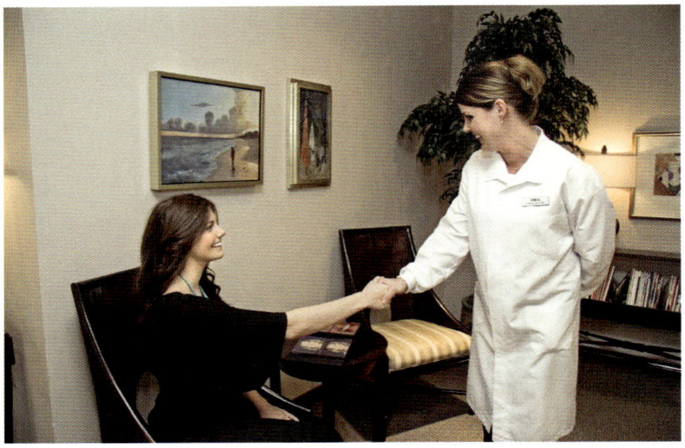

Fig 10-7 The clinical assistant greeting the new patient.

Greeting

The person greeting the patient needs to stop what they are doing and stand up to greet the patient (Fig 10-6). Introductions are appropriate. Personalize this time so that people feel comfortable and welcome. Let them know that you are ready for them.

> **Business administrator:** "Rachel, it's a pleasure to meet you. I'm Pam. I spoke with you on the telephone. We're glad you're here. Thank you for sending your information to us. The dentist has reviewed your information and is ready for you. Have a seat, and his assistant will be with you in just a moment."

You continue to build the relationship with the patient when they actually enter the dental practice.

The next person to meet the patient would be the clinical assistant or nurse. The clinical assistant should also introduce herself to the new patient (Fig 10-7). Remember, the assistant will be placing her hands on the patient, in the patient's mouth, or, at least assisting the dentist with treatment. The patient must have a good relationship with her, too.

Address the person in the following manner:

> **Clinical assistant/nurse:** "Rachel, my name is Erika. I'm Dr Hamlett's clinical assistant. It's a pleasure to meet you. I will be working with you today, along with Dr Hamlett. You may come with me now."

The patient is then escorted to a non-clinical area for the initial interview. The clinical assistant/nurse could review the health history form, patient information form, and smile evaluation, making note of anything that needs to be brought to the dentist's attention (Fig 10-8). Of course, if the material has been received digitally prior to the patient's appointment or if the patient has mailed in the information in advance, the dentist will have already reviewed the information.

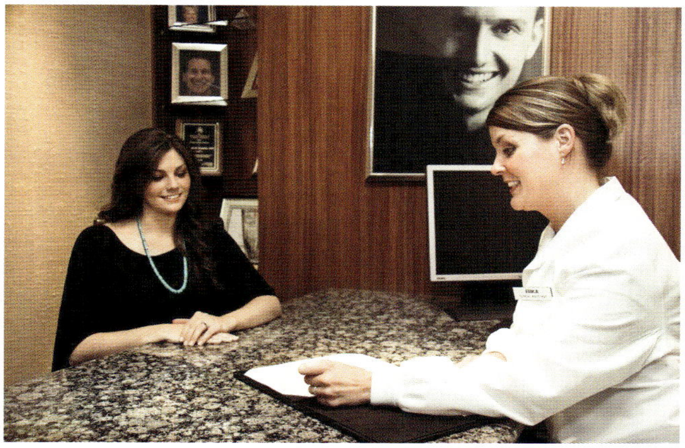

Fig 10-8 The new patient interview.

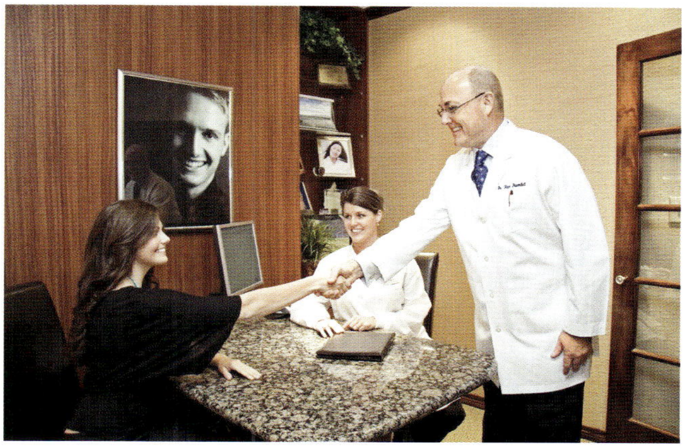

Fig 10-9 The dentist greeting the new patient.

The clinical assistant/nurse makes sure that she notes the referral source, if there is one, in order to establish a point of immediate rapport with the person. She will also inform the new patient about the procedure of the initial appointment. The patient will be more relaxed and comfortable if they are informed.

When you know in advance that a patient is interested in aesthetic care, including a smile makeover, show them a patient information video or a photo album of your dentistry. People will become even more excited when they can see the possibilities that are available. A patient education video can answer many questions that may be on the patient's mind.

When the dentist arrives, the clinical assistant makes an introduction or the dentist can introduce him or herself to the patient (Fig 10-9). The initial interview begins.

After the initial greeting, the dentist reviews the information with the patient and may carefully refer to comments made by the patient on the smile evaluation form. Their answers will give the dentist important insight and could open the door for aesthetic conversations.

Step 2: Establish the need

Now it is time to establish both the perceived or "felt" need and to establish the clinical need. Begin with an initial interview. Perform the initial interview in a non-clinical area, if possible (Fig 10-10a). You do not know how a patient might feel once they are seated in a dental chair: they may be anxious or nervous. If this is not possible due to facility constraints, do the initial interview in the clinical area, but keep the patient sitting upright in an adult-to-adult position (Fig 10-10b).

Most people make a buying decision emotionally and will back that decision up with logic. In order for you to help a person make a decision to proceed with care, including any aesthetic care, you need to be clear about their own "felt" or perceived need. People will buy what they want long before they will buy what they need. Your responsibility in your initial interview is to determine that "felt" need. You do this by asking questions and listening. Use all four of the listening skills discussed in Chapter 7 to give the patient a

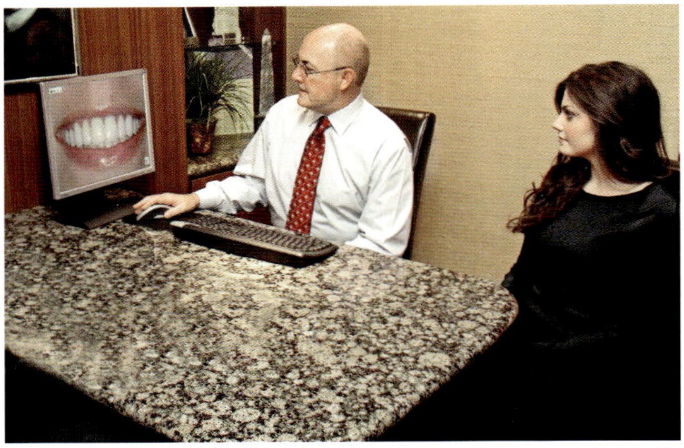

Fig 10-10a Initial interview, ideally in a non-clinical setting.

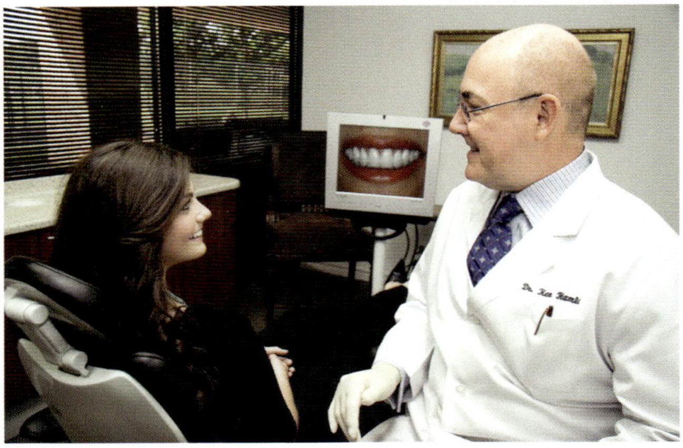

Fig 10-10b Initial interview in a clinical area, with the patient sitting upright.

chance to provide information, give you insights, get comfortable talking to you, and to establish trust in you.

As you are listening, be careful not to jump in and start recommending treatment. In addition, do not place your own values or thought processes on the patient. Listen without judgment. Use open-ended questions that do not stimulate a simple "yes" or "no" response. Listen carefully. Use passive listening to encourage them to continue until you understand what they are seeking. When the patient is finished, use active listening to reflect what you think they have said. They will tell you what kind of dentistry they want. Know that the better you listen to a patient, the better they will listen to you when it comes time for you to present your recommendations.

Ask questions and listen

During the initial interview, open-ended questions relating to a person's feelings about their teeth and smile need to be gently and caringly asked. An open-ended question cannot be answered with "yes" or "no". It is an invitation for the patient to talk, give you information and begin sharing their feelings with you.

Many negative emotions that people have about dentistry can be resolved when a patient realizes that you and your team are willing to listen to their point of view. The best way to dissolve fear or anger is to listen. There may be no communicative skill more important than the skill of listening.

Below are some examples of open-ended questions or statements.

- *"Mr Smith, on your smile evaluation form, you note that you are not happy with your smile. Tell me about that."*
- *"Mrs Wright, on your questionnaire, you have noted that you are happy with most aspects of your smile. The exception is the color of your teeth. You say they are yellow and you wish they were whiter. Tell me more."*
- *"Rachel, if you could change the appearance of your smile, how would you change it?"*

- *"If you were to tell me what you want most for your mouth, your teeth, and your smile, what would that be?"*
- *"Ms Johnson, tell me what your goals are for your mouth, your teeth, and your smile."*
- *"Mrs Jones, tell me your hopes and aspiration for your mouth and your smile."*

The latter question opens the door for amazing conversations with a patient regarding their oral health and their appearance. If a person cannot answer that question at the outset, tell them that you will revisit that question at the end of the appointment. But encourage them to think about your question. You want them to tell you what they want, since people buy what they want long before they buy what they need. Record the patient's responses. You will build your consultation presentation around their response to this question. You are identifying their main motivator or their emotional "hot button." This will become the focus of your consultation.

Now that you have completed the initial interview, escort the patient to the clinical area for the comprehensive oral evaluation. Provide a thorough evaluation on each new patient or on all returning patients (see Chapter 9), and do so in the same way every time.

An example of the protocol for a comprehensive oral evaluation might be as follows:

1. greet
2. seat
3. review of health history and patient information
4. initial interview, including a review of the smile evaluation
5. blood pressure screening
6. necessary radiographs
7. periodontal evaluation
8. oral cancer screening
9. head and neck evaluation
10. occlusal evaluation
11. recording of missing teeth and existing/defective restorations
12. tooth-by-tooth diagnosis
13. tour of the mouth with the intraoral or digital camera (Fig 10-11)
14. cosmetic imaging, if you use this technology
15. invitation to come back for a consultation (treatment planning takes place between the evaluation and the consultation).

At the end of your comprehensive evaluation, set the patient up, roll your chair around, establish eye contact and invite them back for a consultation (Fig 10-12).

Dentist: "Rachel, we have collected a great deal of information about your situation today. You've given me some important information regarding your expectations. I need time to evaluate this data so that I can design a treatment plan that is ideal for you, and one that would support your

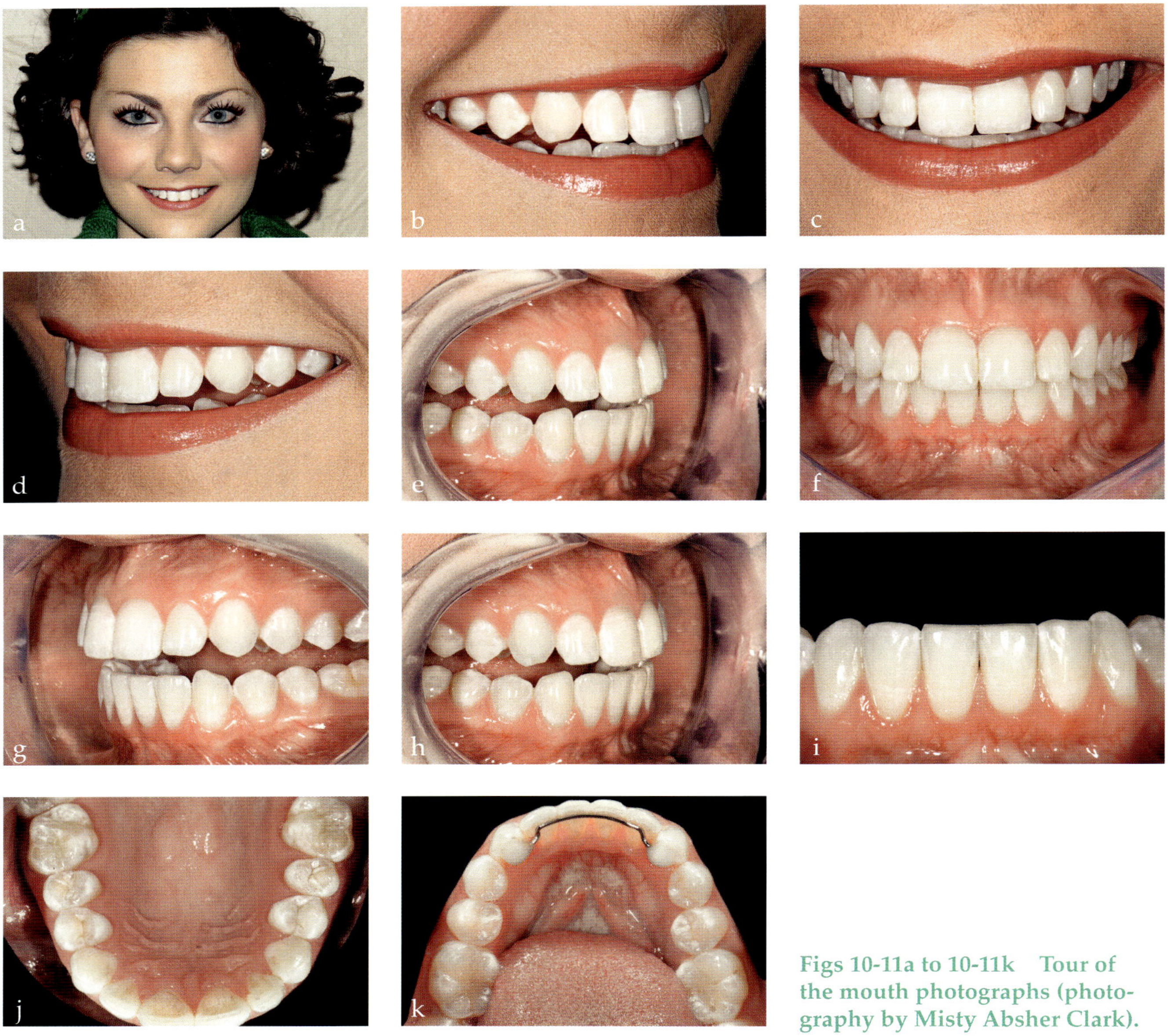

Figs 10-11a to 10-11k Tour of the mouth photographs (photography by Misty Absher Clark).

goals. I'd like to invite you back to the office in about a week so that we can sit down together uninterrupted to discuss my recommendations. Would that be acceptable to you?"

Once a person says yes to the consultation, ask them one more very important question:

Dentist: "Rachel, other than yourself, who will be deciding how you proceed with your treatment?"

Find out if there are other decision makers involved. There is no reason to call for a decision if the decision maker is not there. Determine the decision makers and make effort to schedule your consultation at a time when both

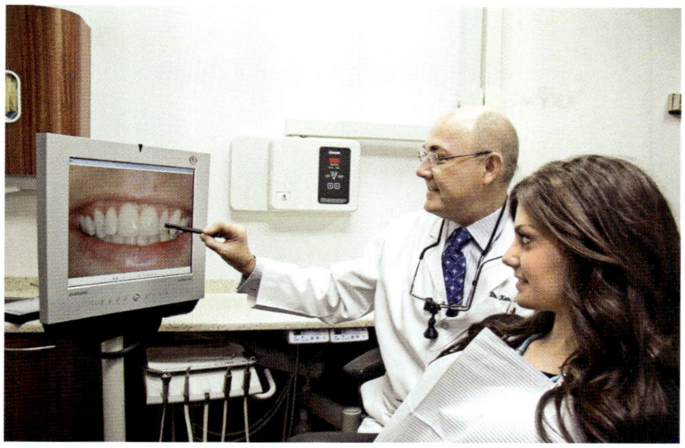

Fig 10-12 Return consultation invitation.

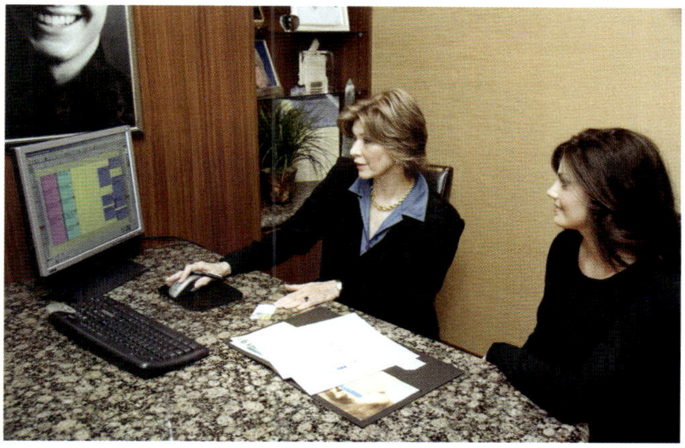

Fig 10-13 Scheduling the consultation appointment.

parties can be in your office. Dental decisions are not made sitting around the dining table, they need to be made at your dental practice where you have the visual aids and the professional information. However, if you cannot get all decision makers at the consultation and if you have used our protocol for Digital Case Presentation© (see Appendixes 10-1 and 10-2), the resulting CD can provide visual and written support of your treatment plan if decision makers are not present.

Don't think that people will not come back for a consultation. They will be happy to return. You are going to change their smile. They are going to make a significant investment, and so need to be informed. They will come back. Give yourself and your patients the time and attention needed to make this major decision. A quick discussion at the chair is not the avenue to gaining high levels of case acceptance.

Schedule the consultation appointment within one to a maximum of two weeks following the initial evaluation (Fig 10-13). The patient's interest will be at its highest level. Letting too much time pass before the consultation could lead to waning interest.

Treatment planning

Once you have completed the comprehensive evaluation, schedule time to design a treatment plan that is optimal for the patient. Plan your cases while the information is fresh in your mind and before the patient comes back for their consultation appointment. Careful planning and documentation will support your care of the patient throughout their time with you. Your team can only perform well in all of their roles if a carefully designed treatment plan is a part of the patient record. Team members cannot make excellent financial arrangements nor can they schedule appointments properly if they don't have a carefully documented treatment plan. Failing to plan will reduce your rate of case acceptance.

Refer to the chapter on the treatment coordinator (Chapter 11). The development of this role in your dental practice can lead to higher levels of case

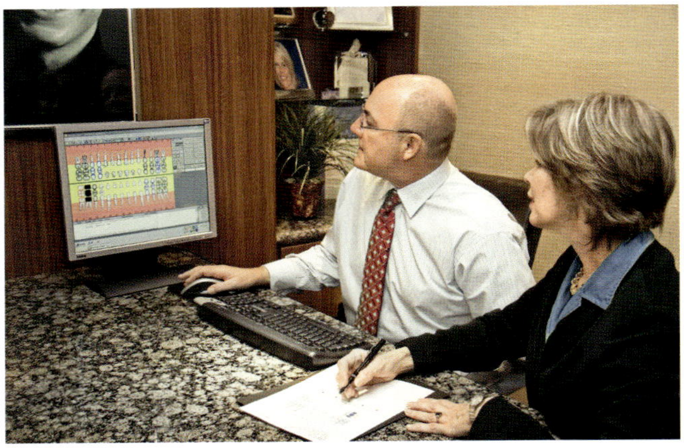

Fig 10-14 Planning the case with the treatment coordinator.

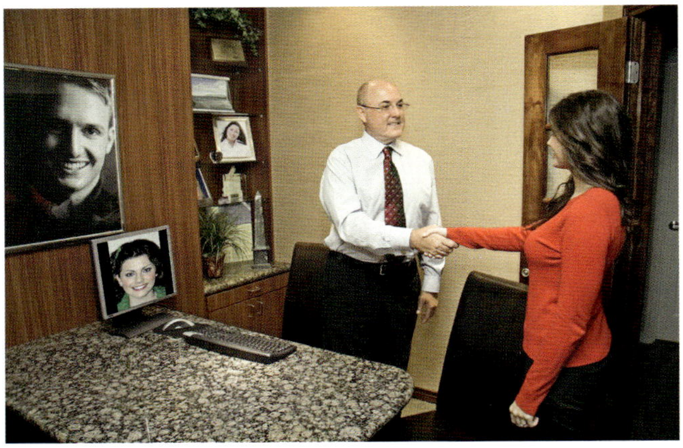

Fig 10-15 Welcoming the patient back for consultation.

acceptance. The treatment coordinator needs to schedule time for the dentist to plan the case. It is his or her responsibility to have all diagnostic information and data ready for the dentist to review as he/she plans the case. Please make this important note: the treatment coordinator needs to be present while the dentist plans the case so he/she knows what the dentist wants to do, where the dentist wants to start and progress through treatment, how many teeth will be treated at each appointment, and the type of procedure to be provided, including materials (Fig 10-14). Only then can financing and scheduling be coordinated properly. Again, the *team members can only perform their individual responsibilities if a comprehensive treatment plan has been designed*.

Step 3: Educate and motivate

The comprehensive evaluation has been completed, the case has been planned, the treatment coordinator has been informed by the dentist about the planned treatment, and they have organized their financial presentation. Now it is time for the patient to come into the dental practice for the consultation appointment (Fig 10-15). You have planned, prepared, and now you are ready to present. You are now going to educate the patient about what is going on in their mouth at the present time and what you are recommending that you do to restore the mouth to health again, change the smile, or both.

Case presentation is an important system. The goal of presenting your recommendations is to gain acceptance of the recommendations you are making.

The treatment coordinator will have the room prepared for the consultation and all necessary material for both she and the dentist will be in place. The treatment coordinator will join the dentist for the consultation and will be present to listen and watch for visual and verbal buying signs from the patient (Fig 10-16).

While the dentist may present the clinical aspects of treatment, the treatment coordinator will give the dentist third-party back-up support, will make the financial arrangements, and will schedule the first appointment.

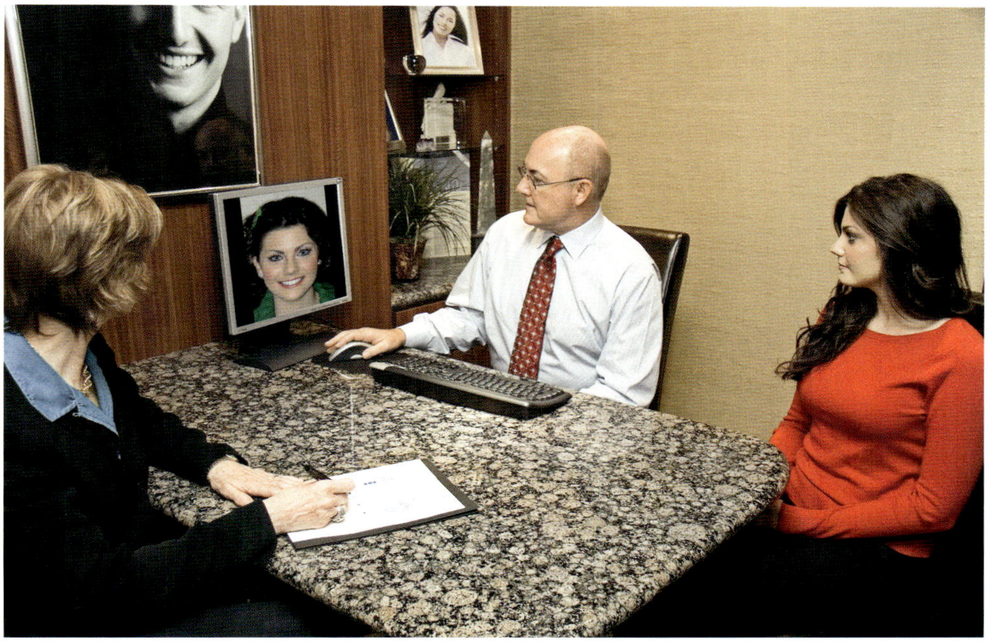

Fig 10-16 The presentation appointment.

At the consultation, patients want to spend quality, uninterrupted time with you. Do not schedule treatment with other patients opposite your consultation. You must not be pulled away from this critical time with this patient.

The consultation gives you the opportunity to perform a review of findings and to present your recommendations. You want patients to make their decision at this appointment. There is a danger in a patient going home to "think about it". Your goal is to present the case well enough so that all questions are answered and so that the patient is motivated to proceed.

Visual aids

Approximately 83% of a person's learning takes place visually. Only about 11% of learning takes place through auditory methods. If all you do is "tell" someone what they need and what you intend to do, you will have very little success. Patients do not know about dentistry. You need to "show" them what is going on in their own situation and "show" them examples of similar situations, or "show" them a digitally produced example of what they could look like through cosmetic imaging.

All behavior is driven by "what's in this for me?" (LeBoeuf, 1985). People need and want to know how the treatment will impact them, how treatment will affect their health, looks, wallet, and schedule. The major motivator of the patient was discovered at your initial appointment. Now it's time to engineer your presentation to respond accordingly.

Be careful not to engulf the presentation with clinical dialogue that loses the patient in dental lingo. Dental professionals get so involved with describing the clinical technique that they totally lose the patient. The patient becomes confused. A confused person cannot make a decision. Keep the presentation patient friendly. Practice your presentations. Film and record yourself doing a case presentation. Evaluate your body language, listening skills, educational ability, and excellent use of visual aids.

During your consultation, nothing will be as powerful as photography of your own cases. Create excellent visual aids, such as beautiful "before and after" photographs of your cosmetic dentistry, so that people can visualize what you are explaining. Develop your own photo album and video library.

▶ *"Good photography is critical in case presentation to show the patient their problems and to explain how we achieve their goals. People never see themselves from the sides. Instead of doing 6 front teeth show the patient a side view and they will most likely do 4 or 6 more teeth. Digital X-rays [radiographs] are helpful to be able to view the hard tissue."*

Dr Ken Hamlett (interview)

Aspects of your presentation

During your clinical presentation, you will need to address the following four things:

1. Tell/show the patient what they have now. Show them the photographs on the monitor that is in the patient's direct view.
2. Tell/show the patient examples of treatment that you are recommending to restore their mouth to health again or to change their smile. Use your visual aids here. Show them a similar situation, using before-and-after photography that is as close to their situation as possible. Have this similar situation ready to show the patient. Remember to pre-plan this presentation (see Fig 10-14).

Dentist: "Rachel, this patient had a situation similar to yours. Can you see the similarity? (Listen to her response) I feel confident that once we complete your treatment, your smile will look much like this. Does this look good to you?"

3. Tell/show them the benefits of the treatment you are recommending.
4. Tell/show them any negative factors or risks that might occur if they choose not to proceed with treatment, if this is appropriate.

Suggested ways to use photography effectively

1. Include taking a tour of the mouth with an intraoral camera in each new patient appointment. Take the photographs as suggested and illustrated in this chapter, as well as arch views so that you can focus upon individual teeth that may be problematic using your software.
2. For example:
   - ☐ Full face, smiling. No lip retractors. Capture the lip line for your laboratory.

- ☐ Smile with lip retractors.
- ☐ Right and left lateral with lip retractors.
- ☐ All four quadrants. (Take photographs of individual teeth within each quadrant where a tooth indicates a need if your software does not allow you to view individual teeth or quadrants with the software itself.)
- ☐ Upper and lower arch. (Again, most software today will let you focus upon individual teeth within the arch or quadrant, see Fig 10-11.)

3. Show both the upper and lower anterior views to the patient. Let the patient focus on the maxillary anterior teeth and ask, "What do you like most about the teeth in the front of your mouth, on the top? What do you like least? If you could change anything about the teeth here, what would you change?" Then, go to the mandibular anterior teeth, and do the same thing. Let them begin seeing their teeth in a new way. Let them tell you what they want. Store these images in your software, in the patient record. You will want to use these images during your consultation appointment.
4. Use the photography as a way to communicate with your ceramic specialist. When the ceramic specialist from your laboratory can actually see the situation and discuss the case with you, they will be much better able to achieve the desired result in their preparations. You will then have a visual prescription, as well as a written one. Most of the laboratories today allow for digital transportation of the images.
5. Develop a library of before-and-after photographs. Take "before and afters" of every single case you complete. Then, as you are planning your cases and your presentations, you will be able to use these sets of photographs to show similar situations to patients who are considering treatment. Seeing the features of porcelain laminate veneers, realizing the benefits of this type of treatment, and obtaining proof that you can access results is powerful in your presentations.
6. Consider gathering the same series of photographs on your regular patients who may be coming to the dental practice for a hygienic appointment. Give the patients the smile evaluation form. Then, if any interest in aesthetic or cosmetic dentistry evolves, invite the patient to receive a complimentary cosmetic consultation.

Cosmetic imaging systems

Cosmetic imaging systems are excellent and are a part of most major software packages. The process requires a learning curve and a commitment to practice. Once you master the program, then the issue for many dental practices is to just do it! Review the section on Digital Case Presentation© (Appendixes 10-1 and 10-2). This process has proven effective in organizing and presenting your cases. There is a substantial increase in case acceptance

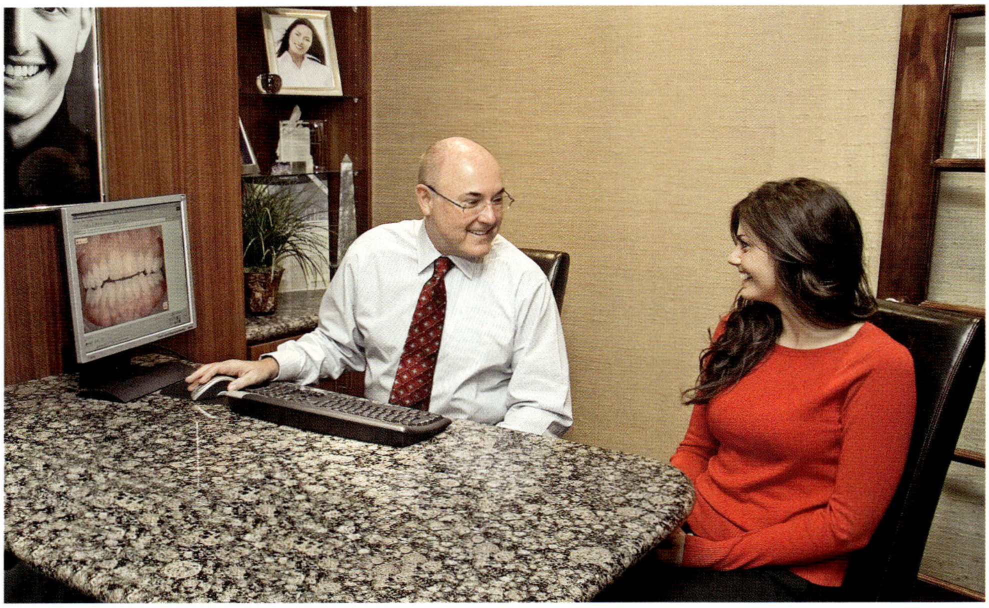

Fig 10-17 Ask for the patient's commitment.

when you take the photographs, using images to illustrate a possible smile makeover to a patient and doing so in such a professional, beautiful manner that the patient is not only impressed but motivated to move ahead.

With our recommended process of Digital Case Presentation© you can send the proposed smile makeover home with the patient for contemplation and discussion with family members. You can enhance your educational and motivational presentation to the patient about the smile change.

> *"Get focused on excellent case presentation with your team on board! Get the process smooth and streamlined so your patients want to say "yes". Implement digital case presentations into your practice with careful instruction on how to do this process excellently. Take quality, consistent digital photographs. Perform cosmetic imaging. Create powerful PowerPoint case presentations. Package your treatment plan on a CD for your patient to take home. Work together, as a team, to create a smooth, positive process and ensure the highest retention rate possible."*
> *Misty Absher Clark, VP of Creative Services, Jameson Management, Inc.*

As is true with any system in a dental practice, comprehensive understanding and use of that system by the entire team is necessary to insure its productivity and profitability.

> *"Taking photographs and effectively using a cosmetic imaging system is an investment in time and money. But, it is a part of every one of our new patient appointments because this works!! The excitement it will generate for the doctor [dentist], for the team and for the patients is unparalleled."*
> *Dr Larry Rosenthal (interview)*

Step 4: Ask for the commitment

Now you have presented your clinical recommendations, ask the patient if they have any questions regarding the treatment itself. Answer any clinical questions. Then, ask for a commitment (Fig 10-17). You will not know whether or not the person intends to proceed unless you ask them! You must ask for a commitment or you may have a lot of people walking out the door, having not made a decision about going ahead.

By asking for a commitment, you determine whether or not a person has agreed to go ahead with treatment or if there are issues that may be causing hesitation. You want to identify these so that you have a chance to work through them. If you never understand a person's issues, you never have a chance to work through them. Of course, you may not be able to work through every problem, but being aware they exist enables you to have a chance to resolve them and move ahead.

Below are examples of how to ask for a commitment:

Dentist: "Rachel, do you have any questions about the treatment I have recommended for you?"
Rachel: "No. I'm pretty clear on what you need to do."
Dentist: "Then, if you have no questions about the treatment, tell me, is this the treatment you would like to receive?"

Dentist: "Have I explained the treatment that I am recommending so that you are comfortable with my explanation?"
Rachel: "Yes. I'm quite clear about what we need to do."
Dentist: "Good. Then, is there any reason why we shouldn't go ahead and schedule an appointment to begin your treatment?"
Rachel: "No. Please book me in."

Dentist: "Rachel, you indicated that you were unhappy with your teeth and wanted a more beautiful smile. The recommendations I am making would give you just that. I've shown you an image that will be similar to what we will obtain for you. Is this the kind of smile you would like to have?"
Rachel: "Yes, I hate my teeth the way they are, and I would love to smile without being embarrassed."
Dentist: "Then, let's get started! Are mornings or afternoons better for you?"

By asking for a commitment you give the patient a chance to ask questions and express their concerns. You may find that they are ready to schedule the next appointment (see Fig 10-13). Remember a person would not have come to you in the first place if they were not interested in something. Your job is to clarify their motivator, present to that motivator and eliminate any reasons why they cannot proceed.

If they have objections or reasons why they might not go ahead, do not be upset by that. An objection is a gift to you. Remember the following (Jameson, 2004):

- An objection is a request for further information, indicating that the person is interested in your proposal.
- If a person doesn't present an objection or obstacle, it probably means that they are not interested.
- Objections are the steps necessary to clear the way for a commitment.

Once all clinical questions have been answered, financial arrangements are made. All clinical questions must be answered before a discussion of money takes place.

As will be discussed in Chapter 12, "Financing Aesthetic Dentistry", the barrier of cost is the overwhelming reason why people postpone needed or desired care. However, it is important that you keep the money questions where they belong. A person must make a commitment to the treatment and acknowledge that this is the type of care they would like to receive before the financial discussion takes place. If you present the fee too early – before you have even shown a person what you intend to do – they will not know what they are buying. They become so overwhelmed with the fee that they cannot hear what you are saying. The human mind can only think of one thing at a time, so if a person is focused on money, they will not hear your presentation at all.

If a patient asks, "How much is this going to cost?" answer their question with a question so that you know what they are asking, for example:

Dentist: "Rachel, I hear your concerns about the fee for the treatment, and I appreciate that. However, let me ask this: are you concerned about the total investment or finding a comfortable method of payment?"
Rachel: "Well, I don't have any idea how much this is going to cost, so I need to know that."
Dentist: "I can certainly appreciate your concerns. I am going to have Pam, my treatment coordinator, discuss the total investment you will be making and the excellent options for payment that we offer here in our dental practice. Pam is very experienced and will be able to explain these thoroughly. But for now, Rachel, I would like to present the treatment that I believe would help you get the smile you want. But, please know that you are in total control here. You get to say if you want to proceed or not. But, for right now, if it's ok with you, I'll present my recommendations, answer the clinical questions and then turn the discussion over to Pam. Does that work for you?"

The dentist recognizes the patient's expressed concern but does not get involved in making a financial arrangement. Certainly the dentist can quote the fee (as long as he/she is absolutely sure what that fee may be!) but we would rather have the treatment coordinator make all financial arrange-

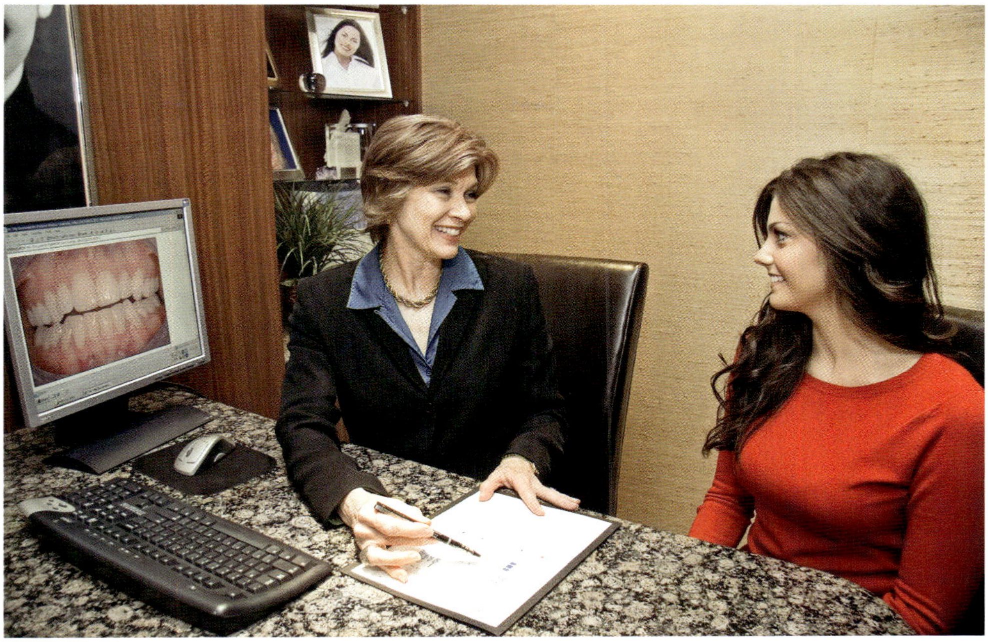

Fig 10-18 Making financial arrangements.

ments (Fig 10-18). However, remember that quoting a fee too early may be more problematic than not quoting the fee at all. If you quote a fee before the patient sees your recommendations, they won't have any idea of what their investment will do for them. Coming to a financial agreement may take longer than the explanation of treatment. That's ok. If the patient doesn't say "yes" to the financial responsibility, no appointment will be scheduled. Give the treatment coordinator time to find a financial solution for the patient. This is critical and productive time. Do not rush this valuable time in the patient journey.

Step 5: Financial arrangements

The financing of aesthetic dentistry can be a major objection and has to be handled with care (see Chapter 12, Financing Aesthetic Dentistry). It doesn't matter how much a person would love to have a beautiful smile, if they think they can't afford it, they will not schedule the appointment. This objection is not one to avoid. It is real. Take a potential negative and turn it around to a positive. Your challenge is to help people want what you believe they need.

Offer the best you can to each patient, make the financing as comfortable as possible, and then let the patient make their own decision. Do not "judge the book by the cover." Give people the opportunity to improve their appearance, find a financial solution, and you may be amazed at who is the next person in your before-and-after album!

Step 6: Schedule the appointment

Once the treatment coordinator has completed establishing a financial agreement, the first appointment can be scheduled (Fig 10-19; see Chapter 13). Financial arrangements always precede the scheduling of the first appointment.

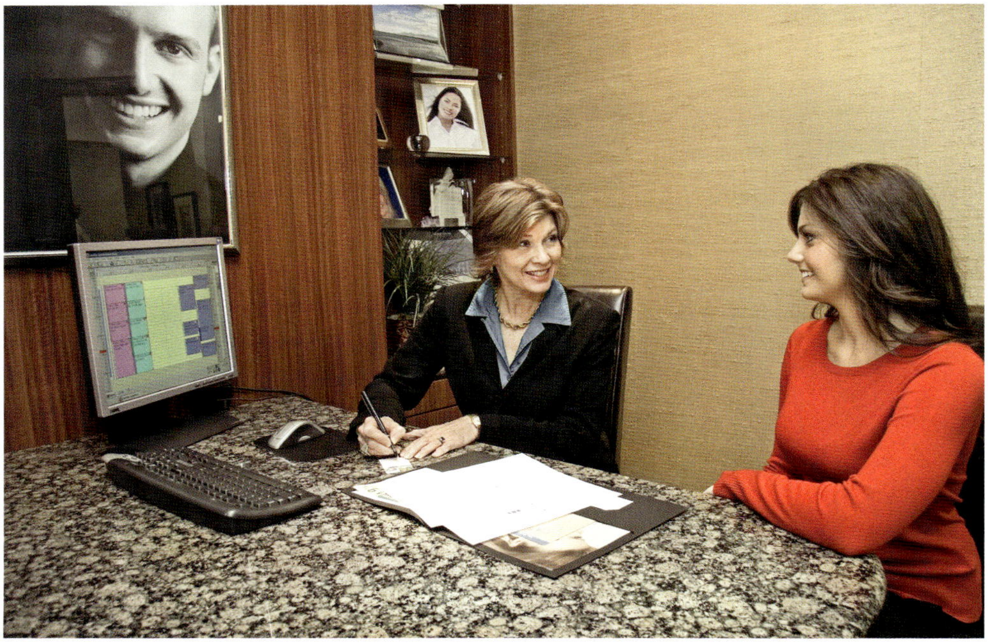

Fig 10-19 Scheduling the first appointment.

In summary

The six steps of the case presentation are as follows:

1. build the relationship
2. establish the need
3. educate, motivate, activate
4. ask for a commitment
5. make financial arrangements
6. schedule an appointment.

Following this six-step process will lead to an increase in case acceptance. The key to dental practice growth is having more people accepting treatment. If even one more person proceeds with a smile makeover each month, the increase in your productivity and in your enjoyment of dentistry will be substantial.

Help a person feel comfortable in your dental practice. Build and maintain a relationship of trust and confidence. Ask questions and listen. Use visual aids. Encourage people to become involved with the decision-making process. Ask for a commitment to identify a patient's intention or challenges. Make good financial arrangements and then, schedule the appointment to begin.

The bottom line to your successful case presentations or consultations is great communication.

Action steps

1. Read and study this entire chapter as a team.
2. Review your present new patient experience and determine which steps of those recommended that you are doing at the present time.

Then, identify the steps that are not being done and organize a plan to integrate each of the six steps into your case acceptance system.

3. Practice the verbal skills that have been recommended in each of the six steps. Spend extra time practicing the verbal skills of asking for a commitment.
4. Make sure that each person in the team is clear about their role and responsibility in gaining high levels of case acceptance.
5. Determine the fee for your average aesthetic case. Multiply that number by 12 to see what kind of financial difference it would make in your practice to perform one more aesthetic case per month. As a team, brainstorm three ways that you can make that happen.

References

1. Hopkins T. Selling. New York, NY: Hungry Minds Press, 2001.
2. Jameson C. Great Communication Equals Great Production. Tulsa, OK: Pennwell Books, 2004.
3. Jameson J. Educate, Motivate, Activate. Lecture. Oklahoma City, OK: JCE Publications, 2009.
4. LeBoeuf M. GMP: The Greatest Management Principle in the World. New York, NY: Penguin Group, 1985.

Appendix 10-1

Digital Case Presentation© by Misty Absher Clark, from Jameson Management, Inc.

The YES plus the exclamation point…

Digital Case Presentation

Getting the "YES!" out of treatment presentation to our patients is what all dental teams want. More importantly, we want the enthusiastic "YES!" (all caps and exclamation point included). It's this kind of "yes" that results in a patient PAYING for treatment, SHOWING UP to the appointment, THANKING US for the beautiful smile, and then REFERRING friends and family to our practice. Is this what you want? Did I hear a "YES!"?

Then, take your case presentation to the next level by incorporating digital elements to your existing consultations. Adding photography, digital imaging, and even PowerPoint to the mix *the right way* can drastically increase the results you get from your already successful consultations. It can mean the difference between the "yes" and the "YES!"

The What?

What does Digital Case Presentation (DCP) mean? DCP is a way of combing great verbal skills with digital tools to support the message. This includes using digital extraoral photos as well as PowerPoint and in some cases, cosmetic imaging. The result is a beautiful PowerPoint presentation filled with the patient's concerns, dentist's diagnosis, treatment considerations, photos, and for cosmetic patients a digital rendering of what he or she *could* look like with cosmetic dentistry.

The Why?

Why do Digital Case Presentations (DCP) encourage the exclamation point and quite often secure a yes when otherwise it would have been a no? The answer is multifold. In an information age, people want – you guessed it – INFORMATION! First, they desire to see photographs that support the diagnosis. In fact, they expect it. The more the patient sees the areas of concern that need treatment, the more they value it and want it. It builds TRUST. Trust between you and your patient.

It also builds strong patient RAPPORT. The patient is hearing their own concerns relayed back to them. They know you are hearing them because you are showing them the photos of the area with which they were concerned. You are showing them the diagnosis and treatments for that concern. They can visually see that you get it. In addition, they know you have taken time to put all this information together. It builds value in the additional appointment to go over your findings. All of this results in a stronger relationship.

DCP acts as a DOOR OPENER to a wider variety of treatment. For patients who express some concern regarding the appearance of their teeth, cosmetic imaging is a great way to sell the case. You read that right – sell. Cosmetic imaging is digitally altering a photograph to render potential results from cosmetic dentistry. It gives the patient an idea of what he or she could look like with porcelain veneers, for example. By showing them this image, they can imagine how they would look without that ugly gap in the middle of the two front teeth. Or how more youthful the patient could look with lighter teeth. The result? Taking the guessing out of the game and creating a patient who WANTS the treatment!

The door opener is not just for cosmetic dentistry, this applies to general and advanced restorative dentistry as well. Jane Doe may have come to you because she is experiencing pain in the upper right portion of her mouth. Upon a thorough evaluation, you discover several other areas that are in distress, which will eventually cause her more pain. Presenting her with radiographs and a diagnosis, may not convince Jane. However, if you show her a presentation with clear photos to which she can relate, she will be more likely to say yes.

It eliminates buyer's remorse. When scheduling larger cases, patients will often times say yes and book the appointment. Then when they leave, their spouse or other influencers will tell them that it isn't worth the money. With the DCP burned onto a CD, the patient can show friends and family members what she learned in the consultation. More often than not, it will result in an outpouring of support for the desired treatment. In addition, when the patient reflects on the consultation, if she has questions, she can simply pull out the CD and be reminded of why she made a GREAT decision.

Involve other decision makers by incorporating DCP. Too often the spouse or other decision maker cannot be available for the consultation. As a result, the patient leaves without making a commitment. We are asking our patients who have very little knowledge of dentistry to go home and sell the dentistry. You already have a challenge doing that one-on-one with your patient. Now we want our patient to do that for us. The CD with DCP is meant to recreate that appointment as best as possible so that proper information in layman's terms with photos can be relayed to other decision makers.

Increase your new patient flow. YES! It increases new patient flow. That is a phenomenon that we did not even anticipate until our practices started to tell us about it. Because patients want the support of those closest to them, they share the CD. When others see the level of detail and effort that went into the CD, they are blown away, prompting them to find out more about this fabulous dentist! You are essentially equipping your patient with the tools to talk about YOU!

Finally, it is motivational for the team. Teams love to be challenged and to take on new endeavors. DCP is no exception. The practices with whom we have worked get excited about learning new technology. The enthusiasm carries over to the patient consultation. The team member is excited to show the patient what can be done and is proud of the format. Patients feel the excitement and energy, realizing it is genuine, and are motivated to say "YES!"

The How?

Now that you are convinced, let's talk about how you put together a Digital Case Presentation. You need five things to make this happen: digital photos, PowerPoint 2003 or 2007, cosmetic imaging software (OPTIONAL), a CD burner, and a willing TEAM!

You start a Digital Case Presentation by taking quality, consistent images with a professional digital SLR camera. There are many great cameras on the market. We recommend the latest Nikon digital SLR (eg, Nikon D90) or the latest Canon digital SLR (eg, Canon 60D). Clear photos that are properly framed will yield you the best results. Patients need to know that you pay attention to the details. Clear photos also help to showcase the teeth more appropriately. To take great photos, you need to allocate approximately 5-10 minutes, based on the team's skill level and the photos you wish to take. With advances in technology, downloading the photos should only take 1-2 minutes.

Does your patient want cosmetic dentistry? If yes, then cosmetic imaging is a great add-on to your Digital Case Presentation. Simply image the photos using software such as Adobe Photoshop, Dentrix DDO, or Envision-A-Smile. There are several different types of software; the aforementioned are a few that our clients like. When imaging a smile, you can invest 5 minutes, 10 minutes, 1 hour, or 24 hours into it. Note that the smile looks just as good at 5-10 minutes as it does at 24 hours! Remember earlier we stated that this is a sales tool – not a diagnostic tool. It is not and should not be used to show the patient EXACTLY what she will look like. Instead, it is meant to give a patient an idea of what is possible.

PowerPoint is the software to use to create a presentation. By using a pre-made template with your logo and color scheme, you can simply insert photos and text. Once you are finished, save the presentation. By going into presentation mode (full screen), the computer screen will be filled with the presentation only. It neatly displays your pictures and includes objects pointing out concerns. Follow up the photo with treatment recommendations. Remember that you are showing this to patients, people without dental degrees. So always use layman's terms. That way the patient can comprehend it even if you are not there to translate. With the template, you need to budget approximately 5-10 minutes.

Once the presentation is created, burn it to a CD. This allows the patient to take it home to share with important decision makers and influencers. This greatly increases the YES!, reduces broken appointments and no-shows, and increases word-of-mouth referrals.

With a willing team, you can incorporate DCP into your routine for general dentistry, advanced restorative or cosmetic treatment. The total amount of time (on the high side) that you need to create a winning DCP is 35 minutes. Like anything, practice makes perfect. The more you do, the more efficient your team will become. Is this worth it for a $10k, $5k, or even a $2,500k case? You bet it is!

Implement DCP today. Start by taking small pieces at a time such as taking digital photographs. Then move into working on PowerPoint. Finally, add cosmetic digital imaging. Once you have those pieces in place, simply burn onto a CD. Print a label with your logo and contact information. Then adhere it to the CD. Voila! You're done. Remember, you should invest approximately 35 minutes into each DCP.

Appendix 10-2 Digital Case Presentation© Tips by Misty Absher Clark, from Jameson Management, Inc.

Tips to making Digital Case Presentations great

- Invest in a quality digital SLR camera system, such as the Nikon D90.
- Take consistent, quality digital images.
- Primarily use smile and portrait images as much as possible.
- For cosmetic cases, alter the image using imaging software such as Photoshop, Dentrix DDO, or Envision-A-Smile, to show the patient what he or she could look like with a smile makeover.
- Use PowerPoint or other digital imaging software to present your cases to the patients.
- Use layman's terms in the PowerPoint.
- Use your logo and color scheme in the PowerPoint design to further your branding efforts.
- When making your PowerPoint presentation, remember less is more.
- Place the digital version of the case presentation onto a CD.
- Make sure your logo and contact info are printed on the CD.
- Print the before-and-after smile and portrait images for the patient to take home.

Things to remember when creating Digital Case Presentations

- Less is more. Too much animation, sound effects, objects, text etc., can overwhelm your patient.
- The total amount of time you or a team member should invest into one Digital Case Presentation is approximately 35 minutes.
- Use PowerPoint templates to minimize the time you put into creating the presentation. Why reinvent the wheel?
- When altering an image to show potential cosmetic results, remember that it is to give the patient an *idea* of what he or she would like with cosmetic dentistry. It is not a diagnostic tool.
- The patient photos need to show his or her teeth: sounds simple and like common sense. However, we see photos being used all the time where the patient is not smiling.

11 Developing the Role of Treatment Coordinator

Cathy Jameson and Linda Greenwall

> *You can do anything if you have enthusiasm. Enthusiasm is the yeast that makes your hopes rise to the stars. Enthusiasm is the spark in your eye, the swing in your gait, the grip of your hand, the irresistible surge of your will and your energy to execute your ideas. Enthusiasts are fighters, they have fortitude, they have staying qualities. With it, there is accomplishment. Without it, there are only alibis.*
>
> *Henry Ford*

Gaining high levels of treatment acceptance

Enthusiasm can become your hallmark. Your patients and your community will become a reflection of your own enthusiasm. Does your enthusiasm and belief in your aesthetic dentistry come through loud and clear in both your clinical and financial consultations, in your follow-up and follow through, and in your practice-building protocols, both internally and externally?

Do patients seem to be falling through the cracks in your dental practice? Are you diagnosing the dentistry but not completing cases? Do you think that you might have a practice within your practice? Is there dentistry sitting in the charts waiting to be done? Do people ask you about aesthetic opportunities but never go from the question to the completion of treatment? Do you have notes in your charts that indicate a patient is interested in tooth whitening or some other kind of aesthetic treatment, but you never follow up on those questions or interests?

An answer of "yes" to any of the above-listed questions would place you in a fellowship of dentists who find that the same thing is happening to them. If what you are presently doing in your dental practice is leaving a great deal of the dentistry diagnosed but incomplete, it may be time to discover the benefits of a treatment coordinator.

Once the role of treatment coordinator is developed and integrated, productivity and collections increase to record levels. Dentists often express surprise and delight at the results accomplished when an outstanding team member is placed in this position and nurtured in this role. The difference in dental practice productivity is measurable.

▶ *"When my management coach, Dr Cathy Jameson, asked me to schedule time in the office for treatment planning with my treatment coordinator present I said, 'Are you kidding – give up production time to plan? This is non-productive time,' I adamantly and almost laughingly demanded. She really had to convince me because I swore it would be a waste of time. Honestly, the only reason I proceeded with the implementation of this seemingly ludicrous suggestion was because in all of our years with Jameson Management, they have never recommended anything that didn't pay back dividends.*

"So, in the following weeks, Cindy Butler, my treatment coordinator and I went in the consultation room on a regular basis to bring up all of the digital photos and go through the case tooth by tooth. We talked about the patients and what we perceived as the patients' primary goals for their health, their teeth and their smile. Then we went through the problem areas and tried to incorporate everything that was needed from firstly a restorative standpoint, and then a cosmetic standpoint. I would, many times, be more conservative than my treatment coordinator. I took good notes and am a good listener, so I felt good about the information I was capturing. But, I was surprised at the details my treatment coordinator and even my assistant could sometimes add to the treatment plan that would make all the difference! My clinical assistant was also involved from time to time for the cosmetic phases because she remembered little phrases about the patients' wants or needs.

"When all was said and done, the system worked. We had more well-rounded treatment plans and, from an emotional standpoint, we were much more accurate about what our patients really wanted from their visit to our practice. They felt listened to and cared about and we found this to be much more fulfilling.

"Our acceptance rate skyrocketed, reaching almost 100%. Not only was that impressive but we were also pleased to see that what we diagnosed went up as the treatment coordinator and the assistant picked up on other aspects of a potential case that would make the patient happier. The entire system really has worked out phenomenally well. We began doing more large cases in excess of $20,000 – which is especially impressive for our small Wisconsin town. People come in, write us a check and it's done. They're thrilled with the result, so obviously we are too. My dream practice is becoming a reality one system at a time. Take my advice on this one – you will be pleased!"

Dr Charles Puntillo (interview)

▶ *"Diagnosing, planning, presenting and implementing optimal care in a busy dental practice has never been more challenging. A well-educated*

> *treatment coordinator is a must if one is to thrive during abundant or turbulent times. Be prepared."*
>
> *Dr Mark Hyman (interview)*

In fact, the role of treatment coordinator may be one of the most productive roles within the dental practice.

You may not need to hire a new person or add a new salary to your dental practice in order to develop this role. Most dental practices have a wonderful, talented person already on the team who would be motivated by the challenge of this high-level position. This person may be right under your nose. Let your team know that you are interested in developing this role, and see if someone on your team would love to maximize their talent and step into this exciting role. You may see the talent within a particular person and a conversation may reveal interest. For most dental practices, this is not a full-time position (although for a large or multi-dentist practice it could be). You would carefully schedule this person's time just like you would schedule the dentist, assistant, or hygienist.

The characteristics needed for this person and for this position to be successful are as follows:

- clinical knowledge
- confident personality
- comfortable quoting complete treatment plan fees
- confident in the clinician's ability
- excellent communication skills, especially the skill of listening
- superb organizational, telephone, and follow-through skills.

The benefits to developing this role in your dental practice are many and are significant:

- retention and follow-up for the dentist
- helping people move ahead with necessary or desired treatment
- fulfilling your responsibility to your patients
- increased production and profit for the dental practice
- rewards for work well done
- being able to provide the care that you believe is beneficial to your patients
- increasing the amount of aesthetic dentistry being provided in your dental practice.

Responsibilities

There are numerous ways to integrate the role of treatment coordinator into your dental practice. The following is a description of some of the possible position responsibilities of the treatment coordinator. Each dental practice would, of course, refine this description to fit its own needs. The treatment coordinator could do the following things, or any combination of them.

New patient experience

1. Perform a portion of the initial interview to determine patient desires and concerns.

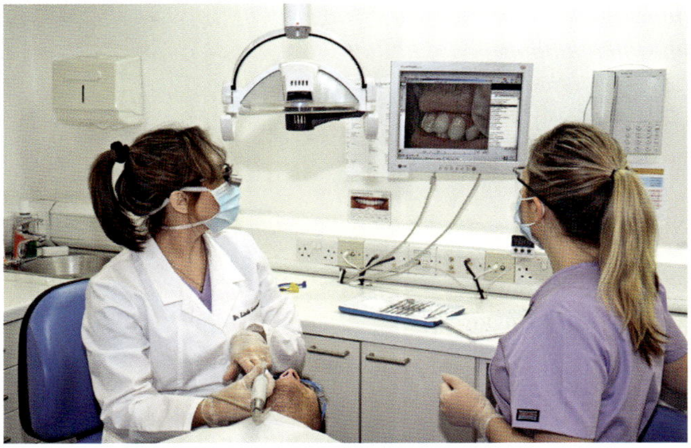

Fig 11-1a Participating in the new patient experience: ensuring the clinical data is entered into the computer.

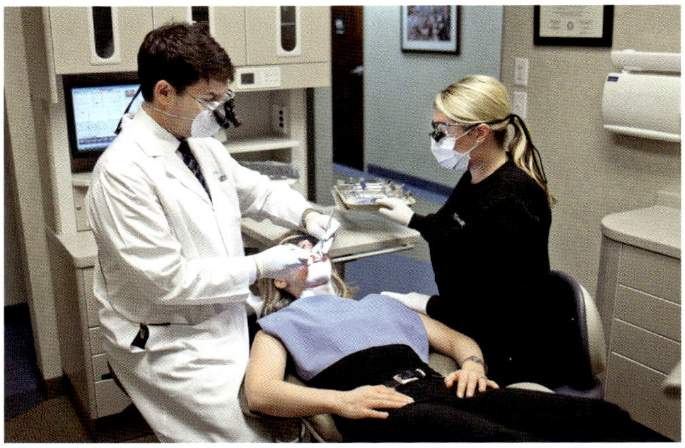

Fig 11-1b A comprehensive oral evaluation on every new patient is an essential step toward excellence in dentistry. Each person on the team has a significant role in the experience. Here Dr Hyman and his clinical assistant provide this evaluation. The gathering of data during this diagnostic appointment provides the necessary information for the treatment planning that will follow.

2. Participate in the new patient experience (Fig 11-1).
3. Take a "tour of the mouth" with the digital camera system, asking relevant questions of the patient to determine perceived need or emotional "hot buttons." Record this photography and any appropriate information from the interview. Bring an image of the full face smile up on the screen and any important information or focal points for the dentist during the evaluation.
4. Make special notes during the dentist–patient initial interview.
5. In some dental practices, the treatment coordinator is the clinical assistant/nurse or the hygienist. At times, the ceramic specialist may participate as well. If this is the case, he/she would, more than likely, join the dentist for the comprehensive oral evaluation, performing the appropriate tasks within that evaluation (Fig 11-2).
6. Schedule the patient back for a consultation appointment.

Treatment planning

1. Join the dentist as they design the specific treatment plan for the patient. Have all necessary data ready for the dentist to review: necessary radiographs, study models, diagnostic sheets, photography, etc. (Fig 11-3).
2. With the dentist, review the radiographs, diagnostic information, and study models (if appropriate) so that excellent presentation will follow careful preparation (Fig 11-4).
3. Listen as the dentist explains what needs to be done and why.
4. Write up the treatment plan on the treatment plan form, or enter the treatment plan into the computer, making sure that the information is complete: tooth number, treatment to be provided (including surfaces

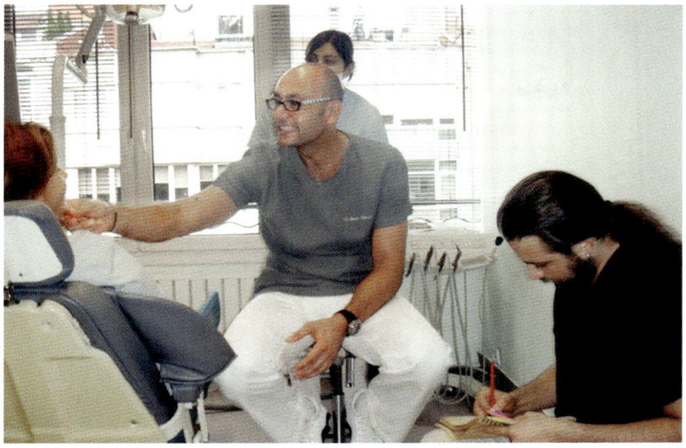

Fig 11-2 Dr Galip Gürel from Istanbul, Turkey with a patient along with his treatment coordinator and ceramic specialist. The treatment coordinator may join the dentist for the comprehensive oral evaluation, performing the appropriate tasks within that evaluation.

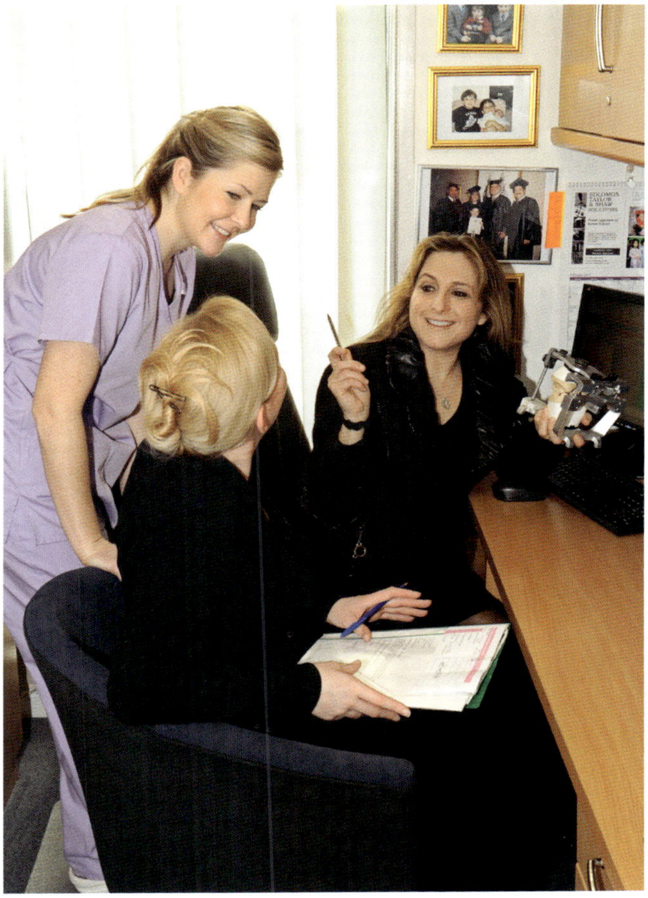

Fig 11-3 The role of the treatment coordinator is essential in the development of an excellent aesthetic dental practice. Here she joins the dentist during the treatment planning stage and prepares all the documentation and visual aids needed to plan and present the recommendations. In this photograph, the business administrator is also providing insights.

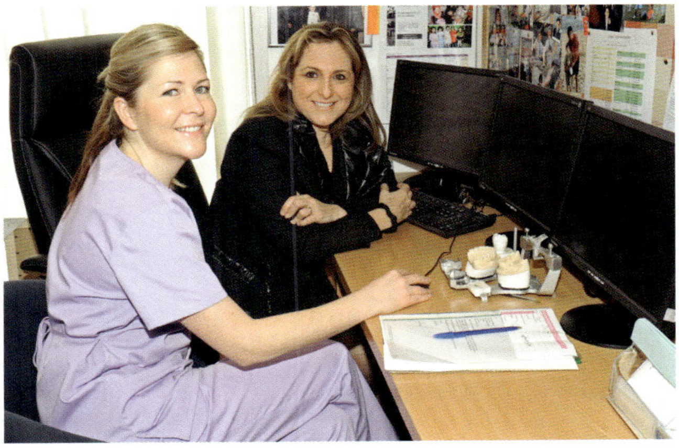

Fig 11-4 The treatment coordinator sits with Dr Greenwall while she plans the case. She makes notes on the proposed treatment and the phases of treatment. The treatment is planned tooth by tooth. Dr Greenwall plans the treatment in her personal office where she has three monitors so that digital radiographs are on one screen on the left, the center screen is for the patient's clinical photographs and the right screen for the CT scan or the computer charting. In this way all data is present when needed for treatment planning.

and material), how much treatment is to be provided at each appointment, the order in which treatment is to proceed, time necessary for each appointment, and the time between appointments. This can be done at the time of the diagnosis, if the necessary treatment is minimal. If this is a larger case, the treatment coordinator may need to write up the treatment plan at pre-blocked time in his/her schedule where coordinating the necessary data from the dentist's instructions.

5. Have the dentist read the treatment plan for approval.
6. Once the treatment plan has been designed, determine the financial responsibilities for the treatment, including expected insurance coverage (when and where this is appropriate).
7. Know which financial options could be made available to the patient. Have any necessary financial information prepared and ready for presentation during the financial portion of the consultation appointment.

Consultation appointment

1. Make sure that the consultation room is ready prior to the patient's arrival, and the necessary radiographs are mounted and photographs are retrievable. Have the patient's full face photograph up on the screen in a consultation room so that when the patient enters the room, they see that you are ready for their presentation.
2. Make sure that any necessary and appropriate visual aids are in the room ready for the educational portion of the presentation. In addition, the treatment plan, models, diagnostic waxups and financial information are all in the consultation room ready for use.
3. Greet the patient in the reception area and escort them to the consultation room.
4. Join the dentist for consultation (the dentist should ask permission from the patient for the treatment coordinator to be present).
5. Once the dentist has made the clinical presentation and has answered any questions that the patient might have about the treatment itself, the dentist excuses him or herself and the treatment coordinator takes over.
6. The treatment coordinator would invite clinical questions from the patient. Many patients will ask an auxiliary person questions that they might not ask the dentist. They may be embarrassed to ask questions of the dentist. They may not wish to look stupid. They may not have had time to think of the questions during the clinical presentation. They may ask some questions for reassurance, ie, "Do you think I need this? Would you do this if it were you?" and so on.
7. The treatment coordinator would refer back to the visual aids (the photographic camera images, specifically) to give back-up support to the dentist and to further the education of the patient. They must have clinical knowledge so that they can answer questions accurately and confidently (Fig 11-5).
8. Once all questions have been answered concerning clinical treatment, the treatment coordinator discusses the financial responsibilities.

Financial coordinator

All consultations are two-fold: the clinical presentation and the financial presentation. The treatment coordinator would be the person who presents the fee and who establishes the financial agreement with the patient. They must have the following skills:

- a clear knowledge of all financial options
- excellent verbal skills for presenting the fees

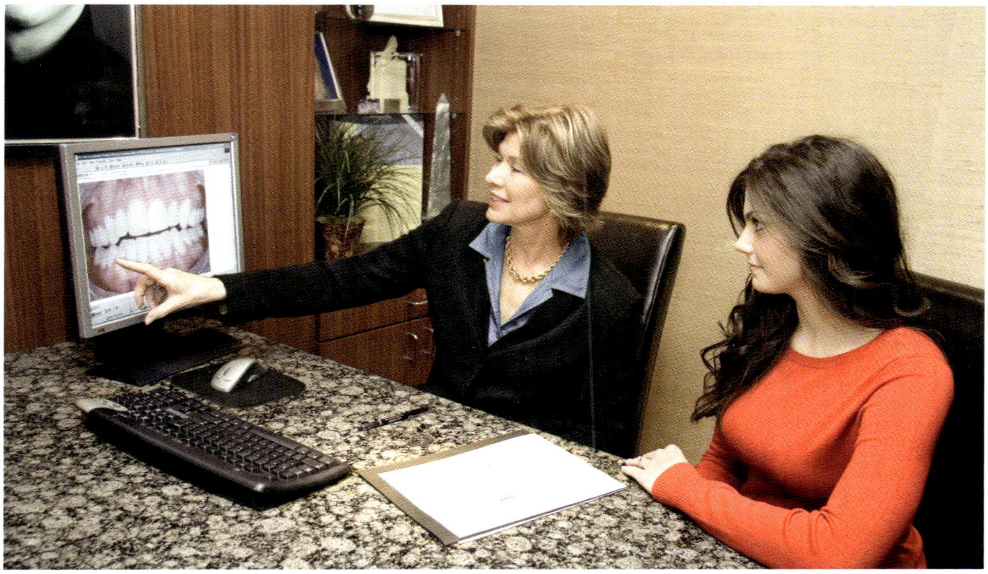

Fig 11-5 Dr Hamlett's treatment coordinator, Pamela, answering questions for the patient.

- the ability to identify objections and to overcome them
- the ability to complete any paperwork
- a belief that the fees for the service are equitable for the treatment being rendered
- confidence in the dentist's ability to accomplish the described results
- a strong belief in the value of aesthetic dentistry and in the benefits of a smile makeover to an individual, when and where appropriate.

Once the questions regarding treatment have been explained, then a discussion of the financial responsibility and the available options takes place (see Chapter 12). The financial consultation may take as long, or longer, than the clinical consultation. If anything is going to get in the way of the patient going ahead, it will probably be money.

Preplanning can make or break this entire "treatment presentation" sequence. Plan to be successful. The treatment coordinator would know the fee for the services to be rendered. They would know the total investment, the investment per appointment, the expected insurance portion, the private pay portion, the monthly investments, and if the patient chooses to utilize a healthcare financing program, what options are available to them. The final close of the consultation appointment comes when there is a financial agreement.

Before the consultation is completed, the patient would (hopefully) have agreed to the treatment and a specific financial agreement. This agreement would include an acknowledgment of the type of financial option that the patient has selected.

Communication skills

The presentation of treatment must be accented by excellent verbal and communication skills. You can say something one way and get a definite "no" or an "I'll think it over" response. But you can say something in a different way and help a person make a decision that is good for them: a decision to go ahead with treatment (Jameson, 2004).

A dentist wouldn't diagnose treatment if the patient didn't need or want it. Therefore, if someone walks out the door not saying "yes" to the treatment, the patient loses the chance to get healthier or more beautiful teeth or, in some cases, both. In a consultation situation, you have an important period of time in which to educate, motivate, and activate a patient. This cannot be done "off the cuff." Your case presentation should be carefully planned and orchestrated. If a patient doesn't accept treatment, not only does the patient lose but also the dental practice and all team members lose, including the dentist. The skills of case presentation and financial presentation can be learned. But this will take study and practice.

Practice

As you begin this process, get together on a regular basis to review how things are going. If things aren't going as well as you would like, or if patients are presenting objections that you were not prepared to handle, go back over everything, refine, perfect, and try it again.

The treatment coordinator must be prepared for almost all situations. As a team, you need to sit down and list the major objections that patients present to you. Then, write scripts or verbal skills of how to handle each of those situations. Then, practice the verbal skills together until the treatment coordinator gets comfortable with them. Work on this together. This person is going to need the dental practice and your support to become highly qualified for this position.

As you begin this process, get together on a regular basis to review how things are going. If things aren't going as well as you would like, or if patients are presenting objections that you were not prepared to handle, go back over everything, refine, perfect, and try it again.

Tom Hopkins (Hopkins, 2001) says that there are 4 Ps of professionalism:

- pre-plan
- practice
- perfect
- perform.

Do these four processes and you will get better at everything you do.

Once the financial discussion has taken place and an agreement has been achieved, the treatment coordinator will make the close by asking the patient to move ahead. If there are no further questions and the financial agreement has been reached, the first appointment will be scheduled.

Follow-up

Dr Lee Manzer (2007), Professor of Marketing at Oklahoma State University, says that "the difference between being average and being fantastic" is miniscule. He suggests that the difference lies in the person or business (or dental practice) that goes the extra mile, does more than is expected, and is willing to follow up. Being able to track the dentistry diagnosed but incomplete will let you do just that.

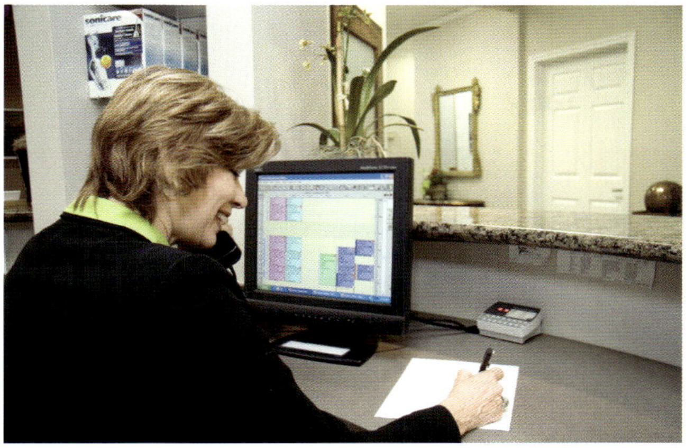

Fig 11-6a Dr Hamlett's treatment coordinator following up and tracking patients who need to schedule for their treatment.

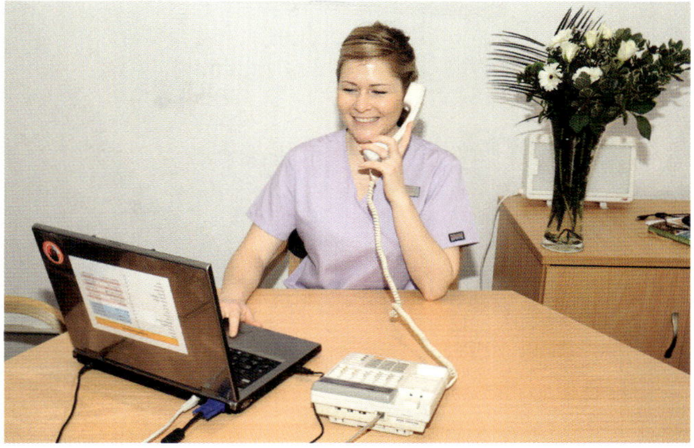

Fig 11-6b Dr Greenwall's treatment coordinator following up and tracking patients.

On a regular basis, the treatment coordinator will make follow-up contact with patients who have not completed treatment. The treatment plans must be at the fingertips of the treatment coordinator, and there should be no problem accessing the information needed to make quality telephone calls for follow-up (Fig 11-6).

In many situations, repetitive contact with a patient is required before a decision to proceed with treatment is made. Some people take a long time to make a decision. In many instances, patients who do not say "yes" right away are not contacted again until their next hygiene appointment. Consider a contact, or multiple contacts, long before that.

The treatment coordinator can do that. He/she would be the person responsible for the follow-up on each patient who has necessary or desired dental care, but who is not scheduled. This is the person who would track each patient from beginning to end. This is the person who could take your dental practice from "being average to being absolutely fantastic," as Dr Manzer suggests (Manzer, 2007).

Contacting the patients with a written message will not be nearly as effective as face-to-face contact in the office or by a telephone call. If a patient leaves the consultation appointment without scheduling their first appointment, make them feel comfortable, but ask their permission to call them in the near future.

More than likely the patient will give permission to be contacted. Get a specific date and time to make that ever-so-important followup call. Then, make a note to yourself on your computer to follow up and call the patient again. In addition, make sure that you follow up on your agreement with the patient to make that call.

On the designated day and time, call to touch base with them and make sure that everything is going fine. Then, reconfirm the need for the next phase of treatment. Next, ask questions to determine if there is an objection or barrier to moving ahead. If there is a barrier, you now have an opportunity to resolve the barrier.

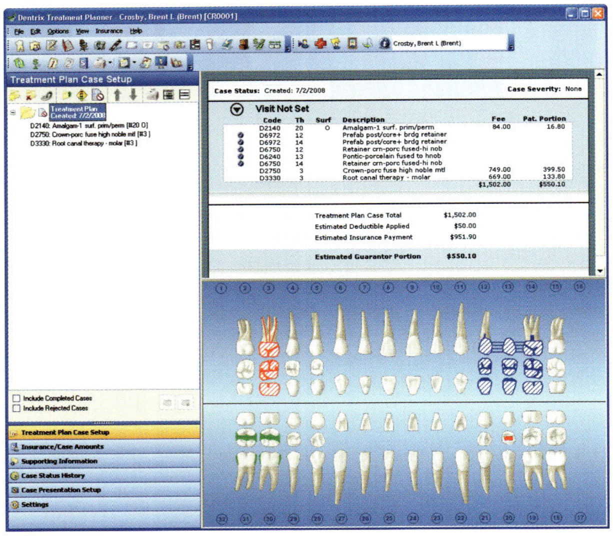

Fig 11-7 Dentrix treatment plan.

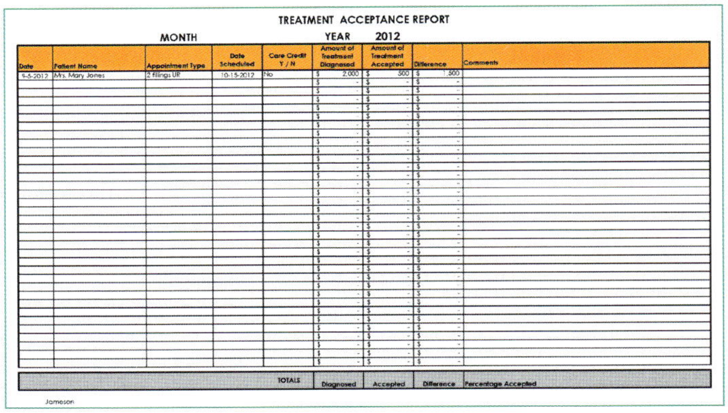

Fig 11-8 Treatment tracking report.

The benefits of carefully planned and well-presented telephone follow-up:

- The patients will know that you are on top of your responsibilities.
- You will be able to answer any questions they might have concerning treatment, finances, or scheduling.
- You will reinforce the need for the next phase of treatment.
- You will fulfill your litigious responsibility to try to complete treatment.
- You will schedule patients, which will reduce the amount of dental care sitting in your charts waiting to be done.
- You will help more people move ahead with dental care that will benefit them now and in the long run.

How to do it

Keep a ring binder with alphabetical dividers. Keep a copy of each treatment plan in the binder – by patient name. The treatment coordinator (or scheduling coordinator) will need to review each day's schedule in order to keep the currency of each treatment plan up to date.

Have computerized treatment plans accessible to the treatment coordinator at all times (Fig 11-7). The list of incomplete treatments must be reviewed regularly, and patients must be called to answer questions. Stay in touch and schedule treatment. Computerization of the treatment plans lets you continuously update the binder of treatment plans. If the treatment is completed, it will be removed from the treatment plan or incomplete treatment list.

When the treatment coordinator reviews a treatment plan that is incomplete, he/she will make a telephone call to that patient. A double-check of the patient's record will be in order to make sure that the telephone call is accurate.

Be sure to track each presentation made by the treatment coordinator (Fig 11-8). Evaluate how much dentistry is being presented and how much is being accepted.

Review of the role of treatment coordinator

Schedule management (treatment planning) time into your appointment book for treatment planning. Remember, you are planning not just the treatment recommendations but also how you will present the treatment, including Digital Case Presentations© (DCP) where appropriate.

Give yourself permission to reserve time each week to sit down and plan your cases. There is no way to do a great job of presenting your recommendations if you haven't spent some time planning and preparing. Increasing case acceptance can be one of the most profound ways to increase the revenues of your dental practice. This cannot happen by magic but rather through continuous improvement of the "fulcrum of your dental practice" (comprehensive diagnosis, complete treatment planning, and well-planned consultations).

Include your business manager/treatment coordinator in the planning of the case. They can prepare for the planning time by having everything ready for the dentist's review and planning of the case. In addition, if they are there while the dentist is planning the case, not only can they provide special insights but will also be better informed and so can give the dentist necessary back-up support following the presentation. Patients will ask team members questions that they won't ask the dentist. The better informed they are, the better the support. This can make the difference as to whether a patient proceeds with treatment or not.

Have the treatment coordinator in the room when the dentist is presenting the case so that they can hear everything that is said between the dentist and the patient. The treatment coordinator needs no surprises when making the financial arrangements. Plus, they can carefully and caringly listen for patient concerns that may be expressed during the consultation. They will then be able to address these concerns. Leaving these concerns unaddressed will give rise to such responses as "I'll have to think about it," "I'll call you," and so on. Get the concerns out in the open and be able to problem solve. This is a key step toward acceptance.

Take case presentation from being an "aside" in your dental practice to being the main focus of your dental practice. Your patients will benefit, your dental practice will thrive, and your treatment coordinator will love the challenge. It's a win-win for everyone.

Does your treatment coordinator add to the cost of the dental practice? No. They add to productivity and profitability; stress will be reduced. Through their efforts working together with the entire team to fully integrate this concept into your office, your dental practice will thrive. Remember that it is not how many patients you see every day that makes the difference, it is the amount of dentistry that you provide. It's not a matter of how many new patients you see every month that matters most, it is how many of those patients accept treatment.

The time and effort put forth in the treatment coordination position will be worth every penny and more. Increase your production and profitability through increased case acceptance. Find the right person to help coordinate treatment presentation and follow-up in your dental practice.

Action steps

1. Write out a job description for the treatment coordinator using the suggestions in this chapter.
2. Present the possibility of developing this role for your dental practice. Speak to individuals already on the team to see if they are interested in assuming this role.
3. Carefully detail the way this position will develop in your dental practice: step by step.
4. Then develop each step of the role until it is fully developed, practiced, and perfected.
5. Evaluate the progress and benefit of the role by tracking how much dentistry the treatment coordinator is presenting and how much is being accepted.

References

1. Hopkins T. Selling. New York, NY: Hungry Minds Press, 2001.
2. Jameson C. Great Communication Equals Great Production. Tulsa, OK: Pennwell Books, 2004.
3. Manzer L. Sales Management. Stillwater, OK: Oklahoma State University Independent and Correspondence Study, 2007.

12 Financing Aesthetic Dentistry

Cathy Jameson and Linda Greenwall

> *By allowing patients to choose the payment option that works best for their situation, this can help more patients improve their appearance and life with aesthetic dentistry.* *Bete Johnson, Director of Business Development, Care Credit (interview)*

The major objection: cost

Rarely does a patient say, "I don't care how much this costs. Don't even tell me the fee. Let's just start." This does not happen. Patients want to know the fee and how much they will be investing before treatment begins. This must always be done. You need to inform the patient of their financial responsibility prior to the rendering of service. Once a person agrees to the treatment that you are recommending, then the financial discussion takes place. The agreement to the total fee and the agreement on the method of payment must be completed before the first appointment is scheduled.

When asked, the majority of people indicate that they would like to change something about their teeth and/or smile. Patients hesitate to ask questions related to a smile makeover because they don't know what can be done, and/or they think it would cost too much. In addition, dentists often miss the opportunity to provide aesthetic dentistry, because they don't:

- continuously inform patients of what is available in dentistry today
- let patients know what type of aesthetic dentistry is provided in their own dental practice
- ask patients if they are happy with their smile
- ask if they would like to change something about their smile
- offer comfortable financing in their dental practice.

In surveys from the *Castle Connolly Consumer Guide* and the Consumer's Research Council of America (Linhart, 2010), the number one reason people do not go to the dentist is money. This is not surprising. This validates what you are probably experiencing in your own dental practice. Knowing what dental consumers are saying in independent surveys is important. You want to know what your consumers/your patients are saying, what they need, what might be keeping them from coming to your dental practice in the first place, or might be preventing them from moving ahead with treatment. Money is the number one barrier.

The barriers, in order, are as follows (Linhart, 2010):

1. Money
2. Not enough time
3. Fear of the dentistry
4. Previous bad dental experience
5. Feel that the mouth is an unnecessary factor for overall body health.

If you, as a team, address each of these barriers and develop programs to respond and overcome these roadblocks for existing or potential patients, you will take the lid off of your dental practice. You will not be able to overcome all of the barriers for all patients. However, when you make small improvements in numerous areas or systems, these refinements can make a significant difference.

The only way to identify and overcome the barriers to treatment acceptance is to listen in order to determine the patient's concerns. Then find a solution to each patient's barriers. If you add one aesthetic case to the existing monthly production that you are experiencing right now, that one case will make a significant and measurable difference in the overall productivity of your dental practice. If you cover your overhead with the existing collections of your dental practice, then adding one aesthetic case increases not only your productivity but also your profitability. If your overhead remains substantially the same and you increase your production, the percentage of overhead drops and the profit margin increases. If you do more cases, then the profitability continues to increase. Track the number of cases you do each month. There is no way to establish a goal of increasing the number of aesthetic cases you are doing each month if you don't know how many you are doing at the present time.

While your new or existing patients may want or need treatment, including aesthetic treatment, they may not agree to proceed with treatment due to money concerns. They may be concerned or even shocked about the total investment. They may want the aesthetic dentistry but need a payment option that fits into their financial situation, whatever that may be.

Dr John Jameson practiced in a small rural town. There are 2,000 people in the community and these are not wealthy people. Many people would believe that it is impossible to do much aesthetic dentistry in such an environment. However, Dr Jameson performed more aesthetic procedures than any of the other dentists in the vicinity.

Why was this possible? The reason was because Dr Jameson decided he wanted to provide this type of care and wanted to focus his dental practice on comprehensive restorative and aesthetic dentistry, and that is exactly what he did. He participated in continuous education courses and worked throughout his entire practicing life to make sure that he was always improving his skills and providing his patients the latest and best.

Once the decision was made to orient the dental practice toward aesthetics, a clear vision was designed of what that would look like. The planned vision had to support the mission and purpose. Then strategic planning or goal setting was undertaken to make sure that the vision became a reality. The management and marketing systems supported the vision. The team was included in the development of the vision and in planning the processes or strategies that would bring the vision to life.

The dental practice had to open its own doors and pave its own way. No one was going to do this for them, just like no one is going to do this for you. The team decided what they wanted to do and made it happen. The strategic plan had to include finding ways to make the financing of their patient's dentistry affordable. They knew that the total investment would be staggering for some people. They introduced patient financing into the dental practice. In this manner, they were able to provide a payment option that made the financing of the dentistry comfortable for patients but let the dental practice firmly uphold their commitment to stay out of the banking business. They applied the same five-step goal accomplishment scenario discussed in Chapter 2 to their vision of building the aesthetic aspect of the dental practice and made it happen.

The team asked people the questions regarding their smile that are suggested in this book. Most people, when they saw photographs of their own smile on the monitor, did indicate that there was something they would like to change about their smile. Dr Jameson would ask their permission to create not only a treatment plan for their restorative care, but also a treatment plan that offered a solution for their smile issues. They always said "yes." They knew that they did not have to accept the treatment he recommended, but he found that people appreciated seeing the options that were available. These were not wealthy people, but working people who felt honored that they were not "judged by the cover" but were offered the very best. The choice of what they did with that offer was totally their own. Dr Jameson says, "You never know what you are going to get unless you ask."

▶ *"Aesthetic dentistry is as much about improving the quality of a patient's life as it is about improving their appearance. We've all seen the differences in before and after photos and how a patient's entire demeanor can change when they feel free to smile without hesitation. When a dental practice commits to offer aesthetic dentistry, it becomes a core offering, which means this level of care is available to all patients, regardless of their age, background, or financial means. Everyone deserves the freedom to smile.*

"It's important to remember that a patient's acceptance of recommended aesthetic dentistry is less about the cost and more about understanding how it fits into their life. This includes convenience of appointments, financial considerations, anticipated benefits, and family support. When

a team tries to 'pre-select' those patients they 'feel' are right for aesthetic care instead of having a face-to-face conversation about what the dentistry may mean in their lives, they do the patient and the dental practice a disservice. Instead, offer appointments that fit a busy patient's scheduling needs, have a conversation about how aesthetic dentistry can improve the quality of their life, and offer a wide variety of payment options."

Bete Johnson, Care Credit (interview)

▶ *"I have followed Cathy's advice on goal accomplishment and strategic planning since I began working with her. I have many projects on my plate and the strategic planning scenario keeps me and my team on track. We decided to provide comprehensive restorative dentistry, including implants and aesthetics. Working on the financial aspect of case acceptance has been one of those major goals. While patient financing is still young in the UK and in other countries and continents, I recommend it as an additional payment option for patients. Even if one patient per month goes ahead with treatment because of this option, then it is valuable for both the patient and for your practice."*

Dr Linda Greenwall (interview)

Making financial arrangements

Dr William Lockard states in his book, The Exceptional Dental Practice, that "approximately 75% of the people who leave a practice do so because of poor financial arrangements" (Lockard, 2007).

One of the most important discussions you will have with a patient is the financial conversation. No matter how much someone may want to proceed with treatment, if they think they can't afford it, they will never schedule the appointment. Thus, you will not get to do the dentistry and they will not have the beautiful smile they want.

Good listening is imperative during this very personal conversation. Identify the patient's wants and needs and identify any objections or barriers they may have to treatment acceptance, including money. You must be able to peel the layers off the problem to determine what is at the core of the problem. Only then can you pave the way for possible solutions. "A problem is only a problem until it becomes defined. Once it becomes defined, it becomes manageable" (Doyle, 1982).

Business experts tell us that people will never buy your product or service unless they have a strong relationship of trust and/or confidence with you. Without question, if people are going to invest in your services, they must have confidence and trust in you and in your services. After all, you are going to be "in their mouth," an intimate zone of the body. In addition, you are going to be discussing a very intimate and personal part of their life, their finances.

▶ *"We cheat our patients if we are not flexible and respectful of where they are at a given time in their lives. Patient financing provides respectful flexibility."*

Dr Mark Hyman (interview)

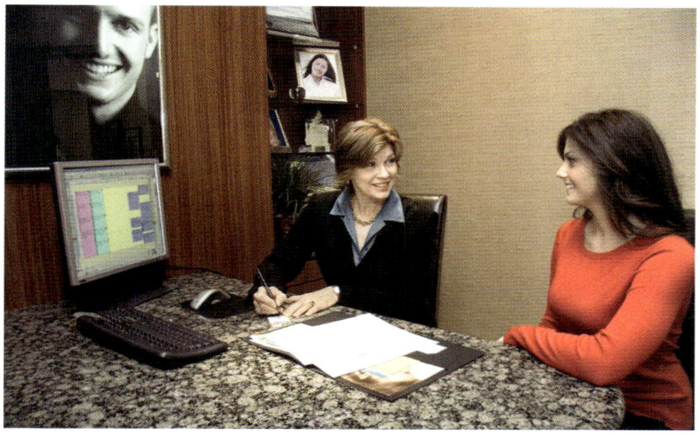

Fig 12-1a Making financial arrangements in Dr Ken Hamlett's dental practice.

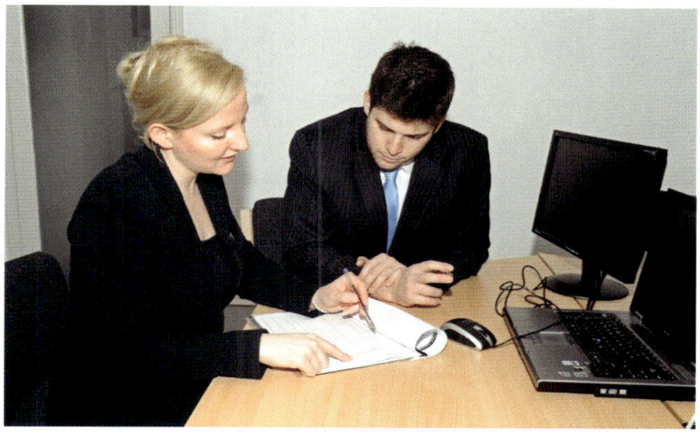

Fig 12-1b Making signed financial arrangements in Dr Greenwall's dental practice.

One of the situations that dental practices are facing in today's busy world is broken appointments and no shows (see Chapter 13). There are times when a patient may schedule an appointment with no intention of showing up because they have not been in a comfortable place to discuss their financial concerns. Rather than be embarrassed they will say "yes" to the scheduling of the appointment but will either cancel or not show up. Thus, it is of benefit to both the dental practice and the patient to have a clear understanding of their financial responsibility and to let patients express their concerns in a private, comfortable environment. Do not make financial arrangements standing at the front desk where other people may hear. First, it is inappropriate according to all confidentiality requirements, and second, you risk an increase in broken appointments. Patients should be seen in a separate office where there can be utmost confidentiality and they can feel comfortable discussing their financial responsibility (Fig 12-1).

Recommendations for increasing acceptance of financial options and for reducing broken appointments are the following:

- Make financial arrangements in private.
- The person making the arrangements needs to be dressed in business attire to convey a professional image.
- If the person making the financial arrangement has not met the patients, introductions are appropriate.
- Use the patient's name frequently during the financial conversation to create comfort for the patient.
- Have all necessary information and mobile credit card terminals at hand so that the patient is not left alone.
- Be prepared so that the patient knows that you are organized and efficient.
- Study and practice specific communication skills related to financial discussions.

Presentation of the fee

Once you have presented the clinical recommendations, the financial discussion will take place. In Chapter 10, the steps of a case presentation were outlined as follows:

1. Build the relationship
2. Establish the need
3. Educate and motivate
4. Ask for the commitment
5. Make financial arrangements
6. Schedule the appointment.

Once the dentist has presented his/her recommendations, he/she needs to ask the following question:

Dentist: "Mr Smith, do you have any questions regarding the treatment that I have just presented to you?"
The patient may have no questions, but more than likely will ask something like the following:
Mr Smith: "Yes, I do. We haven't talked about money yet. How much is this going to cost?"
Dentist: "Are you concerned about the financing of the dentistry?"
Mr Smith: "Of course. I need to know how much this will be. I'm sure this will be quite an investment. I just have to see whether or not I can afford this right now."
Dentist: "I appreciate your concern, Mr Smith. Many patients have felt the same concern until they found out that we do have several excellent payment options available in our dental practice. Jan, our treatment coordinator, will discuss the total investment for your treatment and will discuss the options we have available. We have excellent payment options right here in our dental practice and Jan is very experienced working with these options. She is very competent, and I'm sure she will be able to find a solution that works best for you.
"Let me ask you this, Mr Smith, once you and Jan work out a comfortable financial agreement, if this is the type of treatment you would like to receive?"
Mr Smith: "Yes. I really want to do this. I've hated my teeth all my life. So, there's no question I want to do it. I just have to see whether or not I can afford it."
Dentist: "I appreciate that. Then, I will let you and Jan discuss the financial aspect now. I feel certain that you will find an option that works well for you, and I will look forward to helping you reach your goal of an attractive smile."

The above discussion is a "closing sequence" where the dentist determines if there are clinical questions that need to be answered. The conversation also graciously opens the door for the financial discussion. The dentist respects the patient's expressed concern, clearly defines with whom and how the discussion of money is going to take place, and professionally turns the discussion over to the financial coordinator. Then, leaves! Certainly, the dentist can quote the fee, but the treatment coordinator needs to make the financial arrangements. Please remember that the discussion of financing may take longer than the discussion of the dentistry. That's ok. Let the treatment coordinator have as much time as he/she needs to establish an agreement on the total fee and a method of payment. Without this agreement, the dentistry cannot be scheduled. Your total productivity is related to how well this discussion of financing concludes.

The treatment coordinator needs to sit on the same level with the patient (remember the importance of body language) and there should be no barriers between them like a big desk. She needs to have all necessary paperwork at her fingertips and be totally prepared for the presentation, in advance.

Treatment Coordinator: "Mr Smith, I know that Dr Greenwall asked if you had any questions about the treatment that she recommended and you said no, but I thought that there might be something you would like to ask me before we discuss the financial responsibility."
(All clinical questions need to be answered before a discussion of money takes place. Sometimes patients will ask questions of an auxiliary that they will not ask of the dentist. Make it possible for them to do this.)
Mr Smith: "No. It looks great. I want to do this and I want her to do it. I just need to know how much this is going to cost. I am sure this is no small fee."
Treatment Coordinator: "The fee for the treatment that Dr Greenwall has recommended is $10,000" (or whatever your currency may be). "How would you like to take care of that?"
Present the total fee followed by the statement of the total investment, "How would you like to take care of that?" Give the patient a chance to lead the discussion. Ask the question and listen. There is no need to just start rattling off numerous options. You stay in control of a conversation by asking questions, so ask this question, and then listen to the patient's response. They will give you the direction needed to find an equitable financial solution.
Mr Smith: "Ten thousand dollars! You're kidding, right?"
Treatment Coordinator: "Sounds like you are surprised by the fee."

Keep the lines of communication open and relieve the patient's intense emotion by actively listening. Remember, active listening is reflecting back to the person what you think they have just said, making sure that you have heard them correctly. You need to clarify. But do not overreact. Empathize with their concern and their surprise, but do not sympathize. Certainly it is appropriate to empathize, but present the total fee with confidence and work with the patient to find a resolution to their financial concerns.

Mr Smith: "Surprised ? More than surprised. I'm stunned!! I had no idea that this would cost that much."
Treatment Coordinator: "As you have said, you do want a more attractive smile. And you believe that the plan Dr Greenwall has presented will do just that. But you are overwhelmed by the fee. I know that you came

here prepared to make an investment, but it seems that the investment is larger than you anticipated. Tell me, how much too much is this for you?" (You need to find out if the barrier is the total investment or if the patient needs an alternative way to pay.)
Mr Smith: "Well, it's at least twice as much as I had anticipated. I thought it might be something like $5,000, but $10,000…"
(The treatment coordinator knows that the patient was probably ready to pay $5,000 or so. She needs to acknowledge that and work on finding a payment option for the other $5,000.)
Treatment Coordinator: "Ms. Smith: what I hear you saying is that you were expecting a fee of around $5,000 and were prepared to invest that amount. So, what we need to do is find a way for you to comfortably pay the additional $5,000 that is above what you expected. Is that correct?"
(Actively listen to clarify and to validate what the patient has said.)
Mr Smith: "Well, maybe. I had set aside the $5,000 when I decided I wanted to do this. But, this is, of course, much more than I had expected."
Treatment Coordinator: "Since you are prepared to pay $5,000 from your savings, let's find a way to finance the balance so that you can go ahead with your total treatment in order to get the best results. If we are able to do this, will that make it possible for you to proceed?"

The Treatment Coordinator is reestablishing the patient's goal of a more attractive smile. She is trying to validate the amount of money the patient was prepared to pay but also get the patient thinking about using a combination of payment methods in order to receive the total treatment. Of course, in aesthetic dentistry, depending on the situation, splitting the treatment may be impossible if an excellent result is to be obtained.

Once the patient agrees to this discussion, the description of options can be given.

The person who is presenting the fee must be confident in the dentist, the end results of treatment, in her own ability to discuss financial matters, and in the options you offer. The verbal skills and financial communication skills of financial presentations are specific and critical to acceptance.

Write down (or enter into your computer) the patient's agreement to the total fee and the selected method of payment. You will have a copy of the agreement in your patient's file/chart or, if you are paperless, this will be stored in the patient's record. Make sure that you have digitized signature capability so that you do have a patient's signature of agreement to their financial responsibility. When a person comes to the office, collect the agreed upon amount of money using the payment method that they have selected. If there is a follow-up appointment, reconfirm the financial responsibility for that upcoming appointment before the patient leaves. Figure 12-2 shows a business administrator collecting the fee at the front desk at the time of check out. Figure 12-3 shows a business administrator collecting the fee in a private

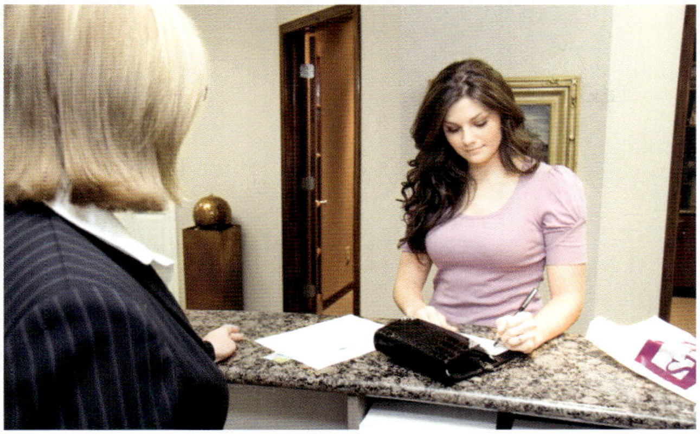

Fig 12-2 Collecting the fee at the front desk at the time of checkout.

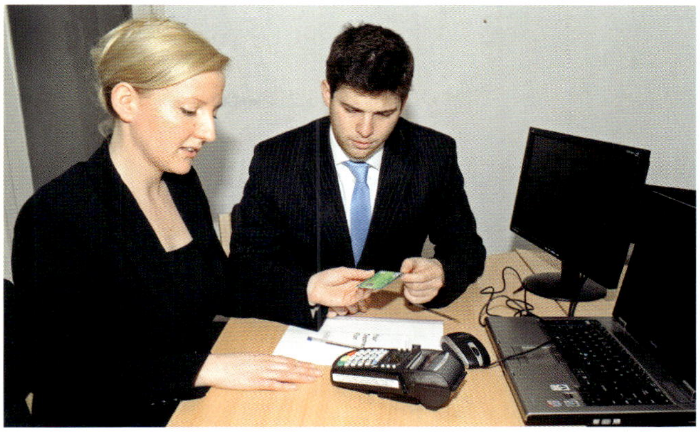

Fig 12-3 Collecting the fee in a private area at the time of checkout. The patient is paying with a bank card in this example.

area. The fee for the upcoming appointment can be written for the patient's preparation for the upcoming visit.

The investment patients will make in aesthetic dentistry will be one of ultimate value. That being said, patients may express concern regarding the size of their investment. Some people may respond to your internal or external marketing and come to your dental practice with an enthusiastic desire for a smile makeover or some aesthetic alteration, but be overwhelmed when they discover the amount of the fee for the treatment. In those countries where dental insurance is a part of patient care, most aesthetic dentistry is not covered by insurance. People may be surprised to discover this fact.

In establishing fees for your aesthetic procedures, you will evaluate your own costs of operation and the time you invest in these procedures. However, no matter where you set your fees, some people will automatically think that your fees are too high. Some of your patients will not give themselves permission to invest this kind of money in their own appearance. This is where your listening skills and presentation skills will prove the most valuable. When people feel comfortable stating why a beautiful, healthy smile is important to them, they may feel more willing to invest in their own care. Be diligent in studying the chapter on case presentation and the sections on financing your patient's care. Having the appropriate financial options in place that meet the needs of the vast majority of your patients will be imperative for case acceptance no matter what your fees may be.

Analysis of fees

Analyze your fees at least every six months and you will—more than likely—need to increase fees once per year. Your fees will go up as your cost of operation goes up. Therefore, it is imperative that you know your own cost of operation, your overhead, and, of course, your margin of profit. If your costs go up, your fees must reflect that increase. Otherwise your margin of profit goes down.

Increasing fees is oftentimes difficult for a dentist or team to implement. The following are some of the reasons why dentists and/or team members hesitate to increase fees:

- don't want to upset patients
- don't like complaints about fees
- don't wish for patients to think that the dentist is interested in money only—not in them as individuals
- have a concern about losing patients to other dental practices whose fees may be lower.

All of these are legitimate concerns or fears. However, a careful analysis of your fees and, perhaps, a slight increase in fees may be appropriate if you are going to pursue impeccable aesthetic dentistry. You may find that even a small increase in fees may help to overcome some of your own increases in costs. For example, if a fee is $500 for a procedure and you increase your fees by 10%, the fee is now $550. The patient may notice this slight increase in fee, but more than likely will not. If they want the procedure, the difference of 10% will not determine whether or not they will proceed. If they would not proceed at $550, they more than likely would not have proceeded at the $500. If they complain about your fee of $550, they would probably complain about the fee at $500. Remember, people may not be as concerned about the total investment as they are concerned about having a comfortable way to pay.

Of course, your fees must be equitable for the service you are providing. You must feel that you are being paid appropriately for the time and money being invested and the patient must feel that the fee they paid was worth the results. Continue to improve your services throughout the lifetime of your career.

Supply and demand

If you are interested in building the aesthetic aspect of your dental practice, you must have the time to focus on the initial evaluation, the planning of the treatment, the presentation of your recommendations, and doing the treatment itself. There is no place for shortcuts if this type of quality care is to take place in your dental practice. If you are so busy seeing huge numbers of patients, you will not have the time necessary to implement the strategies being outlined in this book. Remember that the key to your productivity and profitability is not how many patients you see every day but how much dentistry you do every day. If you are booked out so far into the future that you cannot see patients expediently, you run the risk of a patient going somewhere else for their care. An appropriate increase in fees may cause some people to go elsewhere, but the increase in profitability will allow you to focus on fewer patients, doing more dentistry per patient while maintaining a commitment to being a profitable business. You can be profitable while maintaining an uncompromising commitment to quality care of your patients. Quality care means not only exquisite dental treatment but also exquisite customer/patient care in every area of your dental practice.

If you are so busy that you can't see patients expediently, then the law of supply and demand is in your favor. Consider an increase in fees. Being *too busy* can lead to stress for all members of the team, including the dentist. This can lead to diminished patient time, increased overhead, and reduction of quality. Organization of your dental practice—all systems—is the avenue to quality care, excellent patient relationships, reduced stress and increased production (Jameson, 2006).

Focus on the "fulcrum" of the dental practice: thorough diagnosis, careful and complete treatment planning, and well organized and presented consultations. Doing so will support your goal of increasing the aesthetic aspect of your dental practice and will lead to more comprehensive care, longer appointments, less stress for the patient and the providers. By spending more time with patients, you will see an increase in case acceptance and resulting increased revenues.

As you are organizing your practice, consider what Jameson Management calls the "Model of Success." This model of organizational design will support your goal of being able to provide aesthetic dentistry in a manner conducive to excellent results and enjoyment of your dentistry:

- see fewer patients each day
- do more dentistry per patient (when and where appropriate)
- See those patients for fewer visits
- minimize the number of team members
- maximize their talent
- increase the profit
- share the profit
- decrease stress.

Of course you don't want to lose patients. You don't want patients to leave you to go to another dental practice with lower fees. You don't like to have patients complain about your fees. Nor do you enjoy hearing patients complain about fees. However, if you focus your dental practice on careful and caring attention to your patients and if you commit to uncompromising quality in all your care, clinically and personally, people will not leave you. They will stay. They will agree to treatment. And, if through your internal marketing and patient education people know who you are, what you do, and why coming to you is a good decision, they will want to place their care in your hands. The relationships must be built on trust—trust of the dentist and of each person on the team. If there is an equitable exchange of value, they will pay and pay willingly.

There will be patients who will complain about your fees. As a professional, carefully analyze your fees and make decisions that are good for you and for your patients. Compromising fees could lead to compromising time and quality. This serves no one.

Go into every consultation with a belief that this person will be better served by agreeing to the treatment you are recommending. Your confidence and belief will transfer to the patient. Be confident that the fees you are charging for your services are equitable. Be sure that each interaction a patient has with your dental practice is excellent—every time. Epitomize excellence. Set your fees accordingly. Provide care that makes you proud. Be willing to show the results of your care to anyone and know in your heart that the treatment has been outstanding. Each person who receives either

XYZ DENTAL ASSOCIATES

Financial Options

Thank you for choosing XYZ Dental Associates. Our purpose is to provide the best and most comprehensive dental care possible. As a service to our patients, we offer convenient, comfortable financial options.

Please know that we are here to help you. If you have any questions, please feel free to discuss these with members of our team.

Payment Options:

- We offer a 5% accounting reduction for patients who pay for treatment in full before treatment begins. This option is for those patients whose care is for $1000 or more.
- ½ of the fee to reserve the appointment and ½ of the fee at the time of treatment.
- All major bankcards
- For patients with dental insurance, we will do everything possible to help you maximize your benefits. If, for any reason, we have not received payment from your dental insurance program within 60 days, you will be responsible for the total fee and will need to contact your insurance company to receive your own reimbursement. We will provide all necessary paperwork.
- For any long-term of extended payments, we offer Care Credit, our patient financing partner.

Total Investment:____________________________________

Option Selected:____________________________________

If you have any questions, please do not hesitate to ask. We are here to help you achieve optimum dental health.

____

Patient, Parent or Guardian Signature Date

____

Patient Name (Please Print)

Fig 12-4 Financial agreement form.

restorative or aesthetic care in your dental practice can be an ambassador for your dental practice. Their health and well being, and their beautiful smile, will be a reflection of your technical ability and your commitment to the extraordinary.

Every person in the office should be able to access the financial information on a patient. If, for any reason, the treatment coordinator or business administrator is out for the day or unavailable at the time of check out, the fee still needs to be collected. Cross training is imperative. A written financial agreement form which includes the expected and agreed upon payment for each appointment is imperative. Figures 12-4 and 12-5 provide samples of two different financial agreement forms.

XYZ DENTAL ASSOCIATES

PATIENT PAYMENT AGREEMENT

You have made a decision to proceed with treatment that will support your goal of a healthy mouth and a beautiful smile. We have discussed the total investment you will be making and our options for payment. The following is a description of our financial agreement.
The estimated fee for your treatment is $______________. If additional treatment is required, we will always inform you of such a change, including any alterations in your financial responsibility, before further treatment is provided. __________(Please initial)

Your dental insurance is an excellent supplement to your care. We have estimated that your insurance will cover $______________. You will be responsible for the patient portion at the time of service. If, for any reason, your insurance does not cover the anticipated amount, you will be responsible for the balance in full.
You have chosen and agreed to pay for your treatment fee, including any patient portion not covered by insurance, in the following way:

- Payment in full in the amount of $______________________

  Paid with: ______________________________________

- ½ to reserve the appointment and ½ at the time of treatment: $______________________________

  Paid with: ______________________________

- Bank Card: ____________________________________

If you have questions about your treatment plan or our payment options, please do not hesitate to ask. We are here to support you on your path to oral health and beauty.

We have reserved the following appointment just for you: Date: ____________ Time: ___________.

____
Patient, Parent or Guardian

Signature: ___________________________________ Date: ________________

____
Patient Name (Please Print)

Fig 12-5 Patient payment agreement form.

Everyone who leaves your dental practice should leave with an appointment either with the hygienist for their next continuous care appointment or for restorative or aesthetic treatment or, in some cases, both. In the same manner, everyone should walk out of the door with clarity about their financial responsibility for the upcoming appointment.

Payment options

Here are the financial options that are recommended to all dental practices, in all countries:

- Five percent accounting reduction (or cash courtesy) for payment of the entire treatment plan, in advance (cash or check). (You are not providing discount dentistry, so do not use the word discount.)

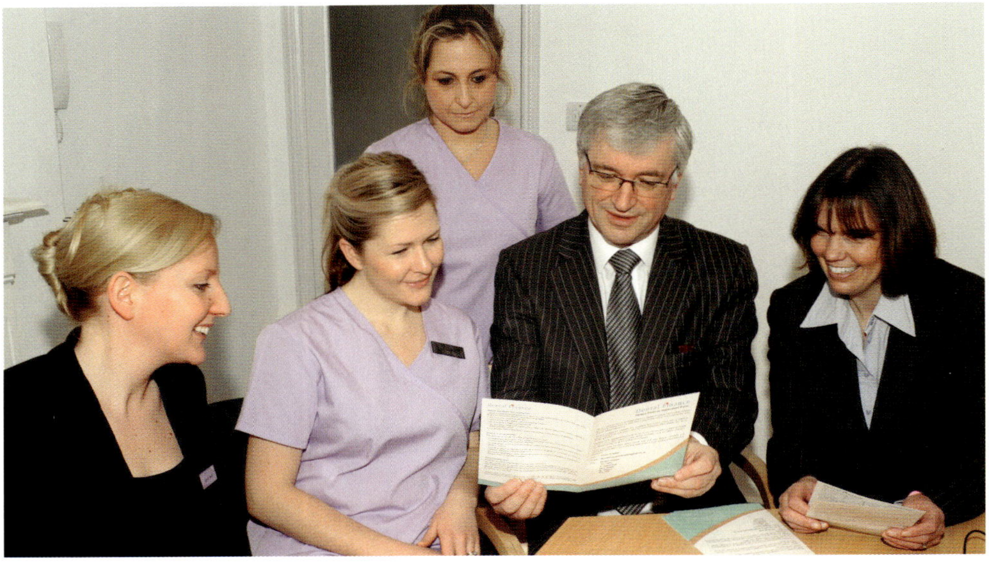

Fig 12-6 Planning the administration for patient finance programs within the dental practice. The dental team is undertaking training in order to offer the financing program effectively and efficiently.

- Half of the total fee paid to reserve the appointment and the other half paid at the time of the treatment. (If this is treatment that involves laboratory produced procedures, the payment is completed by the time of the insertion appointment.)
- Payment by the appointment. (You must have clearly defined treatment plans in order for this option to be viable.)
- All major bank cards.
- For any long-term or extended payments, a patient financing program:
  - revolving payment option
  - interest free option
  - extended payment option.

Patient financing programs

Successful dentists are able to provide the kind of care they wish, including comprehensive restorative and aesthetic care, in the manner they choose. In relation to treatment acceptance and being able to schedule to your desired production goals, patient financing is an essential factor (Fig 12-6). Since aesthetic/cosmetic dentistry is not covered by dental insurance, for the most part, the patient must come up with the entire fee.

When a person does not accept treatment, it is not usually because they don't want a more beautiful smile, but rather because they think they cannot afford it. Your responsibility and the responsibility of your team is to find a financing vehicle that will work for your patients so that more people can proceed with treatment. By offering the above-recommended set of financial options, you can make it possible for almost anyone who wants and/or needs aesthetic enhancement to receive it. People need a way to pay for treatment that fits into their particular financial situation.

▶ *"We approach each situation believing that there is always a way for a patient to obtain the treatment he or she desires. It is all about being able to successfully meet their needs with enough options to make treatment affordable. The more financial options you are able to offer a patient, the higher your case closure rate will be. Options we offer are as follows: (1) Care Credit – interest free program; (2) Care Credit term loans 1–4 years; (3) a courtesy (or reduction) in fee for payment in full upfront at the time that they book treatment; and (4) we offer our patients the ability to make payments with credit cards so they may charge a lump sum and pay for it in monthly installments.*

"These are our major financial options. There are some exceptions to the rule. We have learned to flex in challenging times when the economy has its ups and downs, or when a patient we wish to serve can't afford our fees. We may take the opportunity to offer treatment at a reduced fee to those patients. This is an incredible opportunity for a patient to have the smile they have dreamed of more affordably and is presented as such."

Jacqueline Pastore (interview), Practice Administrator for Drs Larry Rosenthal and Michael Apa

Extended payment plans

In the above statement, Jacqueline refers to "term loans." During the past few years, most of the patient financing programs have added an extended payment plan. This option came because both dentists and patients were seeking treatment that exceeded most of the lines of credit that had been established with the traditional financing plans. Treatment for implants, comprehensive restorative dentistry, and cosmetic cases are big-ticket items. So, the financing companies responded.

These programs where a person can access a line of credit of $1,000–$25,000 or more make it possible for people to receive a large amount of treatment but still keep a reasonable monthly payment structure. The length of time that a person takes to pay off the account depends on how much he or she can pay per month. These programs have been one of the major vehicles for the advancement for aesthetic dentistry. There are many other factors but this is, surely, one of them. No matter how much someone wants a beautiful smile, financing must be possible. Affordability and comfortable financing are a must.

In many countries, third party patient financing is not yet available. However, just as credit card usage has spread universally, we believe that patient financing for healthcare will do the same thing.

Patient financing is one solution to the main reason people do not come to the dentist or do not say yes to treatment: money. People will be better able to accept your aesthetic treatment recommendations if they can handle the investment without feeling financially stressed. Your case acceptance percentage will accelerate.

Verbal skills for handling financial questions or objections

The following are recommended ways for answering questions or objections patients may present.

Situation: You are no longer doing in-office financing.
"We found a better way for our patients to finance their dental care. We have a financial partner, XYZ Financing, who work with us, right

here in our dental practice to help our patients finance their dental care. Certainly, we want to help you with the financing of your new smile and this is why we have a new partner in financing."

Situation: Patient wants to wait until after insurance has paid to make any private payments (for the countries where this is an issue).

"Mrs Jones, we will do everything possible to help you maximize your dental insurance. We have accurate information on your insurance benefits and are able to estimate what we expect insurance to cover and what your portion of the payment will be. Therefore, in order to cover our laboratory and operating expenses, we ask that you take care of your part at the time of the service.

We will file your insurance as a service to you. However, if for any reason your insurance company does not pay what we expect, then you will be responsible for the balance. But we are going to do everything possible to assist you." (This example, of course, represents those practices that are taking insurance on assignment. You will collect the patient's expected portion the day of the service and file insurance as a service to the patient. If you are providing aesthetic treatment that is not covered by insurance, this scenario is no problem for you.)

Situation: Patient doesn't have her checkbook.

"Oh, I see. Well, that happens sometimes, doesn't it? We do accept all the major bankcards. Which would you prefer?"

And, if they don't have a bankcard:

"Then, Mrs Jones, I will give you a statement and a self-addressed, stamped envelope. You can send us a check as soon as you get home. We will look forward to receiving that check in a couple of days. I will make a note to myself that we can expect your check. I will inform the dentist of our agreement." (Make a note in the tickler file. If you don't get the check in a few days, call.)

Situation: You have made financial arrangements with a patient. They come in for their preparation appointment. When they are being excused from the clinical area, they inform you that they do not have the agreed upon payment.

"Mrs Jones, since we had agreed on the payment for today, I am confused. I thought we had come to an agreement that we both accepted. However, I would be able to accept a credit card for payment today."

Situation: A financial arrangement is made for treatment. The patient is in the middle of the treatment but is not abiding by the financial agreement.

"When you are not able to follow through with the financial agreement that we established, that may force us to delay your treatment. I know how important it is to you to have your new smile and that time is of concern for you. Therefore, we need to review the original agreement and alter it so that we are both comfortable with the new agreement."

Table 12-1 Substitutions that change words or phrases from negative to positive.

Negative	Positive
Money, dollars	Fee for the service/treatment
Charge, cost	Financial responsibility, total investment, or monthly investment
Bill	Statement
Discount	Cash courtesy, fee reduction, or accounting reduction
Sign here	Please initial, or may I ask for your signature?
Policy	Financial options, or financial protocol
Deposit	Initial investment
Do you want to pay today?	Mrs Jones, your fee today is fifty-five. Will that be cash, check, or do you prefer to use a bank card?

Communicating financially

Always know that how you say something will make all the difference. You can say something one way and get a positive response and say something another way and get a negative response. There is so much at stake every time you communicate with a patient, doing so with care and excellence is worth the effort. Don't think you can just "talk" in any manner and that you will gain great results. Use positive words and phrases. Table 12-1 shows some examples of substitutions from negative to positive.

In summary

Creating a financial agreement between your dental practice and your patients is a service to both. This is a very special conversation with patients and takes careful and caring communication. You must have a patient's agreement on their financial responsibility before you start treatment.

While you may present your treatment recommendations with excellence, without a clear and comfortable financial arrangement/agreement, nothing happens. People will walk out your door. Having a variety of payment options that meet the needs of your patients opens the door for more people to accept more treatment. Objections may be presented to you. Do not avoid these objections. Rather, learn how to listen and respond effectively to them. An objection is a request for information and indicates that the patient is interested in your proposal.

Action steps

1. Establish a financial protocol that outlines your specific financial options.
2. Study and practice the communicative skills of presenting fees and of overcoming objections.
3. The dentist may quote fees, as long as the quotation is accurate, but the treatment coordinator needs to be the one making the financial arrangement.
4. Make sure that your fees are properly aligned and appropriate for the services you are providing. Set your fees and be confident that they are equitable for the treatment your patient receives.

5. Give the treatment coordinator time to find a financial solution for each patient.
6. Make financial arrangements before treatment is provided. This service will reduce broken appointments and no shows.
7. The treatment coordinator must be confident in the dentist, the dentistry being performed, and the fees. While he/she must be an excellent communicator, being an outstanding listener is of utmost importance.

References

1. Doyle M. How to Make Meetings Work. New York, NY: Berkley Publishing Group, 1982.
2. Jameson C. Collect What You Produce. Tulsa, OK: Pennwell Books, 2006.
3. Linhart J. 5 Reasons Why People Do Not Go to the Dentist. New York, NY: Castle Connolly Medical Ltd. EZineArticles, 2010.
4. Lockard W. The Exceptional Dental Practice. Oklahoma City, OK: Lockard Publications, 2007.

13 Scheduling Aesthetic Dentistry

Cathy Jameson and Linda Greenwall

> *If concentration provides the energy and attention needed for right action to take place and discrimination provides the intention and standards needed to know what action needs to be taken, then organization provides the room for right action to take place. There are three things which can be so organized: time, space, and work.*
> *Michael E Gerber (1985)*

The heartbeat of your practice: scheduling

The scheduling strategies for aesthetic dentistry are the most essential element in a well organized aesthetic dental practice. As aesthetic procedures require focused time, it is essential that these procedures are scheduled effectively. Placing names in the appointment book and filling lines on the schedule does not work if your goals are productivity, profitability, and stress control. In addition, since your goal is to build the aesthetic aspect of your dental practice, managing the schedule efficiently will make it possible to schedule aesthetic cases expediently. In fact, the appointment schedule may become problematic due to your success. You want to control the appointment book rather than letting the appointment book control you. Without careful guidelines, scheduling can become a nightmare. It can become one of the most stressful areas of the dental practice. Control of stress should be a goal, one that receives the attention and commitment of every person on the team. An out of control appointment book can be one of the most stressful systems in the practice. It doesn't have to be this way.

Successful scheduling is the responsibility of everyone on the team. Each person will have specific responsibilities and must be depended upon to carry out those responsibilities. However, you will probably have one person executing the appointment book. It takes specific expertise and commitment to organize days properly. Dr Tom McDougal of Dallas, Texas (1985) coined the phrase, "engineering the appointment book." The team must, "engineer" the appointments, the time frames, and the organization of the day so that production goals are met, people are seen expediently, proper time allotments are incorporated for the unique treatment types, and people are able to function well. The clinical team needs adequate time to perform well, but not have excess time that is wasted. This can be a difficult balance.

The person responsible for the appointment book must have the ability, education, time, and the desire to make each and every day successful. Today's lost production is lost forever.

Eight steps to strategic scheduling

There are eight steps to strategic scheduling that will impact your ability to practice efficiently:

1. Schedule toward a specific daily production goal
2. Determine dentist time and assistant time, then schedule each provider
3. Use the proper appointment book or tool
4. Place the appropriate detail in the schedule
5. Schedule a variety of procedures into every day
6. Pre-block your schedule
7. Organize periodic hygiene evaluations
8. Handle emergencies smoothly.

1. Schedule toward a specific daily production goal

As an astute businessperson, you must know the required monthly costs of operation or outgoings as well as the amount of money coming in. This will help you to determine your production goal. A month that is made up of evenly productive days will be less stressful than a month that is full of high days and low days. This "roller coaster" type of scheduling leads to stress and to concern over financial security.

You need to consider the three following factors as you determine your monthly goal.

- Determine how much it costs to run your dental practice on a monthly basis.
- Add to this the desired amount of dentist salary and compensation.
- Add a percentage of planned profit.

Total these three areas to determine the amount you need to produce every month.

Then, count the number of days in which dentistry will be produced during each month. Divide the production goal by the number of available days. This will give you the daily production goal: the goal towards which you will be scheduling, divided by the number of days' dentistry that will be produced.

Monthly goal	=	monthly overhead + dentist's compensation + profit
Daily goal	=	monthly overhead + dentist's compensation + profit divided by the number of days dentistry will be produced

The monthly goal will not change. The bills will come due and salaries will be paid no matter how many days you are in the office. What will change from month to month will be the daily goal. The daily goal will depend upon the number of days you are working each month. Alternatively, you can determine the total production goal for the year and divide that number by the number of days you will be performing dentistry in the upcoming year. That, too, will give you a daily production goal.

The scheduling coordinator must have specific goals if she is to schedule smoothly and precisely and if she is to integrate your aesthetic cases into your schedule.

	Crown Prep (Molar Tooth)	
8:00	Greet, Seat, Review Health History, Toopical, Anesthesia, Opp. Model, Shade	C•
8:10	Prep	|
8:20	Prep	|
8:30	Pack Cord, Final Impression	|
8:40	Temporization	C
8:50		C
9:00	Dismiss Patient, Decontaminate Room	C
9:10		
9:20		
9:30		
9:40		
9:50		

Fig 13-1 Example of a procedure analysis sheet (•, anesthesia; C, clinical assistant; |, dentist).

2. Determine dentist time and assistant time, then schedule each provider

According to your state or country, delegate everything you can possibly delegate to various members of the team. The dentist should do the things that only he/she can do and delegate everything else. No matter how much or how little the clinical assistants, nurses, therapists, or hygienists can do in your particular situation, be sure to delegate those things. Provide the necessary education and skill development so that the auxiliary persons will be competent, comfortable, and confident with their responsibilities.

Once you have determined what can be delegated and have provided all necessary training for competency, turn those aspects of procedures over to the appropriate team member. Perform an analysis of your major procedures to identify dentist time, assistant time, and decontamination time (see Fig 13-1). Indicate what happens during each phase of the treatment, how long each part takes, and who is doing what.

Place this analysis into the computer so that when you post a procedure you have the correct analysis of time allotments. Certainly, when you are doing combined procedures, the clinical assistant or nurse will need to give the scheduling coordinator any unique time analysis. In each case, he/she needs to let the scheduler know how much time is needed in terms of both assistant and dentist time.

Figure 13-1 is an example of a procedure analysis sheet. Analysis of the procedure indicates anesthesia time, clinical assistant/nurse time, and dentist time. These symbols mean that this person is occupied and cannot be in

8:00	Sam Smith	C•		
8:10	Crn Prep #19	|		
8:20	369-2501	|		
8:30	(0450)	|	C	Mark Moeller
8:40		C	C•	MO #13 MOD #14
8:50		C	|	MO #15
9:00		C	|	369-7718
9:10			|	(0180)
9:20	Susie Hightower	C	|	
9:30	(Emergency)	|	C	
9:40	(broken tooth)	C		
9:50				

Fig 13-2 Example of "interfaced" appointments (•, anesthesia; C, clinical assistant; |, dentist).

another place at the same time. This information needs to be clearly identified in the appointment book. Each appointment has a procedure analysis sheet documented on a step-by-step basis. Produce one of these sheets for each major procedure. Place a formula at the bottom of the sheet for multiple teeth, surfaces etc. For example, for each additional crown add one unit of time for the prep and one unit of time for the temporization. On your aesthetic cases, you will be doing many procedures per appointment, so a unique designation will be appropriate. The clinical team needs to indicate how much time in total they require, as well as defining the dentist and assistant time for each specific appointment. Interfaced appointments can also be scheduled in this way (Fig 13-2). Suitable photographs for the required set-ups may be produced and placed in the sterilization area so that the clinical assistants or nurses can make sure that everything is prepared before the dentist or the patient enter the treatment area/surgery suite (Fig 13-3).

Proper delegation can be developed through excellent training, as outlined below.

- Study your current dental/jurisprudence laws to determine what can be delegated to various auxiliary persons.
- Write down each step of your procedures and complete the procedure analysis sheets for all procedures.
- During an appointment, explain to the assistant what you are doing and why.
- Do some "hands on" training.
- Have the assistant perform the new task on a patient or in the laboratory while the dentist gives direction. (Tell the patient what you're doing and ask their permission to teach during their appointment. The assistant should log at least 10 cases during her training to demonstrate competency and proficiency in that clinical procedure.)
- Let the assistant take over when appropriate.
- Evaluate on a regular basis to make sure things are going well. Feedback is essential. Don't assume that your assistant knows she's doing a good job. Tell her. Or if you want something done differently, tell her that also. She will want to know. How can she get better if she doesn't know what you want?

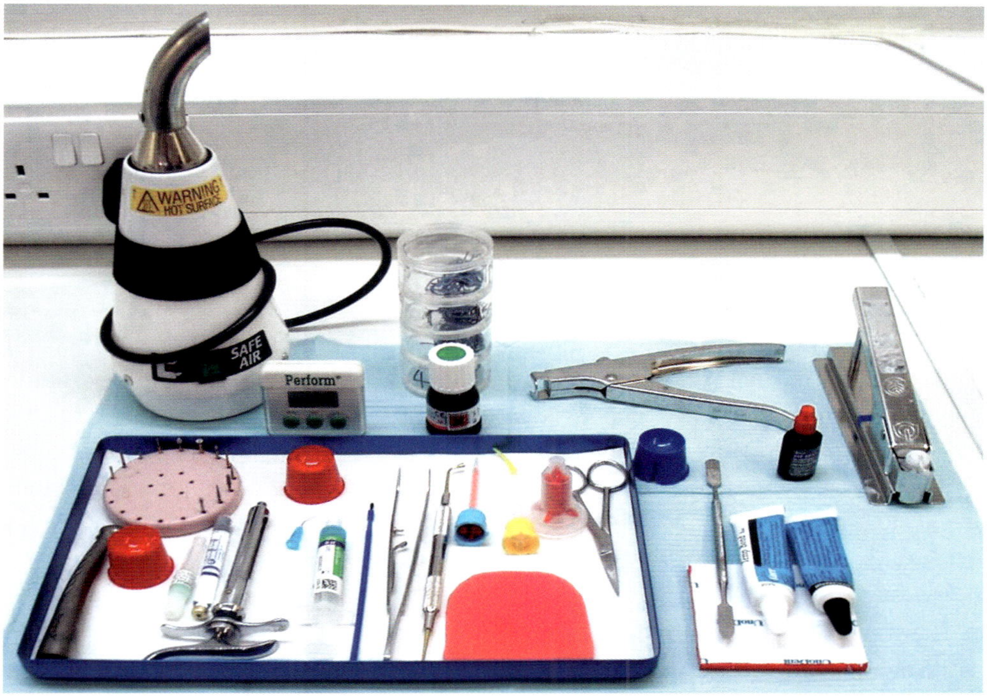

Fig 13-3 The tray set-up for a core buildup and crown preparation to accompany the procedure analysis sheet, which forms part of the practice procedure for the team in Dr Greenwall's UK dental practice.

3. Appointment book or tool

Your appointment book or tool needs to let you do all of the things that are being outlined in this chapter. Most appointment books are computerized in today's world. An appointment book that is broken down into 10-minute units is preferred. Hi-tech/hi-speed dentistry and the ability of talented and skilled assistants make it possible for dental teams to provide excellent care in a time-efficient manner.

Good scheduling means good time management. Therefore, careful use of your time makes good sense. You will be able to schedule for more efficient management of time with a 10-minute schedule, rather than a 15-minute system.

You will need one column per active chair. You must be sure that each and every day is well scheduled. Trying to "make up for lost time" because of a poorly scheduled day leads to increased stress.

4. Place the appropriate detail in the schedule

Specific information needs to be placed into the schedule. The ability to place accurate data into your schedule will be dependent upon the quality of your treatment plans. Remember, each person needs a comprehensive, detailed treatment plan (preferably with the treatment plan broken down into appointment number). Without complete treatment plans, the scheduling coordinator has their hands tied. The coordinator is a vehicle for the clinical team. The written or digital information that comes to the business office from the clinical team is as critical as any verbal communication. They need to know which teeth, how many surfaces, and what type of restorations are to be scheduled.

5. Schedule a variety of procedures into every day

The variety of procedures needs to be scheduled into most days. This variety is a mixture of primary, secondary, and tertiary procedures (Fig 13-4).

- Primary procedures are the procedures that have a higher financial value attached to them.
- Secondary procedures have lower fees attached.
- Tertiary procedures have no fee: these are the no charge procedures.

In a general dental practice, primary procedures may be crowns, endodontics, dentures and partial dentures, implant restorations, a quadrant of resin composites, and most cosmetic procedures such as porcelain veneers. Secondary procedures would be evaluations, simple resin composites, and extractions etc. Tertiary procedures are those procedures where there is no specific charge attached, for example seating of crowns and fixed partial dentures, suture removals, and denture adjustments. There are other procedures in each of these categories. You identify each within your own dental practice.

There is *no difference* in the importance of any one procedure over another. The insertion of a crown is every bit as important as the day you prep the tooth for the crown. The day you remove the sutures and evaluate a patient's healing is as critical as the day you perform the surgery. However, in terms of smooth, productive days that control stress, having a balance of these procedures is critical.

How do you engineer this variety into the days? The key to great scheduling is pre-blocking.

Primary procedures	Secondary procedures	Tertiary procedures
high financial value, eg, a crown prep	lower financial value, eg, an evaluation and a simple resin composite restoration	no financial value, eg, seating crowns, adjusting a denture
preblocked for half your daily production goal	will fill the rest of the schedule	interfaced with primary and secondary appointments

Fig 13-4 Breakdown of procedures.

6. Pre-block your schedule

Pre-blocking allows you to gain control of your schedule. Reserve specific times in each day for primary procedures. *Pre-block for primary appointments.* Your primary procedures would be the approximate value of a crown, whatever that fee is in your dental practice. Pre-block your days for approximately half of your production goal. This applies to all providers, including the hygienists.

Secondary and tertiary procedures will complete your days. Your computerized schedules allow you to color code your pre-blocked time frames. You will not need to pre-block for secondary and tertiary procedures.

Two to three days in advance of a pre-blocked primary appointment, release the reserved time. Make every effort to fill that primary time. Inform the clinical team of the upcoming available primary time. They can help. However, if you cannot fill this reserved time with a primary procedure, fill it with other types of appointments. Don't get nervous and let it go too soon.

In terms of aesthetic cases, you will need to see a patient in the near future if they have decided to proceed with treatment. If your appointment is heavily booked into the future and someone decides they want to proceed with a smile makeover, don't risk having them lose their enthusiasm because you can't see them for several weeks. It is essential to pre-block your schedule for aesthetic cases. These will need longer time frames, so reserve those. In addition, you may need to reserve some long tertiary appointments for seating/placement of crowns/veneers. Start by reserving one long aesthetic appointment every other week, once per week, or whatever fits your situation. Once you have these reservations or pre-blocks, engineer people into those times. If you build the aesthetic aspect of your dental practice and you see that the number of pre-blocks is not sufficient any longer, add more to your schedule. These large, highly productive appointments make it possible for you to see fewer patients in a day but reach pre-determined production goals. In fact, you will normally exceed production goals on those days.

You will also need to pre-block for your predetermined and appropriate number of new patient evaluations so that you can see your new patients expediently. In addition, if you are seeing more than two emergencies per day, you may wish to pre-block for some emergency time in each day.

7. Periodic hygiene evaluations

The dentist needs to provide the periodic hygiene evaluations at his/her convenience, rather than at the end of the appointment. If the hygienist waits until the end of the appointment to indicate to the dentist that he/she is ready for an evaluation, the dentist may be intensely involved with another procedure and may not be able to get up and leave. Talk about good times for evaluations at the morning meetings. This will ensure time for an effective dentist/hygiene evaluation and no interruptions during your long aesthetic case appointments.

When the hygienist needs to gather necessary data for the dentist to be able to provide the evaluation, such as a full mouth series, he/she needs to make note of this during the morning meeting so that the dentist knows not to come in to provide the evaluation until 20 minutes or so have passed.

Before the dentist sits down at the chair to begin an aesthetic case, the dentist needs to perform hygiene evaluations (perhaps after social graces and after anesthetic has been administered) so that once he/she begins to provide treatment, there will be no need to get up and leave the patient. Even with extremely long appointments, do the hygiene evaluations at the beginning, sit down to provide care, and then do the evaluations during the second hour at a natural break in the dentist's schedule.

8. Emergencies

Patients who are in a true emergency situation need to be seen the day they call. However, they need to be seen in a manner that does not take away from the regularly scheduled patients.

Emergencies for the most part should receive palliative treatment on the day (trauma is, of course, an exception). When a new patient or an existing patient calls with an emergency concern, the person on the telephone needs to gather appropriate accurate information to determine the status of the emergency, such as duration of pain, location, swelling, or broken tooth. Then, that person will be scheduled into a time frame of approximately 40–50 minutes depending on the emergency situation. After the evaluation, the images/photos, and the radiographs, normally 40–50 minutes should be sufficient for the palliative treatment/dressing of the tooth.

The assistant will greet, seat, review the health history, and interview. The dentist will do a quick "look – see" and will prescribe the necessary x-ray, when appropriate. The area of concern is recorded on the intraoral or digital camera.

The dentist will provide the diagnosis and the recommendation, as well as the palliative treatment or prescription. Once the patient accepts treatment, he/she is rescheduled for the necessary treatment and for the appropriate amount of time. This will give the business administrator the opportunity to discuss the financial responsibility and, then, to schedule the appointment.

Do not proceed with treatment on an emergency patient unless two things are in place:

- You have the time to provide treatment without that having a negative effect on your regularly scheduled patients.
- The person needs to understand and accept the financial responsibility.

Respect the time of your patients. Do not abuse their time. Respect your patients enough to inform them of their financial responsibility before treatment is rendered. Do not spend their money without their consent.

Of course, if you do have the time and if the patient is clear and comfortable with the financial responsibility, proceeding with treatment makes good sense for everyone.

As a team, make great effort to convince an emergency patient of the value of getting healthy and staying healthy. Being treated with such respect and caring, you will find that many of your comprehensive cases and aesthetic cases will come from people who may have come to your dental practice as an emergency originally. You can make an effort to change a one-time patient into a 'forever' patient.

When busyness causes scheduling challenges

If you do not control your schedule, the patients do. If the patients control the schedule, chaos results. Chaos breeds stress, and we are trying to control stress.

Controlling your schedule does not mean that you are not going to carefully try to meet the scheduling needs of your patients. However, when you do control the schedule and coordinate your days carefully then everyone wins, including the patients.

Being busy is a compliment to you. It means that you are doing a lot of things right and people are seeking your services. However, being too busy can be a problem unto itself. In fact, busyness and the inability to schedule an aesthetic case expediently can become a detriment to your goal of building the aesthetic aspect of your dental practice.

You want to make sure that your appointment book does not work against you, but rather works with you to provide scheduling opportunities for your patients while not stressing your dentist and/or your team. Jacqueline Pastore of the Rosenthal Apa Group in New York City manages one of the largest and most successful aesthetic dental practices in the world. When asked about scheduling their large aesthetic cases, Jacqueline provided the following insights.

> *"Many of our cases take several hours at either the preparation appointment and/or the insertion appointment. I think it is best to have a schedule template for our larger cases to avoid unnecessary stress and to provide our patients with the time and attention needed for these cases. Everyone on our team knows that our dentists prefer to schedule large prep appointments in the mornings on Mondays and Tuesdays and large insertion appointments are scheduled in the afternoons on Wednesdays and Thursdays when it is less hectic. We pre-block our appointments to make sure we can schedule as desired."*
>
> *Jacqueline Pastore (interview),*
> *Practice Administrator for*
> *Drs Larry Rosenthal and Michael Apa*

Scheduling is a critical part of building the aesthetic aspect of your dental practice. Difficult but important decisions must be made in relation to how you are scheduling, if aesthetic cases are going to become a part of your dental practice. Do not let busyness and a full schedule make it impossible to engineer an aesthetic case into your schedule.

Seven elements for control of busyness

1. Manage your schedule
2. Delegate
3. Patient financing programs
4. Fees
5. Associates and/or additional dentists
6. Refer
7. Insurance.

1. Manage your schedule

Organize your treatment plans to do a quadrant or a half-mouth per appointment (or more in some cases). Try to treat a patient in as few appointments as possible. Both you and the patient win. Your appointment book will not be so clogged with numerous small appointments.

2. Delegate

As mentioned above, delegate when and where possible, according to the laws of your state or country. The dentist should do the things that only a dentist can do and should delegate all else. Delegation becomes an important time management principle.

3. Patient financing programs

(When and where available, see Chapter 12.) Many patients ask for "one tooth at a time" dentistry, or many dental practices find themselves offering this kind of treatment because of the investment. In order to do more dentistry per patient on fewer patients per day and see the patient for fewer visits, a patient financing program is a major asset. Being able to fit the payments for their dental care into a patient's personal budget can pave the way for treatment acceptance and efficient scheduling.

4. Fees

The law of supply and demand may indicate that raising your fees is appropriate. If you lose some patients from your dental practice due to fee increases, you may find that the profit margin of the dental practice remains steadfast, while you see fewer patients and spend more time with them. You will have more time to do exceptional new patient evaluations and consultations, and can do quadrant, half-mouth, arch, or full-mouth cases, whether restorative or aesthetic. Certainly, your fees must be equitable to the services being offered. A reasonable and appropriate fee increase may give you freedom not previously allowed when the schedule is overly crowded.

5. Associates and/or additional dentists

If the first four suggestions have been met or exceeded, you may need to consider an associate. This is a major decision and needs much consideration, planning and advice.

6. Refer

As a dental practice that is too busy, consider referring as much as possible. Focus your dental practice on the type of dentistry you love, and refer everything else. You will replace the production of the referred dentistry by carefully organizing your treatment planning and scheduling.

7. Insurance

In countries where dental insurance or national healthcare systems exist, if you are too busy, and if you are on any managed care programs, this may be the time to decide whether or not you wish to remain a provider.

List all of the programs in which you are enrolled. Analyze these to determine which ones generate the most revenue. As you build the fee-for-service or private part of your dental practice, begin eliminating the managed care programs starting with the least productive and go up from there.

This is neither an easy choice nor an easy decision, nor is it appropriate for all dental practices. You have to decide.

Broken appointments and no-shows

Prevention is the best way to reduce broken appointments and no-shows, and communication skills are the key to reducing these scheduling glitches. When the entire team practices excellent communication skills, the impact is astounding. Communication is fundamental to your success, no matter in what aspect of patient care.

The reduction of broken appointments and no-shows begins in the clinical area when the clinical team stresses the significance of the next appointment. "Linkage communication"© between the clinical team and the business team is imperative for scheduling success.

There are six strategies for reducing broken appointments and no-shows:

1. The verbal skills of scheduling
2. Reason to come back
3. Confirming appointments
4. Rescheduling
5. Advance collection of fees
6. No-shows

1. The verbal skills of scheduling

The appointment coordinator must stress not only the importance of that next appointment, but he/she must also indicate the amount of time being reserved for the patient in the dentist's schedule. The appointment is the responsibility of the patient and you can help the patient accept that responsibility by the way you schedule in the first place. Your aesthetic cases will be long and will demand your ultimate attention. Careful scheduling of these appointments will relieve any anxiety that you may have about reserving long appointments.

Appointment coordinator to patient: "Mr Bailey, Dr Greenwall will need 2 hours to provide the treatment that you have accepted. In order to reserve this much of your time and of Dr Greenwall's time, we need to make sure that we find a time that is good for both of you. We need to make sure that we can count on you to be here for this very special appointment. Rescheduling this much of the dentist's time on short notice would be impossible. So, let's find a time that is good for you and good for the dentist. Which is better for you, mornings or afternoons? Mornings are better? Dr Greenwall has an available 2-hour appointment on Monday, July 21 at 10:00 or on Thursday, July 24 at 9:00. In your schedule, Mr Bailey, which appointment works best? Thursday, July 24 at 9:00? Great. We appreciate being able to count on you. I will reserve this time for you now."

2. Reason to come back

At the end of every appointment, the clinical team member who is with the patient should set the patient in an upright position and stress the significance of the next appointment. You want to plant in the patient's mind the benefits of the next appointment and the possible risks of not scheduling or of not showing up for that appointment.

No matter how wonderful the person in the business office may be, that person will not have as strong an impact on the patient as the clinical team member who has been with the patient during treatment. The dentist, hygienist, or assistant will have a strong effect on whether or not the patient schedules and /or keeps their next appointment.

Hygienist to patient: "Mrs Jones, you are doing a great job with your home care. However, Dr Greenwall and I are still very concerned about the gum tissue on the upper right around those crowns. I'm making a note in your clinical record to evaluate this area again in 4 weeks. It will be very critical that we see you at that time. Can we can count on seeing you at that time?"
Clinical assistant to patient: "Mr Crawford, your root canal has been very successful. Dr Greenwall is very pleased with the results. Now, she is recommending that we support the tooth with a crown in order to prevent the tooth from breaking. The last thing you want is to lose that tooth. So, let's go ahead and schedule your crown appointment now."
Dentist to emergency patient: "James, we need to see you again to do a comprehensive evaluation. Once a complete evaluation has been completed, we can sit down together and discuss your total treatment needs. We're going to take care of this immediate need, then we need to develop a plan of care that will stop this pattern of emergencies. Please know that your best interest is foremost in our minds at all times."

Then, whoever escorts the patient to the business office for the scheduling of the appointment should reiterate the significance of the upcoming appointment, not so much for the business administrator, but for the patient. Remember that repetition is the key to learning.

3. Confirming appointments

Begin confirming appointments in the morning around 9:00. Confirm in a very positive manner, and always stress the importance of the appointment and the patient's responsibility for the appointment.

When you are originally scheduling the appointment, try to make notes in the patient's personal record regarding a particular area of concern. Then, when you are confirming, you can reinforce the need for the appointment relative to this area of concern. The patient will be more strongly motivated to come to the appointment if you stress the benefits of the appointment and certain risks that might occur if they do not come. In addition, you will be showing your patients that you go the extra mile in providing patient care. In other words, you aren't just calling off of a list; you are knowledgeable about their particular situation.

In today's "answering device world," you may be frustrated if all you get is a recorder. Be sure to ask for a daytime number for confirmation when you are scheduling the patient in the first place. Otherwise, you are setting yourself up for frustration. Do not leave a message and think that you have confirmed. A message left on an answering device, a text, or an e-mail is not a confirmation.

The digital world lets you confirm via e-mail, text, cell phone, etc. Find out how a patient wishes to receive confirmation and access the electronic capability to do so. You can confirm an appointment a day or two in advance and also send a text one hour before an appointment for that last minute "heads up" to a busy person.

If you have called at 9:00, then again at noon, and you are beginning to panic over the patient you cannot reach, then leave a message. However, in your message, ask the patient to call you to confirm his/her appointment. Ask them to call by a certain time. Thank them for their cooperation.

Appointment coordinator: "Mr Bailey this is Nicola from Dr Greenwall's dental office. I'm sorry that I have been unable to reach you personally. Mr Bailey, I am calling regarding your appointment with Dr Greenwall on Thursday, July 24 at 9:00. Please call our office by 12:00 tomorrow – that's Tuesday – about that appointment. I'll look forward to your call. Thank you."

If you are having a great deal of trouble with no-shows and broken appointments, you may want to start confirming your appointments two days in advance. This will give you a little extra time should you have unavoidable changes of schedule. You will reduce your stress by doing this. Nothing can be more stressful than to have a change of schedule at 4:00 in the afternoon and have no time to fill that void. Don't put yourself in this type of compromised position. Pre-plan. Engage in preventive management.

If you have been confirming one day in advance and change to two days, be sure to let your patients know that you are making this change. Otherwise, you will have two day's worth of patients showing up at the same time.

Appointment coordinator: "Mr Bailey, in the past we have confirmed our appointments one day in advance. However, today, I am calling two days in advance to give you plenty of advanced notice. I am calling about your appointment the day after tomorrow – that's Thursday, July 24 at 9:00. Do you have your calendar with you? Check to make sure you have that on your schedule."

Recording devices

If you are having a lot of changes of schedule left on your recording device during the night, you may want to consider changing your message. Some people will call you at night, and leave that type of message because they do not want to "face the music." This leaves you in a terrible mess because you have no chance to convince them of the need to come to their appointment or no chance to reschedule them.

Consider the following message. You will maintain much better control with this recording.

Recorded message: "You have reached Dr Greenwall's dental office. Our office is presently closed. Our regular working hours are Monday through Thursday from 8:30 to 5:00. If you are calling regarding a dental emergency, you may reach Dr Greenwall at 405-231-5467. If you need to speak with us regarding your dental appointment, please call during our regular working hours. We ask that you do not leave a message regarding changes of schedule on this machine. However, if you are calling to confirm an upcoming appointment, you may leave the message now. Thank you."

You will find that people will respect your request and they will not become perturbed by this message.

You may be thinking, "Well, then when we come in the next morning, the phone will ring with patients needing to change their appointments." Great! This will give you a chance to speak with the patient directly. Thus, you will be able to try to convince them of the benefits of coming to the appointment. If you cannot convince them to keep the appointment, then at least you have them on the phone and can reschedule the appointment.

4. Rescheduling

If a person does call to make a change of schedule, obviously your goal is to reschedule them while you have them on the phone.

If you say, "Oh, that's OK. Call us when you think you can make it," or if you allow a person to just call at their convenience, then you have just committed "appointment suicide."

Rather, when a person calls to tell you that they can't make an appointment that you carefully scheduled, say the following to the patient.

Appointment coordinator: "Oh, Mrs Jones, that is very difficult. As you recall, we have reserved 2 hours of your time and 2 hours of Dr Greenwall's time for this appointment. At this late notice, I would not be able to fill the void left by your absence. This, of course, would be very difficult for us. I'm sure you can understand the dilemma. Is there anything we can do to make it possible for you to come on for this appointment?"

If the person is ill or has some other unsolvable problem, obviously you would accept that situation. Your responsibility is then to reschedule the appointment. If, for any reason you are unable to get that appointment rescheduled, ask the patient for permission to call them back.

Appointment coordinator: "Mrs Jones, I can understand your inability to reschedule at this time, and I appreciate your offer to call me at a later date. However, it is our responsibility to make sure that we keep you on

> a program of regular care, so may I ask your permission to call you in the near future to reschedule this appointment? Thank you. Tell me, Mrs Jones, should I call in 2 weeks or would you prefer that I call right after the first of the month?"

You are staying in control by asking the patient to let you give them a call. In addition, when you do call, you will not be intruding since you've obtained permission beforehand.

Notice that you give the patient two choices, either of which you accept. This is called an alternative of choice. Most people will respond positively to this request, to call them one time or the other. Make sure that you make a note of when you are to call. Then, do it! Always do what you have told a person you will do. Use a tickler system to remind yourself, either a manual system or a computerized system. Use it, and follow it.

5. Advance collection of fees

Using the recommended payment options as suggested in Chapter 12, collect the fees in advance. This will certainly reduce many of your broken, cancelled appointments and no-shows. For your large aesthetic cases where you are reserving a significant amount of time, insist that the fee for the treatment be paid before services begin. You cannot afford to reserve large blocks of time and not have a patient show up. The prepayment will assure the patient's commitment to treatment. You will respect their time and all you are asking is that they respect your time, as well.

6. No-shows

There is nothing worse than a no-show: the person who agrees to the appointment when you call to confirm, then does not show up! What can you possibly do?

There is no question that this is the most challenging of all scheduling glitches, and it is the one that is most difficult, if not impossible, to rectify.

Here are a few tried-and-true strategies for handling this type of difficult situation:

- Call the patient if he/she is 5 minutes late to see if they are on their way or if you need to reschedule. If you are unable to reach them or if they indicate that they are not coming, try to contact your "quick notice" patients who live or work nearby to see if they can come in with this last minute notification (always keep a list at your fingertips or on the computer).
- Put the no-show patient data in the tickler file or on the computer if you are unable to reach them. Don't let them slip away. If you are unable to reach the person, make sure that your tickler file moves their name forward until the point that you do get them rescheduled.
- If you are unable to contact the patient, send them a letter or e-mail expressing your concern over the missed appointment. Stress your commitment to their health and well being. Let them know that you have tried on multiple occasions to call and reschedule the appointment. Invite them to call you for that rescheduling.

In summary

In order to manage a productive, profitable dental practice in which stress is controlled, excellent scheduling is essential. Now that you are going to perform more aesthetic procedures, your scheduling must support that goal. Each of the scheduling strategies outlined will be beneficial to your aesthetic dental practice.

How you communicate your scheduling parameters to patients makes all the difference. Patients feel comfortable about almost anything when communication is clear. When patients know you have their best interests in mind, they normally respond well to your requests. Spend time, as a team, practicing the verbal skills suggested in this chapter. Practice improves almost anything, including communication.

Action steps

1. Utilize your appointment book, computer, or scheduling tool to the maximum. Full understanding of this tool is important for the entire team.
2. Determine your yearly, monthly, weekly, and daily production goals.
3. Analyze your major procedures to determine the dentist time/assistant time so that you can schedule all people on the clinical team. Pre-block every day and every provider for approximately half of their daily production goal. Pre-blocks will be for primary procedures, emergencies, and new patients.
4. Do the research to find out what can be delegated in your state or country. Provide the training necessary for each team member to maximize their time in the dental practice.
5. Analyze your situation to determine your level of busyness. Study the 7 steps of controlling busyness and do what is necessary to organize your dental practice to make sure that busyness not become a barrier to building the aesthetic aspect of your dental practice.
6. Spend time, as a team, practicing the verbal skills suggested in this chapter.

References

1. Gerber ME. Power Point. New York, NY: HarperCollins, 1985.
2. McDougal T. Commitment to Excellence. Dallas, TX: TexasGP, 1985.

14 The Hygienist's Role in Promoting Aesthetic Dentistry

Cathy Jameson and Linda Greenwall

> *One of the main responsibilities of any dental professional is to educate patients about the needs that exist in their mouths and about opportunities that are available in dentistry today, including aesthetic treatment options. There is no one on the team who has a closer relationship with a patient than the hygienist.*
>
> *Dru Halverson, RDH (interview),*
> *Director of Quality Assurance and Senior Hygiene Consultant,*
> *Jameson Management, Inc.*

The lifeblood of the dental practice

The hygienist spends long, quality appointment time with a patient, is able to converse during most appointments, has a confident level of trust with patients and is a qualified dental educator. The hygienic care of the patient is an integral and essential part of getting patients healthy, keeping them healthy, insuring restoration longevity, and introducing advanced types of care, including aesthetics. Your mission and/or vision of your dental practice probably include a commitment to total care of your patients, which includes comprehensive hygienic care.

► *"Key to patients joining and staying on a journey to oral health is comprehensive diagnosis and treatment planning as well as effective communication and patient education. We must not only stay true to our goal of evidence based individualized care, but we must help the patient understand the reasoning behind our recommended plan. This requires a systematic team approach to comprehensive care and patient education.*

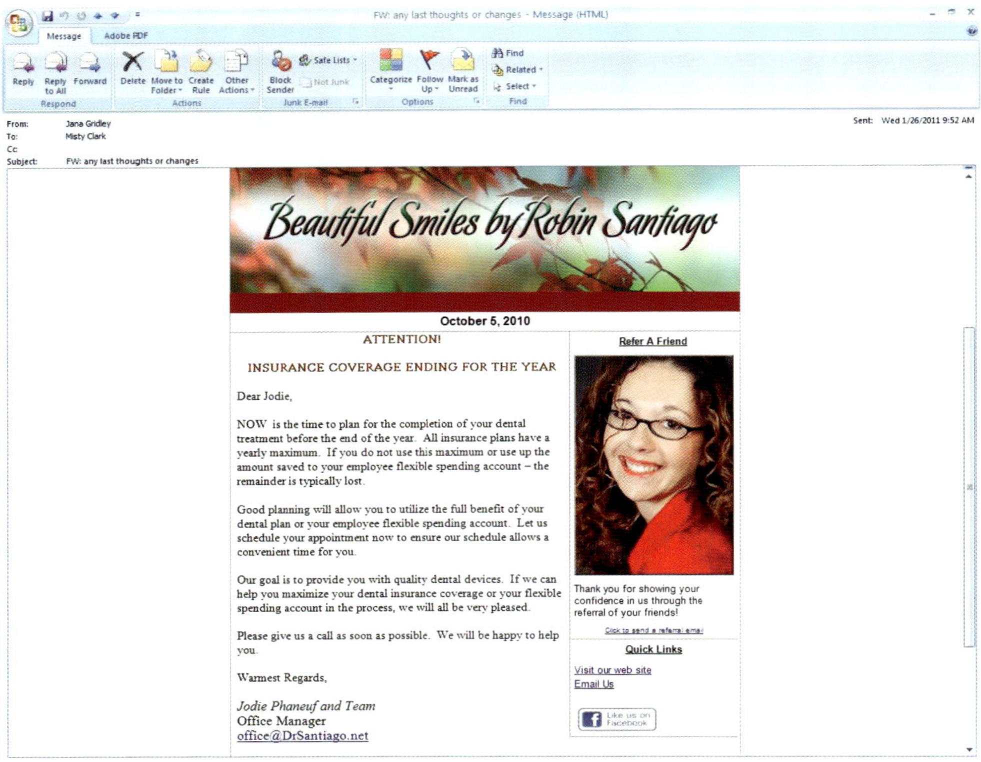

Fig 14-1 Smile reminder sample e-mail.

Everyone must have the same itinerary and be following the same map. Once you can effectively communicate evidence-based care, patients gain an entirely new understanding of your recommendation for what is in their best interest. They are genuinely appreciative. The original trust they had in you as a dental professional is only enhanced."

Nancy Dukes, RDH (interview), Senior Consultant and Director of Hygiene for Jameson Management, Inc.

Most people do not know what is available in aesthetic dentistry. When asked to describe porcelain laminate veneers, for example, very few lay persons are able to do that. Sometimes we, as dental professionals, think that people know more than they do about our field and are often amazed to realize the low dental IQ of the average person. Thus, constantly educating patients in multiple ways helps the patient by letting them know what might be available to them. This helps to build the dental practice by opening the door for additional treatment for new or existing patients.

The hygienist as educator

The following are some suggestions about how the hygienist can be a proactive educator, one who opens the door for aesthetic possibilities within the dental practice:

1. Send brochures or letters with appointment notices
2. Send brochures to all patients
3. Frame photographs

4. Take photographs
5. Digital education programs.

1. Send brochures or letters with appointment notices

When sending hygiene notices, eg, confirming a pre-scheduled appointment or a past due letter for their hygiene appointment, include an informative letter and a brochure about one particular cosmetic procedure that your dental practice is providing. Change this letter and brochure every 3 to 6 months so that your patients are continually informed about different types of cosmetic procedures. You never know which type of procedure is going to stimulate someone's interest. If you are using e-mails or texts, these messages can be modified to be sent electronically (Fig 14-1).

2. Send brochures to all patients

Send a letter and a brochure about a particular procedure to the entire patient family (Fig 14-2a). Then, when patients are flowing through the hygienic area, ask if they have received the information and if they have any questions. Show them before and after photographs, either in a photo album or video library.

Example of a proactive hygienist

A dentist client wanted to do more whitening/bleaching in the dental practice. He had attended a course on whitening, had purchased a whitening system and was ready to go. The dental practice sent an advertisement (Fig 14-2b) and letter to the entire patient family along with a brochure (provided by the whitening system). In the letter, the patients were invited to call for further information or to schedule a consultation appointment to discuss the possibilities. The phone rang off the wall and they were able to schedule many patients for this most requested procedure.

The hygienist in this dental practice bleached her maxillary teeth, leaving the mandibular teeth for a later time. They took photographs of her teeth before and after the bleaching. They stored these photographs so she could pull her photographs up on the monitor during appointments, and also printed them so she could easily show them to patients.

Each time a patient came into her area, the hygienist asked people if they had received the letter about their new bleaching system. Then she showed them her own before and after photographs. She enthusiastically shared her feelings of joy over the change in her smile and asked if whitening the smile would be of interest to the patient.

The response was amazing. So many people did the bleaching process that the dentist was amazed.

If this type of promotion is of interest to you, but there isn't a hygienist who wants or needs bleaching, do this on any member of the team, or a patient who gives you permission to use their before and after photographs for educational purposes. Written permission is, of course, essential.

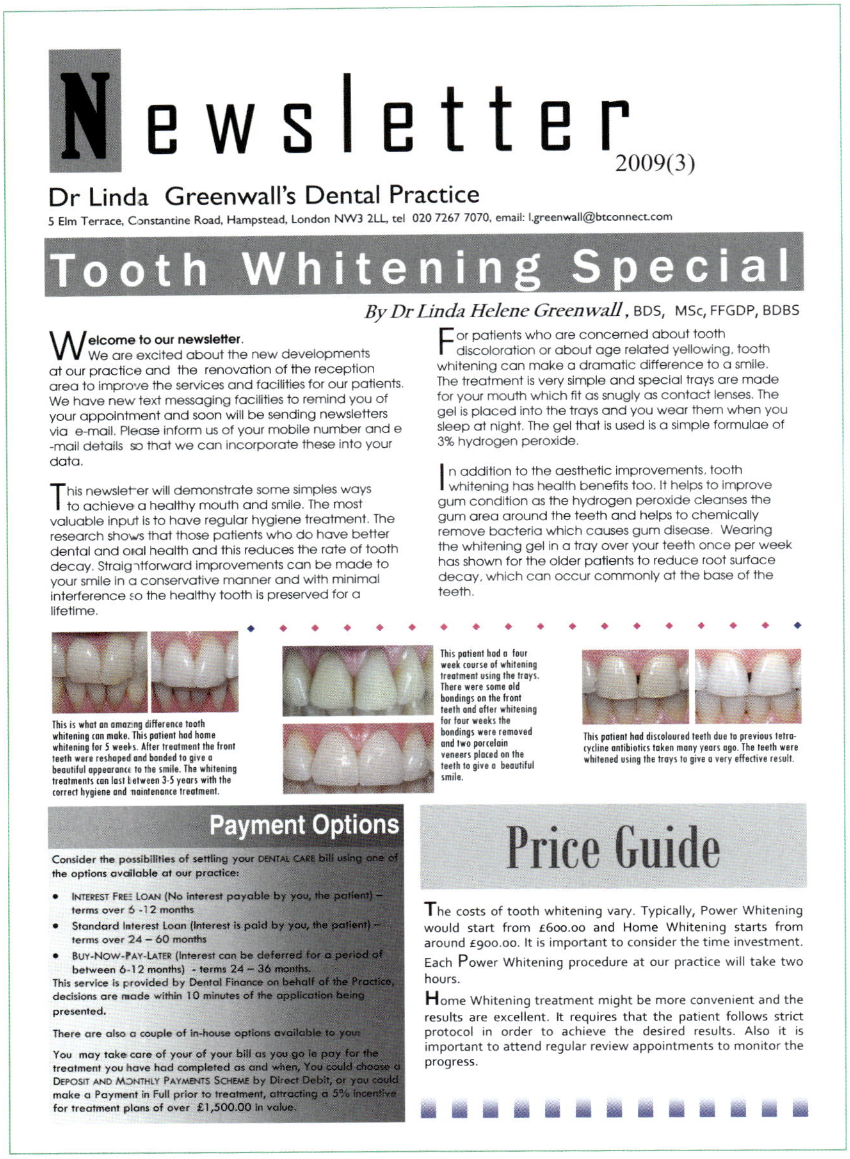

Newsletter 2009(3)

Dr Linda Greenwall's Dental Practice

5 Elm Terrace, Constantine Road, Hampstead, London NW3 2LL, tel 020 7267 7070, email: l.greenwall@btconnect.com

Tooth Whitening Special

By Dr Linda Helene Greenwall, BDS, MSc, FFGDP, BDBS

Welcome to our newsletter. We are excited about the new developments at our practice and the renovation of the reception area to improve the services and facilities for our patients. We have new text messaging facilities to remind you of your appointment and soon will be sending newsletters via e-mail. Please inform us of your mobile number and e-mail details so that we can incorporate these into your data.

This newsletter will demonstrate some simples ways to achieve a healthy mouth and smile. The most valuable input is to have regular hygiene treatment. The research shows that those patients who do have better dental and oral health and this reduces the rate of tooth decay. Straightforward improvements can be made to your smile in a conservative manner and with minimal interference so the healthy tooth is preserved for a lifetime.

For patients who are concerned about tooth discoloration or about age related yellowing, tooth whitening can make a dramatic difference to a smile. The treatment is very simple and special trays are made for your mouth which fit as snugly as contact lenses. The gel is placed into the trays and you wear them when you sleep at night. The gel that is used is a simple formulae of 3% hydrogen peroxide.

In addition to the aesthetic improvements, tooth whitening has health benefits too. It helps to improve gum condition as the hydrogen peroxide cleanses the gum area around the teeth and helps to chemically remove bacteria which causes gum disease. Wearing the whitening gel in a tray over your teeth once per week has shown for the older patients to reduce root surface decay, which can occur commonly at the base of the teeth.

This is what an amazing difference tooth whitening can make. This patient had home whitening for 5 weeks. After treatment the front teeth were reshaped and bonded to give a beautiful appearance to the smile. The whitening treatments can last between 3-5 years with the correct hygiene and maintenance treatment.

This patient had a four week course of whitening treatment using the trays. There were some old bondings on the front teeth and after whitening for four weeks the bondings were removed and two porcelain veneers placed on the teeth to give a beautiful smile.

This patient had discoloured teeth due to previous tetracycline antibiotics taken many years ago. The teeth were whitened using the trays to give a very effective result.

Payment Options

Consider the possibilities of settling your DENTAL CARE bill using one of the options available at our practice:

- INTEREST FREE LOAN (No interest payable by you, the patient) – terms over 6 -12 months
- Standard Interest Loan (Interest is paid by you, the patient) – terms over 24 – 60 months
- BUY-NOW-PAY-LATER (Interest can be deferred for a period of between 6-12 months) - terms 24 – 36 months.

This service is provided by Dental Finance on behalf of the Practice, decisions are made within 10 minutes of the application being presented.

There are also a couple of in-house options available to you:

You may take care of your of your bill as you go ie pay for the treatment you have had completed as and when, You could choose a DEPOSIT AND MONTHLY PAYMENTS SCHEME by Direct Debit, or you could make a Payment in Full prior to treatment, attracting a 5% incentive for treatment plans of over £1,500.00 in value.

Price Guide

The costs of tooth whitening vary. Typically, Power Whitening would start from £600.00 and Home Whitening starts from around £900.00. It is important to consider the time investment.

Each Power Whitening procedure at our practice will take two hours.

Home Whitening treatment might be more convenient and the results are excellent. It requires that the patient follows strict protocol in order to achieve the desired results. Also it is important to attend regular review appointments to monitor the progress.

Fig 14-2a Whitening newsletter that was sent to all patients with a seasonal time-activated special offer to motivate the patient into taking action to get their teeth whitened.

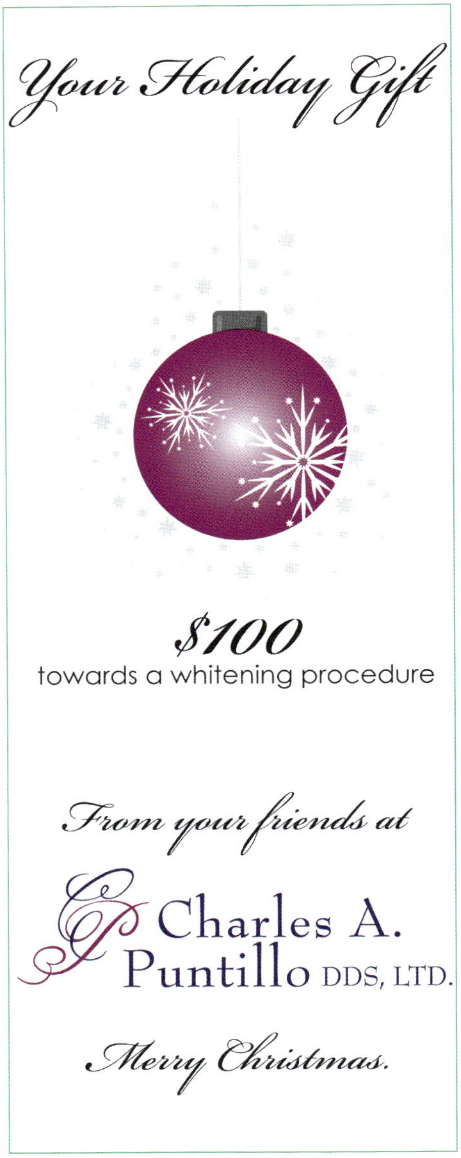

Fig 14-2b Example of a whitening advertisement sent to patients.

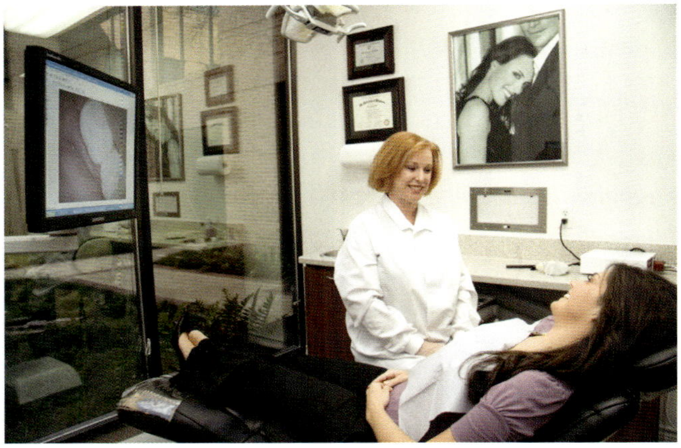

Fig 14-3 Change the photographs and feature a different procedure every 3 to 6 months. Alternatively, change the photographs from one area of the office to another. Be sure these are professional, quality photographs. Have them matted and framed. Remember, everything in your office needs to send the same message, one of aesthetic excellence. Either black and white or color photographs are appropriate. The décor of your office may dictate which would be best.

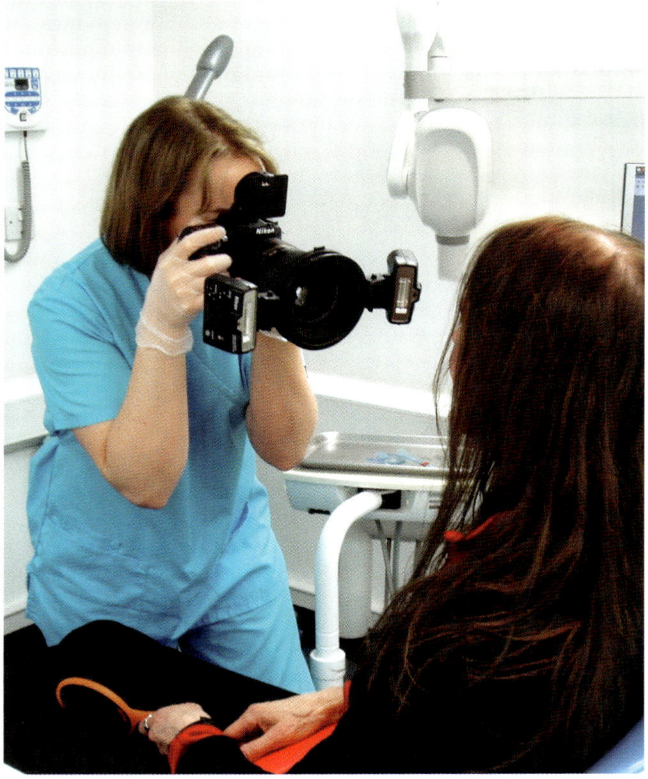

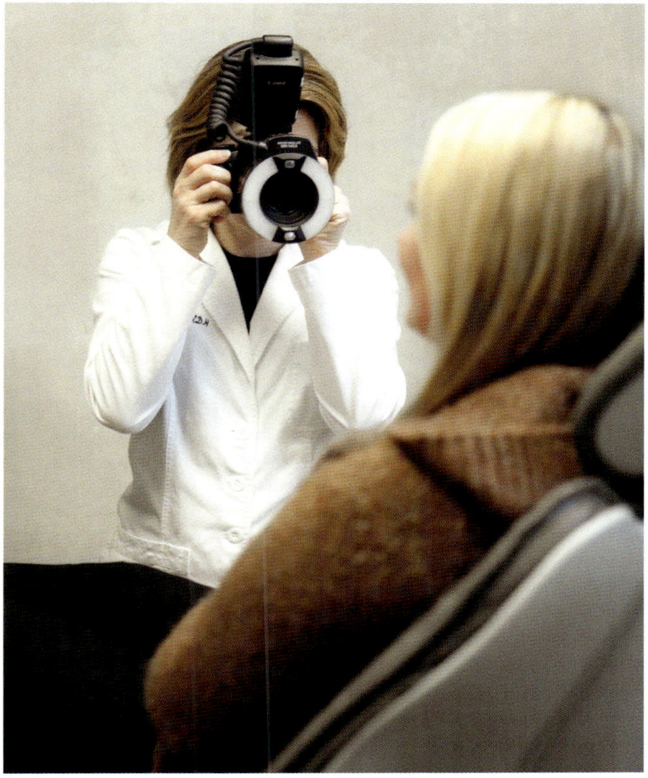

Figs 14-4a and 14-4b These figures illustrate hygienists taking photos to demonstrate to the patient the situation in their mouth and the shade of the teeth prior to whitening. Note: If wearing gloves while taking photographs, always use fresh clean ones.

3. Frame photographs

Matte and frame beautiful photographs of an aesthetic case. Place these in the hygienic treatment room and change them regularly (Fig 14-3). Make sure brochures are kept in a drawer or cabinet away from aerosol spray. The exposure of these beautiful smiles to hygiene patients will stimulate interest. If a patient doesn't mention the photographs, ask questions such as, "Did you notice these new photographs of some of our patients? So many people want to have this kind of beautiful smile but weren't even aware that this type of treatment was possible. Is there anything you would like to change about your smile?" Open the door for conversation by asking questions and then listen.

4. Take photographs

Use the intraoral or digital camera constantly (Fig 14-4). While the hygienist may think she doesn't have time to use the camera or to retrieve and view historically taken photographs, if this is a mandatory part of every appointment, it can be arranged. Organize your hygiene appointments to include the taking or review of photographs (Fig 14-5) showing:

- dentistry diagnosed but incomplete
- new areas of concern since the last appointment

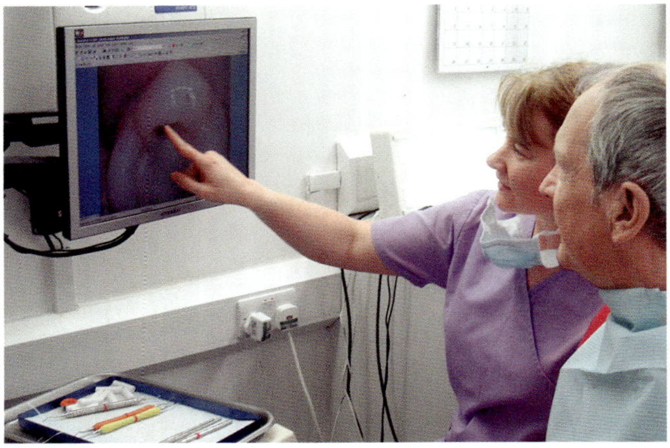

Fig 14-5a Use digital photographs to demonstrate to a patient the situation in their mouth.

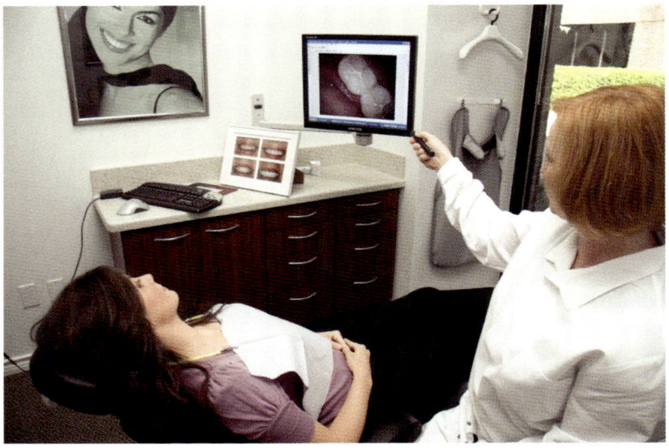

Fig 14-5b The hygienist showing a photograph from the intraoral camera to demonstrate a problem with an existing restoration.

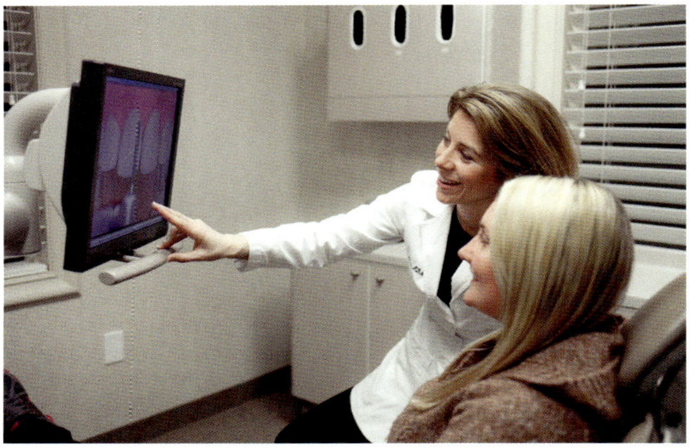

Fig 14-5c The hygienist can point out new areas of concern since the last appointment and show the patient about possible smile changes through aesthetic alteration.

- periodontal concerns
- areas where advanced restorative care would be beneficial
- views that show their present smile, to talk about (or show them) what can be done through aesthetic alteration.

Your cameras and photography are your most important diagnostic and educational tools. Get the camera out of the cabinet and use it on almost every patient almost every day.

When you start taking photographs to illustrate cosmetic possibilities to your hygiene (or restorative) patients, tell the patients that you have a new diagnostic tool in your dental practice for the purpose of taking even better care of the patients and so that you can let them know what is going on in dentistry today.

Refer to the smile evaluation form that the patient has completed and make special note of areas for potential treatment or smile enhancement that they may have indicated. This will give you additional guidelines for photographs that would be appropriate to take and show.

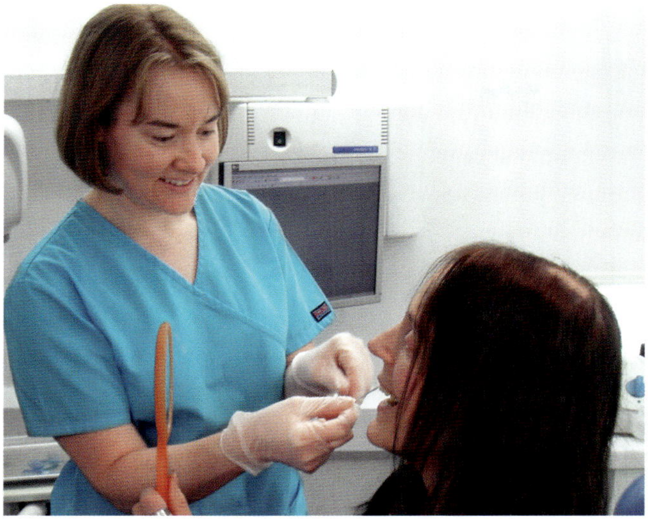

Fig 14-6 The hygienist participating in the bleaching procedure by taking the shade of the patient's teeth. This can stimulate an aesthetic discussion about tooth shade and tooth lightness.

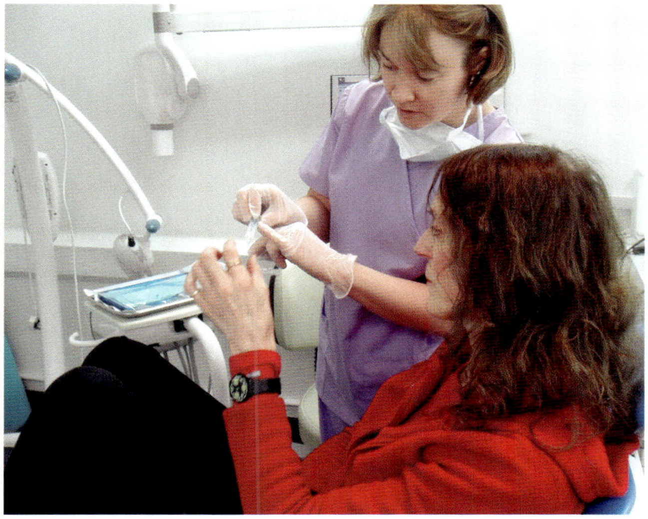

Fig 14-7 The hygienist explaining the home bleaching method of whitening to the patient by demonstrating the amount of gel to use in the trays. It is essential that the hygienist spends time with the patient to demonstrate exactly how much gel to use and where to place the gel in the bleaching tray. Patients should have written instructions as well. However, the best method for patients is actually showing them their own bleaching tray and how to use it.

Then, take a photograph of the patient's maxillary teeth. Ask what they like most about the teeth in the upper area. What do they like least? If they could change anything about the teeth in the upper part of their mouth, what would they change?

Next, shift to a photograph of the mandibular teeth and ask the same questions. A photograph from the lateral views will stimulate unbelievable interest. People are not used to seeing their teeth from the side. Give them a look at this view and listen carefully to their questions. They will begin asking about cosmetic changes. Adding the lateral views to your photographs will lead to an increase in both anterior and posterior aesthetics (see Fig 14-4). In addition, the hygienist can take the existing shade of the patient's teeth (Fig 14-6). This can stimulate a discussion about the color of teeth and whether they are happy with their existing shade or whether they might like to have the teeth whiter. If the legislation permits it, the suitably trained hygienist can conduct and manage the bleaching programs within the dental practice. The hygienist can explain the home bleaching process to the patient and go through the consent forms and paperwork prior to commencing treatment. The hygienist can demonstrate to patients how to place the bleaching gel (Fig 14-7) in the tray and how to use it, whether this is for night time or day use.

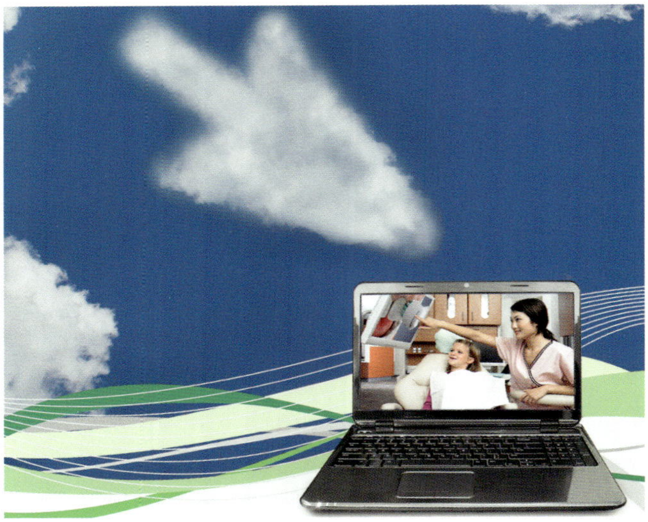

Fig 14-8a Digital patient education.

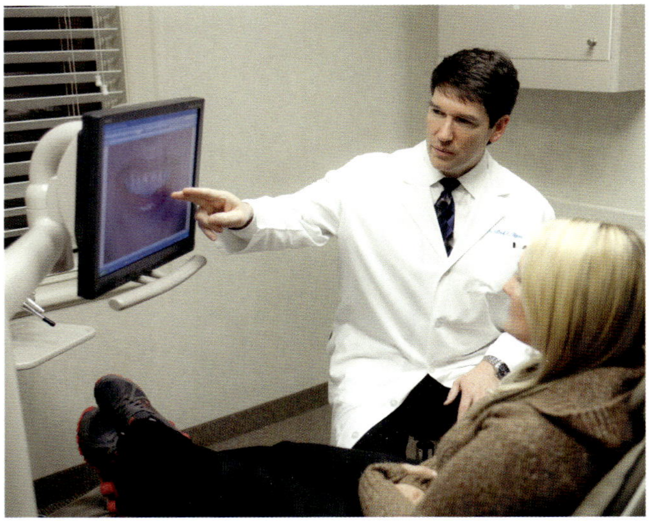

Fig 14-8b Dr Hyman using patient education programming to visually illustrate his recommendations.

5. Digital education programs

Digital patient education systems are a great way to show patients what is available in dentistry. This can stimulate questions and interest. They can be used chairside by any of the clinicians to provide additional visual education or to introduce dental/aesthetic possibilities. These systems can be placed in the reception area and can play in an ongoing manner. They can be placed in the consultation area for back-up support of your recommendations.

These programs are patient friendly and very accurate. Since approximately 83% of learning takes place visually, you will save time and get better results if you use visual aids to support your presentation or to answer questions (Fig 14-8).

These are five powerful ways for the hygienist to be an educator about cosmetic dentistry. Set a goal to develop this exciting part of your dental practice. Accept the role and responsibility to be an educator about the new and wonderful services related to cosmetic dentistry. You will love the results, your patients will be happy dental patients, and your dental practice will thrive. That makes for a fulfilling and rewarding environment.

The hygienist's role in promoting dentistry

Ask yourself this question: "How much dentistry do you have sitting in your charts waiting to be done?" You may believe that you have more dentistry sitting in your charts waiting to be done, than you have ever done in your practicing life.

This doesn't mean that you have done anything wrong or are not doing a good job. It means you have an amazing opportunity to get the dentistry out of the charts and into the mouths of the patients. Most dental practices can double their production by nurturing that which they already have: their existing patient family. Supporting this kind of educational process in the hygienic area can make all the difference. Hygienists, in most countries and states, can participate in numerous procedures, such as tooth whitening or bleaching. They are not only educators of this excellent procedure but can participate in parts of the procedure itself (see Fig 14-6).

As noted in Chapter 3 on Critical Factors of the Business of Dentistry, set a goal of having 40 to 60% of your restorative or aesthetic dentistry coming right out of the hygiene area. In order for that to happen, you have to give the hygienist the time, training, equipment, and trust to carry out the educational processes, including the photography.

Patients have a very special relationship with their hygienist. He/she helps them to get healthy and stay healthy, plus she helps to insure the health of any restorations they may have already received. She listens to them as they express their joys and concerns. Patients see the hygienist as a concerned "third-party" and develop a very personal and trusting relationship with him/her. As we discussed in the chapter on case presentation, a patient will never purchase your product or service if there is not a level of trust and confidence. The hygienist has the trust and confidence of the patients.

This is not to infer that the patient doesn't have a similar level of trust and confidence with the other members of the team, including the dentist. However, there is a continuous interaction that is healthy, gentle, supportive, and informative between the hygienist and the patient. Plus, she/he usually interacts with the patient more than anyone else does. Familiarity leads to comfort.

The hygiene system: an educational system

The success of your dental practice is in direct proportion to the success of your systems. Synonyms for the word "system" are organization, arrangement, structure, coordination, method, and orderliness. Consider the value and benefit of having systems in your dental practice that epitomize those words. This makes good sense.

Your hygiene systems need to be organized in such a way as to provide for excellent care and to provide time and armamentarium for the hygienists to educate patients on any dentistry diagnosed, but incomplete, areas of concern, and new opportunities for improved health or appearance.

Go through each of your hygiene appointment types: adult prophylaxis, child prophylaxis, all the periodontal appointments, sealants, tooth whitening/bleaching: whatever type of appointments that are handled in your hygienic department. Analyze each appointment type to determine what is being done, how long each aspect of the appointment takes, and the total time needed to provide an "ideal" appointment without compromise. Indicate how much time would be needed to include education in the appointment. As you go through each appointment, look for areas where you could be more efficient and more effective, always paying close attention to time management. Add in time for the inclusion of taking and reviewing photography. Determine how you will incorporate visual aids (including video dentistry) into each and every appointment in order to get the dentistry out of the charts and into the mouths of your patients. Make sure that each hygienist is supporting the system in the same manner. Certainly, they can individualize their interaction with patients, but the system needs to be consistent.

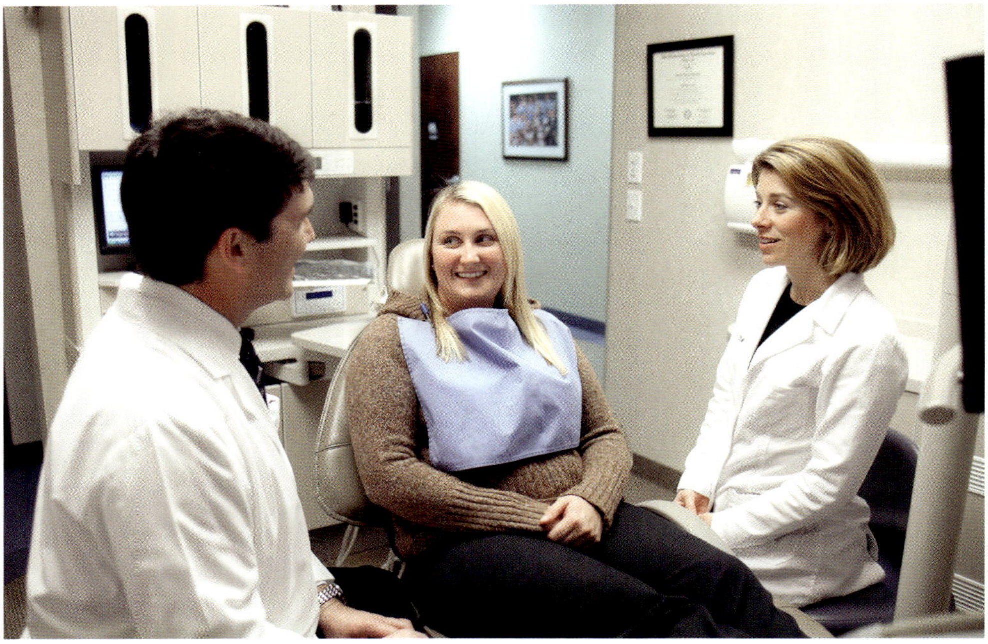

Fig 14-9 The periodic hygienic appointment which includes the dentist's periodic oral evaluation. This is an excellent time to evaluate, motivate, and activate a patient toward comprehensive and aesthetic care.

Include time and space in each appointment for patient education about home therapy or co-therapy and new opportunities for treatment. "How much time will this take?" you may be asking. Do a time-in-motion study. See how much time you need, on average, to provide a good service. This would be the appropriate amount of time to include in each appointment. This procedure should be written down for each hygiene appointment (Fig 14-9). Take a photo of the tray set-up to be included in the procedure manual for the training and education of the hygienist and whole team. Each procedure is documented for a time allocation and consistency.

When you add up the time that you need for the ideal appointment, you may be stunned to find that you need more time than is being scheduled at present. If so, ask yourselves, "Would we give up one hygiene appointment per day to give our hygienist more time per appointment, if this time were dedicated to patient education?" Put a pencil to it. Consider giving your hygienists the freedom and the respect to schedule the appropriate time for each patient. If you dedicate more time for the hygienist to introduce or educate patients about opportunities, this becomes more than a suggestion on the part of the dentist: it becomes a required part of the appointment, just like necessary radiographs.

In addition to the increased revenue, your patients will be better served. You wouldn't diagnose something unless a patient needed or wanted it. So, if a patient walks out your door not proceeding with treatment, both you and the patient lose. You would be able to do more of the kind of dentistry you believe in, and your patients would be healthier and/or more beautiful, or both.

Once you have outlined what you consider "the ideal" for each type of hygiene appointment and you have determined the time you need to add education to your hygiene appointments, begin developing the system of education that you wish to incorporate into your dental practice.

Repetition is the key to learning. So, just because someone has heard something once doesn't mean that they will "get it" or that they will "buy into" the proposal. Repetition not only answers questions, but also solidifies the benefits of the proposal. All behavior is driven by "what's in this for me?" So, it becomes essential that you focus your repeated conversations and presentations about treatment recommendations on the benefits and end results of treatment. Be sure to outline and "show" the person how your recommendations will enhance their health or their appearance, or both. Stress the end results of treatment. Do not hesitate to point out any risks that might occur if a person fails to schedule an appointment or even thinks about canceling their appointment.

Example of the hygienist's role as educator

For example, let's say that a patient has come to your dental practice for a comprehensive oral evaluation. The dentist diagnosed caries in two different quadrants and recommended that the patient have the carious lesions removed and then the teeth restored with resin composite restorations.

The patient comes to the office for a hygiene appointment and it is noted (during the morning meeting) that the patient has dentistry diagnosed but, at this time, incomplete. The patient proceeded with one quadrant but not the second one. The hygienist shows the patient a photograph of the area that has already been treated. She shows the patient what the teeth looked like prior to and following treatment.

Then, the hygienist goes to the next area of necessary treatment and takes or retrieves a photograph of this area. She then shows the patient the next area to be treated. She addresses the patient in the following manner: "Mrs Jones, this is a photograph of the upper left area of your mouth that the dentist evaluated at your last appointment. He has asked that I retake a photograph and radiograph of the decayed area that has not been restored yet to see if further deterioration has occurred. He will re-evaluate that area when he comes in for his exam today."

Dentist performing hygiene evaluation

One of the most important appointments you provide for your patients is the periodic oral evaluation performed during the hygiene appointment. During this appointment, you have the opportunity to diagnose and recommend treatment on new areas of concern, reinforce the importance of proceeding with the next phase of diagnosed dentistry that has not been completed, and introduce people to new options, like aesthetic changes. In addition, the dentist can support the hygienist in his/her efforts to get a patient healthy and keep them healthy (Fig 14-10). Make sure that you give the time and attention that is necessary for a patient to understand the value of proceeding.

Below is an example of communication between the dentist and hygienist (this conversation follows social graces).

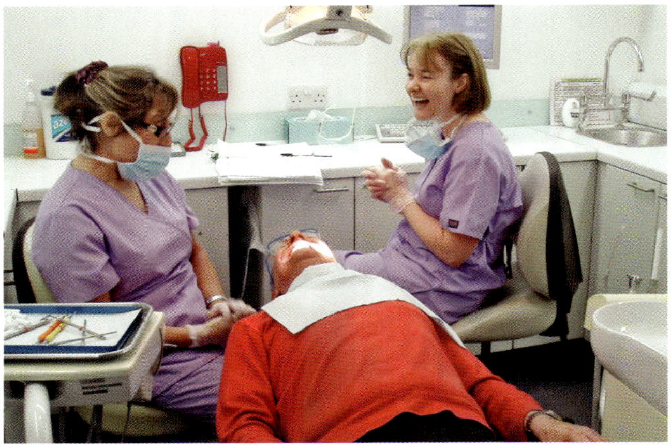

Fig 14-10a The dentist and the hygienist together with patient in the hygienic area. Cross linking communication with the hygienist and dentist.

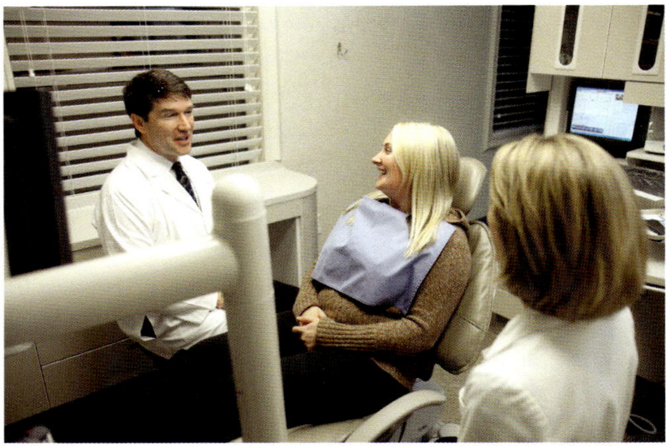

Fig 14-10b The periodic oral evaluation is a critical time of interaction between the patient, the hygienist and the dentist. Here any necessary treatment is re-evaluated and reinforced. Re-education takes place. New aesthetic and restorative opportunities can be introduced and revisited. Do not compromise this valuable time with your patients. Here Dr Hyman and his hygienist discuss treatment benefits with their patient.

Dentist: "Mary, is there anything you would like to bring to my attention about Mrs Jones?"
Hygienist: "Yes, Dr Greenwall. The last time you saw Mrs Jones you indicated a concern about two teeth in the upper left area of her mouth. You discovered decay in those teeth and recommended that we remove that decay and restore those teeth to health again before the decay progressed. She has not received that treatment at this point. So, at your request, I have taken photographs and a radiograph of those two teeth so that you can re-evaluate the situation."
Dentist: "Thank you, Mary. Yes, I do want to see those photographs and radiographs and will see what is happening at this time."

From there, the dentist will re-evaluate, re-educate, and re-motivate the patient to, hopefully, proceed with the needed care.

When the dentist leaves, the hygienist can provide third-party support.

Hygienist: "Mrs Jones, as Dr Greenwall indicated, you have two teeth that have decay in this area. Let me show you. We need to schedule an appointment, so you can have the decay removed from these two teeth and so that they can be restored to health again. Putting this necessary treatment off is difficult. It isn't going to get any better and you risk the decay getting much worse and the needed treatment being more extensive. What questions do you have that I might answer for you?"

A patient-education video could be shown here for back-up support.

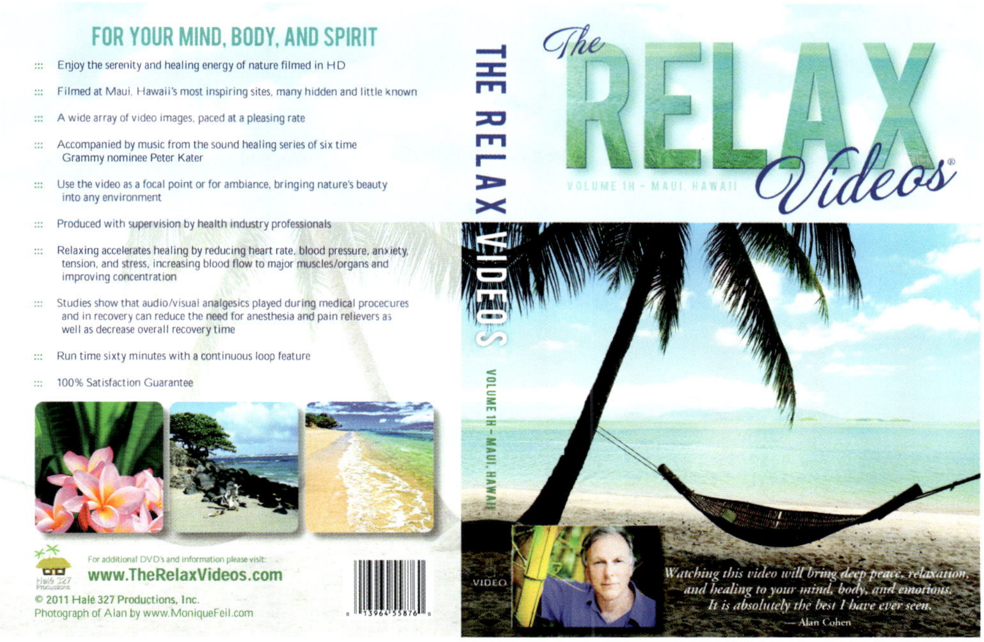

Fig 14-11 Creating a relaxing environment, using both auditory and visual aids, calms the patient and promotes healing. This video series, The Relax Videos, were produced for the purpose of supporting a healing environment.

Have patient education programming in your hygiene rooms. Turn the TVs off that are showing negative news, "soap operas," or other interfering messages. The patients are there for the purpose of dentistry. If you are going to have your TV monitors playing during an appointment, play messages regarding beautiful smiles. It is irritating to have multiple sources of "noise" coming from every direction: music, TVs, videos, etc. Try to calm the patient, not irritate the patient. Creator and producer Dee Winn has developed a video series entitled Relax Videos (Fig 14-11). These can be played as a calming interlude between your patient education programming.

The hygiene system: retention

Coordinating your hygiene retention program with your aesthetic marketing program can be beneficial: (1) you may be able to motivate patients who otherwise have lapsed in their hygiene program, and (2) you may be able to stimulate interest in your aesthetic procedures.

The hygiene retention system in your dental practice is vital to the health and well-being of both your patients and your dental practice. The retention program should be so well defined and administered that patients become involved with your hygiene program and stay that way. This will stop patients from falling through the cracks. Not only do you maintain patients' health in this environment, but you can also introduce them to the latest and best in dentistry, including new and exciting aesthetic opportunities.

It is best to schedule patients for a dental appointment when they are face to face with you. However, if someone doesn't schedule an appointment, or if they fail to attend an appointment and do not reschedule, then you need to make every effort to contact them to reserve an appointment. If you have made regular, carefully orchestrated contacts, both written and over the phone to patients but they have not scheduled, then you may need to take a different approach.

If a patient has not responded positively to scheduling a hygiene appointment, try to "ring their bell" by offering another service like aesthetics. Send a great letter or special notice along with a beautiful brochure to all past due hygiene patients. Introduce the "new" procedure to them in this mailing.

Then, make a follow-up telephone call to answer any questions, and to see if they are interested in "whitening their smile" (or whatever you have introduced).

Appointment coordinator: "Mrs Jones, a couple of weeks ago I sent you a notice regarding your appointment with our hygienist, Dru, for your professional dental cleaning and oral health evaluation. At the same time, I sent you a brochure about a new procedure we are offering in our dental practice: smile enhancement through tooth whitening. Did you receive that information? ... Do you have any questions? ... Is this something that would be of interest to you?"

During your morning meetings or as you audit your charts, pay special attention to your health history questions, smile evaluation forms, or special questionnaires regarding aesthetics. If anyone has alluded to any interest in cosmetic/aesthetic change, speak to them while they are in the dental practice or make note of this during any hygiene retention telephone call or written piece. Make sure that people know you are listening to them and make sure that you walk through any door that a patient has opened for you.

Keep careful records of all contacts made with a patient, including telephone calls and specifics about letters, etc., that have been mailed. It will be imperative that you know what information a patient has given to you, what their interests may be, and if a follow-up call has been promised.

Action steps

1. Make sure that your hygiene retention program is established and working well. Remember your goal needs to be 85 to 90% of your active patient family involved in hygiene.
2. Analyze the various types of hygiene appointments. Determine if you can refine those appointments to make them more efficient in terms of time and motion.
3. Establish a protocol for looking at each patient to determine if they have treatment that could be provided beyond today. Spend time educating them about the next area of potential treatment, including aesthetic opportunities.
4. Use patient education programs in the hygiene department.
5. Use the five suggested methodologies to market aesthetics to your existing patients as they flow through the hygiene area.

15 The Use of Technology in Building the Aesthetic Aspect of a Dental Practice

Cathy Jameson, Linda Greenwall, and John Jameson

> *What is high tech? Future advancement, innovations, progress—control. What is high touch? Embracing that which acknowledges all that is greater than we.*
>
> *John Naisbitt (1999)*

A digital world

- *"Yes. We have an intraoral camera system but we don't use it very much. We don't seem to have time to use it."*
- *"We've considered digital radiographs, but we're so used to the old way we just haven't made the upgrade yet."*
- *"I haven't been able to do much patient education at the chair because I haven't put clinical work stations into the practice."*

Dental practices around the world make statements like these every day about the technology they want, or worse, the systems they have already bought. When it comes to the technology you want or the technology already available in your dental practice, ask yourself a question: "What is your goal for having a system in your dental practice?" Does your answer sound something like, "We want patients to see what they need, so that they will go ahead with treatment. We thought the system would help us to generate more case acceptance. We don't seem to have the time to use it."

Take a look at the technology that you use in your dental practice. The dental practice computers, printer or phone with built-in fax machine, the Internet connection, email-capable computers and texting ability all rely on technology. Technology improves communication, which has an impact on

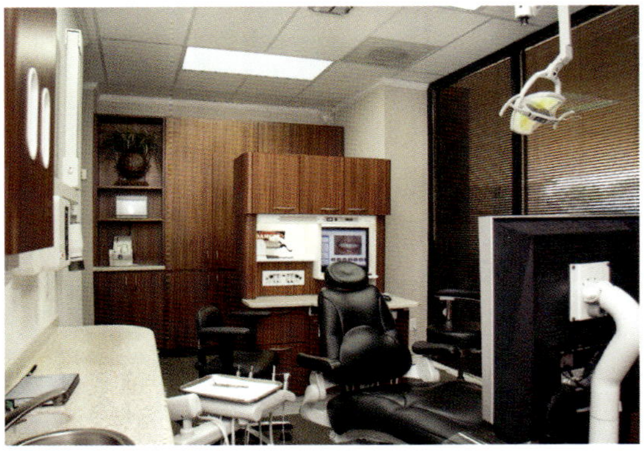

Fig 15-1 Treatment rooms need to be comprehensively and equally equipped.

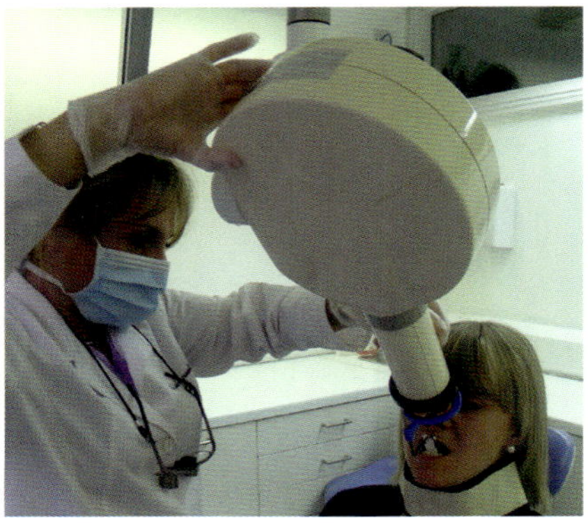

Fig 15-2 Using digital radiography with a beam aiming device for accuracy of periapical radiographs (procedure according to recommended practice by the National Radiological Protection Board [Rout and Brown, 2012]). The digital radiographs are then scanned on a processor and appear on the computer monitor within a few seconds. This assists with instant diagnosis and interpretation of findings on the screen.

the efficiency and productivity of your dental practice. Each new technological invention improves patient communication and service and speed of communication. Without these communication technologies, your patients' experiences suffer.

It is essential to take advantage of technology in building the aesthetic aspect of your dental practice. This will give your patient a complete experience. Proper use of high-tech equipment will accelerate your level of care, your ability to diagnose and plan treatments, and your ability to access a higher rate of treatment acceptance. Your dental practice must use this equipment extensively, every day. With the advancement of computers and digital technology, the ability to gather, save, view, analyze, and display images has developed enough to become a central operation of the dental practice.

Considering the increase in the number of adult patients, you must educate your patients about this high-tech aspect of your dental practice in order to maximize your market share. These visual tools will give your patients an incredibly informative, thorough, life-changing experience, where they understand the benefits of your treatment recommendations and accept your treatment plans. Figure 15-1 shows a technologically advanced dental operatory.

This chapter will discuss aesthetic technologies, primarily intraoral or extraoral digital photography, imaging, and digital radiography, though there are many tools that enhance the visual experience for your patients and you must determine the tools that are right for your dental practice. Consider how you use this equipment, how you integrate the equipment into your appointments and into your days, and how you make the equipment not only pay for itself but also become a profit center for the dental practice.

Diagnostic technology used in aesthetic dentistry includes:

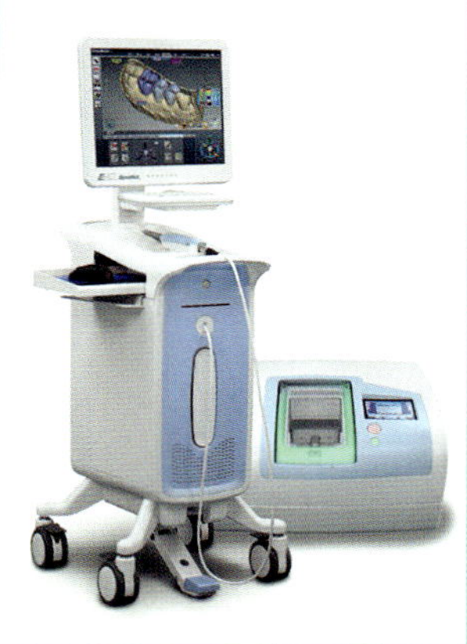

Fig 15-3 CAD/CAM (computer-aided design/computer-assisted manufacture) technology.

1. Intraoral cameras.
2. Extraoral digital cameras.
3. Digital radiography: intraoral (Fig 15-2) and panoramic radiography.
4. CT (computerized tomography) scanning devices. Specially designed CBCT (cone beam CT) scanners can be used in dentistry, which produce adequate imaging with approximately a tenfold reduction in radiation. The cone beam reduces the amount of radiation to the patient. This provides multiple images of the bony structures of the skull so that a three-dimensional (3D) picture can be assessed for the quantity and quality of bone.
5. Digital data scanners CAD/CAM (computer-aided design/computer-assisted manufacture) technology for scanning teeth (Figs 15-3 and 15-4) without the need for a dental impression in a tray and manufacture of indirect restorations.
6. Computerized ceramic restoration fabrication. A 3D computer-aided modeling system (eg, Cerec, Sirona, Bensheim, Germany) records information directly from the tooth and sends it to a milling machine, where the ceramic tooth is fabricated, allowing restoration in a single visit.
7. Magnification: operating microscopes (Figs 15-5 and 15-6) and dental magnification loupes (Fig 15-7) mounted on eye glasses with optional light attachments for better visualization and clinical procedures.

Organization and storage of visual data

As the development of image-based technologies becomes a priority in your dental practice, it is imperative to develop a structure for storage of the data. It is important to be able to capture, store, and retrieve images with great speed. Select a storage format that provides this ability to store and retrieve images quickly. The most common formats used today are digital storage systems. These may involve the use of a CPU (central processing unit), and/or a central server or "cloud" based system to store images. The system must be able to handle a very large volume of data, larger than web-based systems are able to handle at this time. Your hardware must be in-house, but it can take several forms:

- If the dental practice is using a cart system for camera use, the CPU can be located on the cart. Image storage software is used to organize the captured images in individual patient files. This alteration often necessitates the change of monitors and printers.
- If the dental practice has an existing analogue network system, storage can be achieved by placing the CPU in a remote area and capturing and retrieving images there. Again, when making this change, monitors and printers may need to be changed, or wiring altered to create a functional system. One disadvantage of this system is that only one individual can capture or retrieve images at a time.
- In dental practices where clinical computer work stations exist that have CPUs equipped with capture boards or can accept images directly into the management software for storage in the patient's file, images can be captured and stored in the computer network, usually in the server of the dental practice.

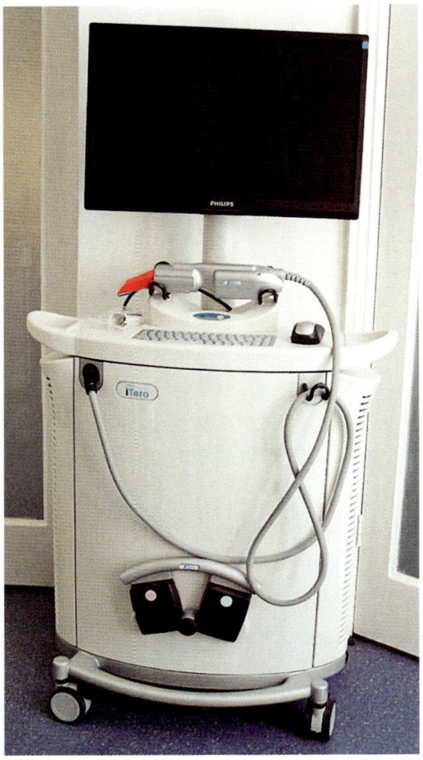

Fig 15-4a Using the intraoral digital scanner will reduce the need for impression taking using trays and impression material. Once the dentist has been trained in using the scanner to record the prepared teeth, this will improve accuracy and speed. The scanner transfers the information via the internet directly to the dental laboratory in order to save time. The picture shows the Cadent iTero scanner (Cadent, Carlstadt, NJ).

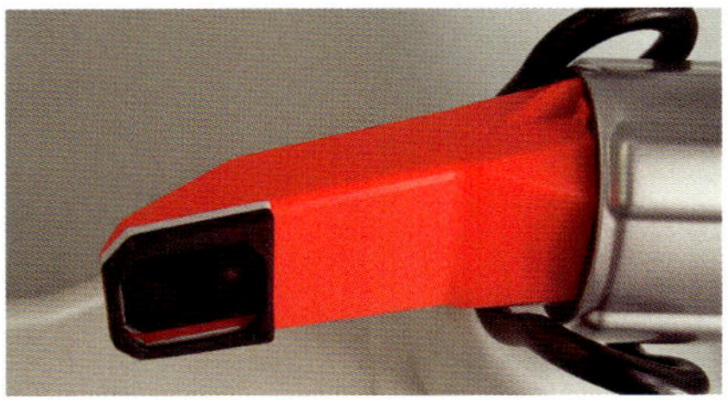

Fig 15-4b The scanner head in close up view. The black part of the head needs to be positioned directly over the tooth and recorded in three dimensions.

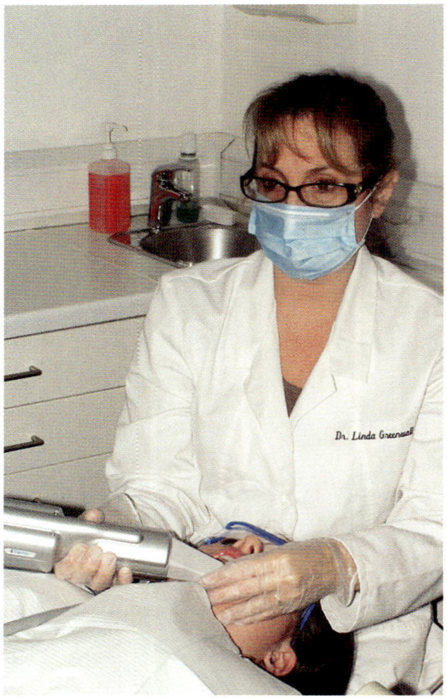

Fig 15-4c The scanner being used clinically. As with all technology, it is essential that further training is undertaken to ensure the best use and full capabilities of the technology.

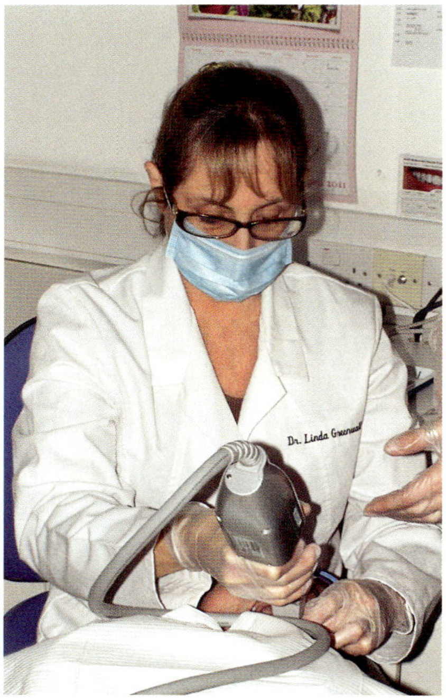

Fig 15-4d Careful positioning of the intraoral scanner is essential.

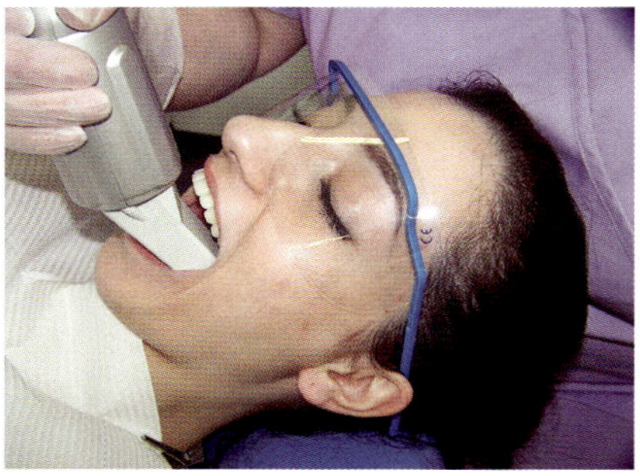

Fig 15-4e The scanner head being placed in the patient's mouth, ready to commence the scanning process.

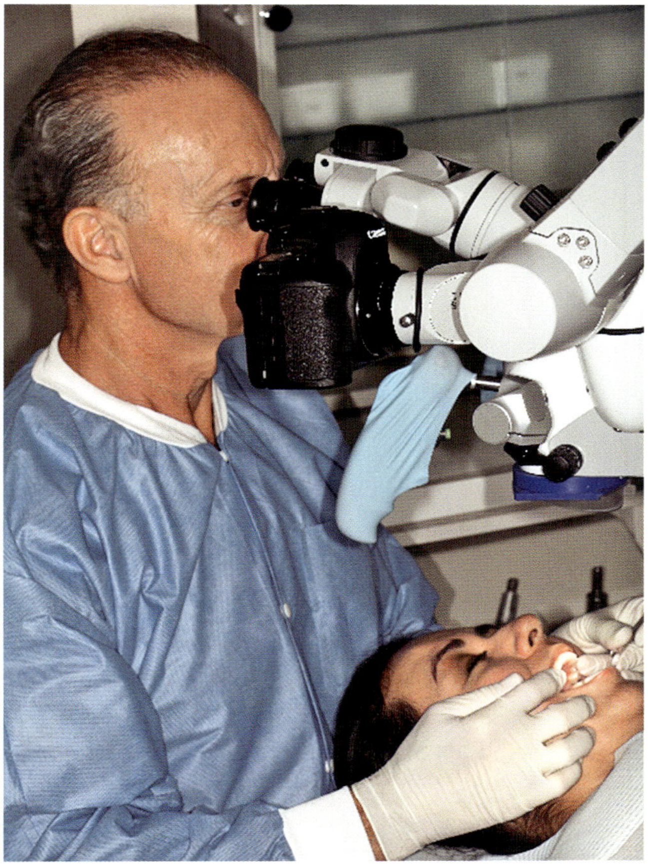

Fig 15-5 Dr Larry Rifkin using the microscope for aesthetic clinical procedures. He has an attachment for the digital camera that fits onto the microscope in order to record clinical procedures. The microscope also has the ability to record videos. This is useful for teaching and for showing to patients.

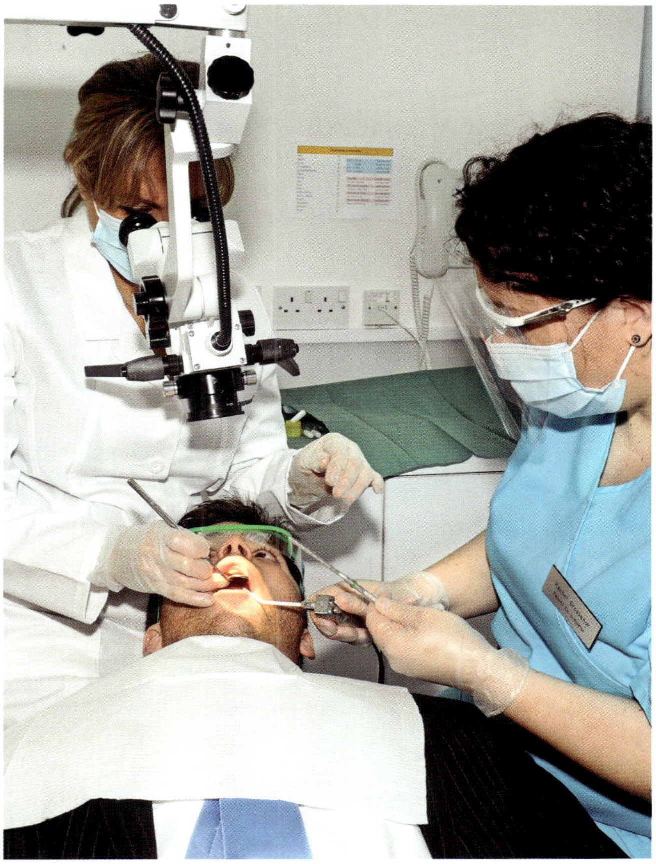

Fig 15-6 Using the operating microscope for aesthetic dentistry procedures improves the quality of the restoration as better visualization is possible. This helps especially when finishing off margins of veneer preparations and the polishing of anterior direct resin composite bondings.

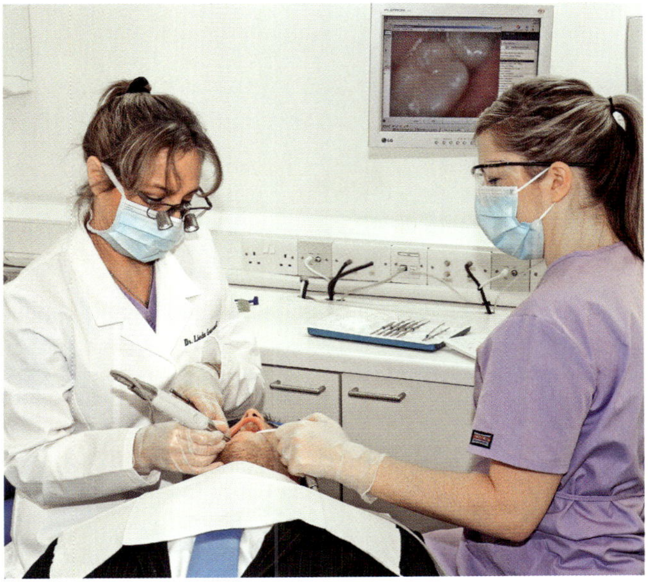

Fig 15-7 The use of dental loupes for magnification is an essential tool for all aesthetic dentists who want to improve their clinical procedures and diagnosis of problems intraorally.

In all cases, special attention should be paid to the software you use to organize and track your patients. Technology has given you the ability to forgo a considerable amount of paper filing, which saves time and money. Choose the software that fulfills your requirements. However, do not neglect to professionally train yourself and your dental team in the proper use of the program. Additionally, wise dental practices will insure their data against loss by using a data backup system (hard disk backup) and off site (or cloud) backup.

The importance of determining the appropriate data storage solution cannot be overstated. Images require large volumes of memory, and systems must be able to retrieve and display high-quality images quickly. People learn visually, and you must be able to recall your patients' images at any moment, showing them their condition and creating a sense of urgency. If your system does not allow for storage and recall of images, and only allows an immediate view of the data, you are not taking full advantage of your tools.

Integrating technology into your dental practice

Purchase aesthetic technologies for the following reasons:

- better diagnostic ability
- better visualization for the patient
- better educational capability for the patient and the dental team
- greater acceptance of treatment recommendations.

This will result in more productivity. The challenge becomes how to integrate your technological systems into every aspect of your dental practice so that everyone benefits, from patient to team member to dentist.

Intraoral camera systems

Ideally, those dental practices that use intraoral cameras adhere to a specific plan to image every patient. Both new and returning patients can benefit from having a visual record of the condition of their teeth from visit to visit. Furthermore, you can specifically document any prior restorations and monitor your patient's condition to prevent future problems. For many patients, seeing their own teeth the way you do is an eye-opening experience. It is essential to take advantage of this educational opportunity.

Proper use of an intraoral camera system demands a significant amount of digital storage. Additionally, those who use a cart system, instead of multiple workstations linked to a server, must coordinate the use of the intraoral camera equipment at each morning meeting. Aesthetic technology should give the patient a feeling of efficient, personalized service, so any waiting should be minimized.

Intraoral camera systems range in price from $6,000 to $35,000 US. Lease/purchase agreements can be arranged that help to make the investment comfortable and affordable. If you integrate the system into your dental practice by appropriately using the camera on each patient, your system will not only pay for itself, but will become a profit center within your dental practice. However, if you buy a system and let it sit in a corner and gather dust, it will be a cost, not an investment.

Study the different systems. Make a decision about the purchase of a system. Then, as a team, determine the ways in which you will use the system.

Extraoral digital photography

The use of extraoral digital cameras with lenses and flash systems appropriate for obtaining excellent dental images is now state of the art. This system is a great add on to intraoral cameras in creating an image library to move the patient to the next level of understanding.

At this time, there are some great cameras on the market. An example of these are the latest Nikon Digital SLR (eg, Nikon D9000) or the latest Canon Digital SLR (eg, 60D). The digital photographs taken must be clear. This allows for excellent viewing of the teeth in before and after treatment images.

These images also lend themselves to the use of cosmetic imaging software. This provides a tool to show the patient the potential aesthetic result of the treatment being recommended. This should not be used to show the patient exactly what the results will be, but rather, give them an idea of what is possible.

Digital radiography (intraoral and panoramic)

Digital radiography allows the auxiliaries of the dental practice to be more productive since computerized radiographs do not require developing or mounting time. The auxiliary can become more productive by using the time saved to provide other functions. The dentist's chair time can be used more effectively as there is no waiting time. Results are immediate. Using digital radiography, the image can be obtained and processed for viewing on the computer monitor in a matter of seconds (see Fig 15-2). There is no down time waiting for the film to be prepared for viewing. In addition, if there is a problem with the radiograph, this problem is immediately discovered and another film can be taken.

There are two different types of systems: The memory phosphor plate and the sensor. The memory phosphor plate (a.k.a. PSP, photostimulable phosphor) is used in place of the film. After the x-ray, the exposed plate (sheet) is placed in a special scanner where the latent formed image is retrieved point by point and digitized, using laser light scanning. This then appears on the computer screen.

The benefits of digital radiography are as follows:

- Time saving, as results are immediate.
- Cost savings, as no film or chemicals (some digital films can be used that will need replacing when they become scratched). As digital radiography use increases in the flow of a dental practice, less film processing chemicals and film mounts are utilized. As we evaluate dental practice overhead items, this saving can be significant.
- Easy, high-quality filing and storage.

Since digital radiographs are stored in a computer and not always on hard copy, the size of the patient file is reduced since it is no longer necessary to store hard radiographic images. The radiographs are stored in the patient's computerized file, with the following benefits:

- Easy retrieval, since all radiographs can be found with the patient record.
- Digitally stored radiographs do not have any decrease in quality over time. The same quality of image can be retrieved from the computer 10 years later than was obtained the day the view was taken.
- Enhanced diagnostic capability. When working with a traditional film-based radiographic system, one can generally obtain various gray levels to view the questionable area. Once the image is obtained, there is then no way of enhancing that image to obtain a better view because it is developed and fixed as you see it. Newer technology shows many more shades of gray, can be inverted from negative to positive view, and can be enhanced with color.
- Magnification "zoom" capabilities of the radiograph units allows the view of the localized area to be enhanced. This gives better diagnosis and patient understanding. Enlargements of 100 to 300% let the clinician examine the detail necessary to make a final decision. Questions are removed when the image is viewed with this type of magnification.
- Decreased radiation exposure. With the onset of digital radiography and the variety of sophisticated intraoral sensors, one can now expect to obtain up to an 80 to 90% reduction in radiation exposure versus the exposure a patient receives from a traditional "D" speed film. This reduction in radiation directly addresses the concern that parents have had for their children as well as themselves about radiation received from dental radiography. Dental practices that have integrated digital radiography have routinely seen an increase in interest and request for use by their patient family when they know that it is available. Patients tend to tell their friends, and the existence of filmless x-ray now becomes a dental practice builder.
- Easy duplication of records. The digital system allows for emailing these radiographs to specialist colleagues for referral and opinions, exchange of radiographic information, digital storage, and compression. Multiple copies can be printed out for patient information, for those patients transferring abroad, and for insurance approval.
- Image manipulation (eg, image enhancement, subtraction radiography, and image reconstruction) and automated analysis may benefit radiodiagnosis (Parks & Williamson, 2002).
- Accuracy of information. Repeatable measurements in digital panoramic radiographs have been shown to be useful for assessing bone density (Toraman Alkurt et al, 2007).

Digital panoramic technologies have the benefit of eliminating errors associated with processing, and providing the opportunities of using digital enhancement and measuring tools. Digital panoramic radiography also ensures a decrease in radiation exposure as it requires a lower dose than conventional radiography. The image quality of digital panoramic radiographs has been researched more extensively, and the overall conclusion is that digital panoramic radiographs are of satisfactory diagnostic performance. Repeatability and reproducibility of the individual measurements for digital panoramic radiographs have been shown to be precise.

Interpreting the digital intraoral radiographic information

There are limitations to using intraoral radiographs. On radiographic images, alveolar crests are usually not anatomical, straight lines, and cementoenamel junctions are not anatomical points: these features represent projections of complex three-dimensional anatomy in two-dimensional images, with their radiographic positions depending strongly on subject-beam-receptor alignments (Hildebolt et al, 2009).

The learning curve

Anything new, especially new technology, requires a learning curve. This learning must occur before the integration of this technology into everyday practice. Dental practices that have incorporated this technology are realizing the positive effects of these and other visual technologies. In order to maximize the profitability of these tools in your dental practice, you must take advantage of daily opportunities to introduce your patients to the technology. If you are consistent, you will realize an increase in efficiency for your dental team and an increase in treatment acceptance among your patients. The learning should include practice sessions and tutorials on how to use the equipment. Practicing together as a team every day helps to integrate the technology into the dental practice so that it becomes easy to use on each patient and readily available. Each member of the dental team needs to know how to use the technology. The 10,000 hour rule can apply (Gladwell, 2009). Gladwell, in his book *The Outliers*, identifies that successful people have had 10,000 hours in their chosen field very early on and thus get 10,000 hours of practice to help them achieve excellence. The same is so for practicing with the intraoral camera so it can be used on every patient with great ease.

Templates and libraries are created to store and file images. Templates are created within the digital software. These need to be set up prior to using the software. Each template is customized directly for the dentist. For example, radiographically we have created templates for full-mouth radiographs, bite wings, periapical radiographs, and the location of where they have been taken, such as maxillary right, maxillary centrals, maxillary left, mandibular centrals, mandibular left, and mandibular right sides. As more images are stored, it is important to have excellent storage systems so that images can be retrieved easily. It is not good enough to save the files under a date without knowing which radiograph and which part of the mouth. Templates for the intraoral camera are used for each shot for easy retrieval.

CT scanning devices

Many dental practices have in-house CBCT scanners, especially those aesthetic dental practices that focus on dental implant placement. The scanners produce accurate and detailed information that allows the area to be assessed from a 3D view and in vertical and horizontal cross section. This helps to see critical anatomy such as the mandibular nerve position and the position of the maxillary sinus. Scanned images are used to monitor bone levels and quantity, infections, and fractures of teeth. These CT scans are essential in treatment planning for dental implants, orthodontics, oral surgery, temporomandibular joint diagnosis and evaluation, periodontal disease, and complex endodontic cases. The 3D images can be shown to patients to help them understand their situation.

Digital scanners: CAD/CAM technology

This technology is becoming more popular in aesthetic dentistry as it has many benefits. It can save impression time and transmission to the dental laboratory and results in a more accurate restoration. The dental surface digitization device can be defined as a device used to record the topographical characteristics of teeth (see Fig 15-4), dental impressions, or stone models by analog or digital methods for use in the CAD/CAM of dental restorative prosthetic devices (Vlaar et al, 2006).

The CAD/CAM systems consist of an optical impression system, design software, and a fabrication machine that have to perform to an accurate level (see Fig 15-3). At present these systems have undergone many versions and the manufacturers need to prove the effectiveness of the system as a whole. These systems continue to evolve and can save chairtime. Some machines scan directly to make inlays, onlays, crowns, and veneers (such as the Cerec, Sirona).

Computerized ceramic restoration fabrication

Using a 3D computer-aided modeling system (eg, Cerec, Sirona), the scanned information is recorded directly from the tooth in the mouth and sent directly to a milling machine, where the ceramic tooth is fabricated within about 20 minutes. Finishing adjustments are made and the restoration can be cemented within an hour. Teeth can thus be restored within a single visit. The cavity preparation is photographed and stored as a 3D digital model and the specifically designed software is used to prepare the ceramic restoration. The dentist then refines the model using 3D software. The information is sent to the milling machine which mills the restorations from a solid block of ceramic. When ready it is cemented into the mouth without the need for a temporary restoration.

Opportunities for daily use of technology

Initial evaluation

As you gather data on each of your new patients, lead them on a "tour" of their mouths with your intraoral photographic system, digital radiographs, and other advanced visual tools. These images will become a part of the patient's permanent record at your dental practice, and you will be able to reference them in the future.

In order to thoroughly utilize your technologically advanced tools, schedule an hour and a half for this new patient experience. The experience should include a comprehensive interview, as well as enough time to gather all the necessary data to make an appropriate diagnosis for the patient. The mindset and intention of the dental team should be to encourage your patient not to be a one-time patient, but a "forever" patient. Using technology, each new patient should walk out of your dental practice feeling that they have received the most comprehensive evaluation that they have ever received. Your treatment rooms need to be comprehensively and equally equipped (see Fig 15-1).

In gathering data during the new patient experience, your team should determine the following:

- What is the patient's current condition?
- What are the patient's goals for their oral health?

Using this information, the dentist and dental team can prepare for the consultation appointment.

Hygiene appointments

During each continuous care appointment, the hygienists should image any particular areas of concern that they detect during their time with the patient. When the dentist enters the treatment area to provide his or her examination, those areas can be easily reviewed on a screen or monitor. The patient will both see and hear about the area of concern. Since repetition is the key to learning, displaying the images will enable you to repeat the concern and discuss possible correction.

Incomplete dental plans

In today's dental practices, most dentists have a significant number of patients who are in the midst of incomplete treatment plans. This is dentistry "sitting in the charts," waiting to be completed. Previously stored images, as well as new images, offer a great opportunity for the dentist to educate the patient and reinforce the need for the next phase of treatment. Many dentists will agree that if they could increase case acceptance among current patients that have outstanding dentistry, they would see a significant increase in productivity and profitability without adding a single new patient.

Emergencies

All patients that come into your dental practice with an emergency situation should be photographed. Once the patient has seen the problem on the screen, they are more likely to proceed with the appropriate recommended treatment. At this time a quick patient "tour" of the mouth can be undertaken. Once you have shown your patient images of their overall dental condition, that patient will be more likely to accept an invitation for a comprehensive examination. This is another example of utilizing technology to turn a one-time patient into a patient for a lifetime.

Insurance

Having a visual representation of a patient's dental condition and treatment comes in handy when sorting out a patient's insurance claim. Detailed digital images give the dental insurance consultant a clear idea of the situation, and they will be able to make a better determination of benefits. Certainly, if an insurance carrier asks for further documentation, these types of visual records will prove to be beneficial for both your dental practice and your patient.

What happens so many times is that dentists just buy equipment with no real plan of how they are going to utilize it. As a dentist begins to think about the technology that they want to implement, they need to develop a plan of utilization to ensure that the system becomes a profit center for their dental

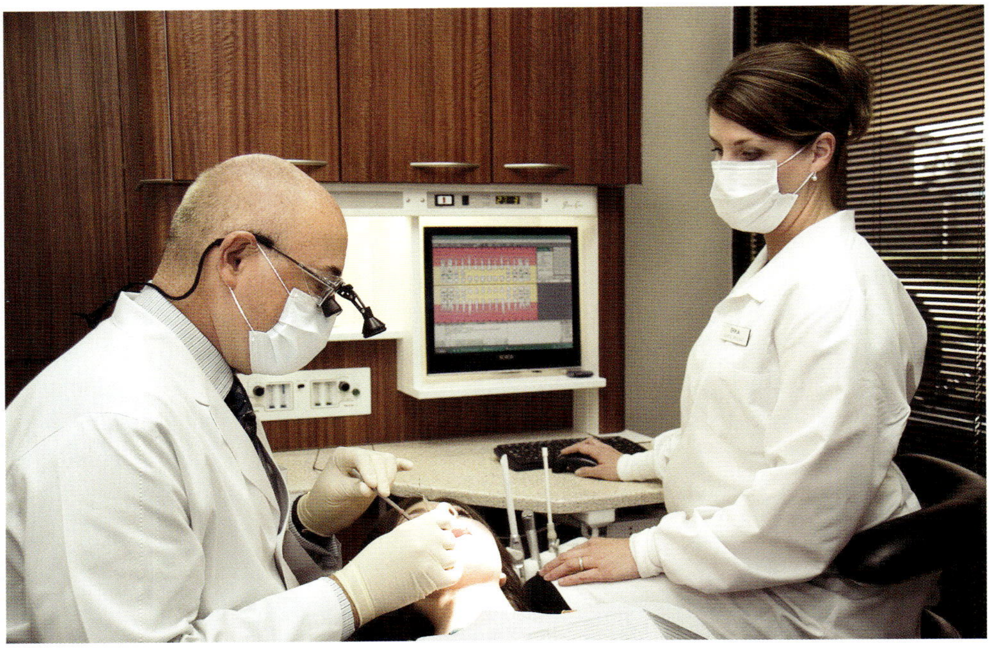

Fig 15-8 The dentist and dental team should make full use of technology.

practice. In other words, there must be a concise plan of how to utilize the system in order to maximize the use of their technology investment.

Too often, technology, such as the intraoral camera, is used sporadically within a dental practice. Many times, the technology is purchased without enough thought to training dental team members about its use or setting up a regular standard for its use with every applicable patient. The temptation is to revert to familiar data collection and diagnostic processes, leaving the new tools to collect dust in a corner. Make full use of your technology (Fig 15-8).

Dentists must develop a protocol for using technology tools on a daily basis (Appendixes 15-1 and 15-2). When aesthetic technology is used on a regular basis, it can be beneficial for all.

Dentists and dental practice administrators must provide appropriate training in the use of aesthetic technologies for the dental team. Just a single day course can be the catalyst that generates profitable and efficient use of a new piece of technology. Most of the companies that supply the technology will provide in-house training and further in-house training for advanced use of the technology.

Utilization of technological tools to increase treatment acceptance

The American Dental Association (ADA, 2004) tells us that the one of the reasons that people do not go to the dentist or do not accept dental treatment is "lack of dental education," or that they consider it "not necessary until a problem occurs." Thus, one of our greatest challenges and commissions as dental professionals is to become educators of dentistry.

Being educators means understanding various teaching methods: methods that get results. Visual learning is, by far, one of the most effective teaching strategies. Approximately 83% of a person's learning takes place visually (Kavale & Forness, 2000). Thus, the use of visual aids during treatment explanation and consultation enhances the learning process, helping people not only to see the situation that exists in their mouth, but also to begin seeing some possibilities for improvement.

The consultation appointment

Because of aesthetic technologies, the consultation appointment now becomes a primary focus in the dental practice since educational and motivational information can be easily viewed and incorporated into the presentation.

The consultation appointment in many dental practices is either unidentified or not scheduled at all. However, this special presentation may be the most important vehicle for using technology to advance the aesthetic aspect of your dental practice. For years, most dentists have offered treatment recommendations by the process of "winging it." Patients are given limited information while sitting in the exam chair. No advanced preparations are made prior to the patient's arrival. It is better to structure a meeting in a comfortable setting, complete with visual aids, all designed to encourage your patient to accept treatment (see Chapter 10).

The traditional "before and after" marketing technique can be well applied during the consultation. Digitally stored photographs of the patient, as well as images of other patients with similar conditions and the treatment results that corrected their problems, can provide powerful motivation for case acceptance (Fig 15-9). These digitally stored photographs provide evidence that your dental practice can provide the treatment that you recommend. Secure a signed release to use patient images for educational purposes. These can then be used to show actual patient cases to motivate new patients or returning hygiene patients to proceed with treatment.

Furthermore, when a patient returns for a post-treatment evaluation, final images of their now-corrected teeth can be taken and stored. If the patient had any reservations about their decision to have accepted treatment, their own before and after images can assure them that they made the right choice. The number one way new patients come into a dental practice is by personal referral. Every effort should always be made to ensure every patient is a raving fan. This post-treatment evaluation can be followed by professional portrait photos with hair and make up for the patient, and sent to the patient as a gift. This photo gift is a good marketing tool for the patient who has completed treatment and for prospective patients, as these photos can be framed and placed in the reception area of the dental practice and used for the website. Video recordings of the final patient interview, once consented and signed for, can be used for the website, social networking, and YouTube websites for further marketing of the services that are provided at the dental practice.

Dedicated aesthetic dentists undertake an extensive amount of continuing education. Many are prepared to provide sophisticated reconstructive, restorative, and cosmetic treatments. However, many of these dentists are suffering financially because of low case acceptance and referral rates. When using visual technology in an organized manner with digital storage for image retrieval, dentists and dental teams can develop a better system for

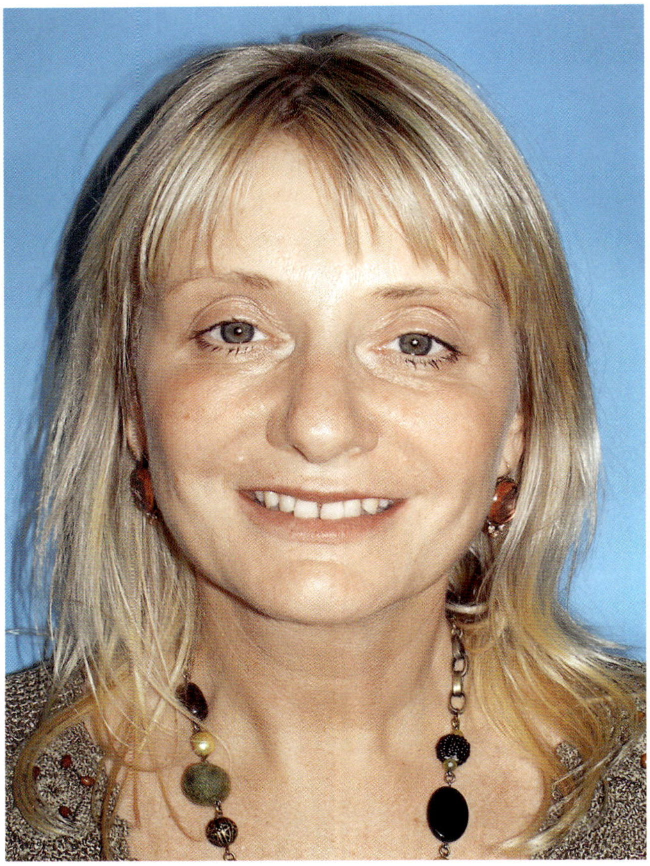

Fig 15-9a Portrait of patient before treatment.

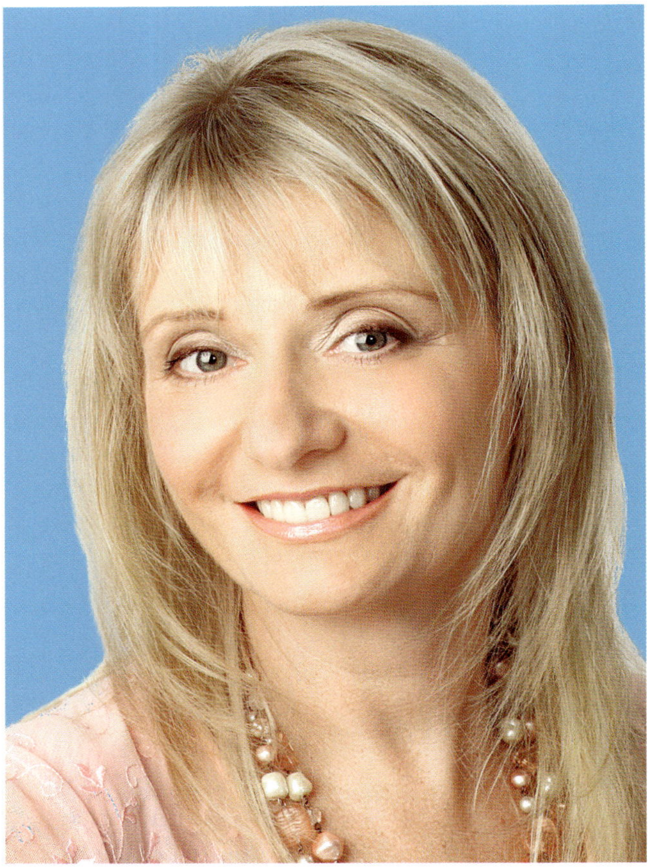

Fig 15-9b Professional photograph with makeover of patient after treatment.

case presentation. They can more effectively educate the patient concerning:

- the patient's current dental health
- available treatment options
- treatment benefits
- the consequences of delaying treatment.

People buy what they want long before they buy what they need (Hopkins, 2001). Many patients floating in and out of your dental practice have diagnosed treatment but incomplete treatment plans. They have not bought into the value of your treatment recommendations largely because they are trying to imagine their existing conditions and treatment opportunities rather than seeing their own dental condition for themselves.

Referral rates in dental practices that use dental photography appropriately in a well-structured program also see significant increase because the patient now recognizes this dental practice as state of the art in providing aesthetic dentistry. Patients are more likely to accept treatment and refer others, and they will also desire a long-term relationship since they perceive that the total experience is of higher quality.

Never before in the history of dentistry has the face of our profession changed as rapidly as it is changing today. Advancements in restorative materials and techniques (Donovan & Heymann, 2011), infection control, diagnostic aids, and treatment planning have created dental practices that are accelerating into arenas not thought of in past years. In these accelerating dental practices, photographic technology is becoming a more important component. The sophisticated treatment options available are of little use without an advanced dental team that is well trained, and helps to instill in the patient a desire for treatment and long-term care because of the data accumulated with these sophisticated dental technological aids.

Suggested clinical applications for digital radiography in areas of the dental practice

Prevention

With the sensor placed at the proper angulation, bitewing exposures can be taken for caries detection interdentally, just as traditional film bitewings are utilized. The problem of root caries detection is better determined by the adjustment capabilities of the software to determine density differences in questionable areas.

Pathology and trauma

Immediate retrieval of data concerning lesions such as abscesses, cysts, and granulomas can be obtained for viewing and evaluation. Questionable locations of bone and root fractures can also be evaluated instantly for consultation with the patient about treatment options.

Endodontics

The multiple image display allows one to follow the stages of root canal therapy step by step. The zoom feature gives a clear view of the apex of the root during each of the utilized steps. The time saved during this process when multiple radiographs had previously been waited upon to develop during treatment is a real benefit in this area of practice.

Oral surgery

Root tip fracture during tooth extraction has always been a difficult problem. With digital radiography, the position and angulation of the fractured tip can be instantly viewed during the procedure.

Implantology

Instant review of implant location during placement can be achieved with digital radiography. Bone healing and density associated with the implant can also be reviewed frequently without the concern of exposing the patient to excessive radiation, as can seating of the impression coping, metal work try-in, and final fit of the implant restoration.

Fixed prosthetics

When post-and-core buildup for crown construction is necessary in endodontically treated teeth, digital radiography gives one an immediate view of the post position in the canal prior to placement or cementation. All crowns and fixed partial dentures can have margins checked prior to cementation or bonding into position to help prevent placement with open margins.

Operative or restorative dentistry

All inlays and onlays, either metal, porcelain, or resin composite, can have their margins viewed prior to placement to prevent open margins. Silver amalgam and direct resin composite restorations can have margins examined for voids or flash prior to appointment completion and patient dismissal. The digital radiography exposure does not negatively affect chair time.

Aesthetics

Digital radiography can be used to check seating margins on veneers.

Action steps

1. Take an inventory of current technology in the dental practice. Determine if the technology is of a current generation, if all upgrades have been purchased, and if each piece of technology integrates with other necessary pieces of technology, including your practice management software.
2. Determine what additional technology you believe would support your vision and your goals of building the aesthetic aspect of your dental practice.
3. Develop a plan of action for each type of patient visit to make sure that appropriate technology is an integral part of that appointment. For example, make sure that photographs are taken as described throughout this book, stored, and retrieved when appropriate.
4. Purchase and participate in continuous education on the use of your technology so that you are maximizing its potential for improved diagnosis, treatment planning, and patient education.
5. Use visual aids during your consultations, remembering that approximately 83% of learning takes place visually (Kavale & Forness, 2000).
6. Consider further training in Digital Case Presentation (DCP) © (Appendixes 10-1 and 10-2) and Microsoft PowerPoint software for the presentation of your recommendations.

References

1. American Dental Association. Survey Center, Public Opinion Surveys. 2003 Public Opinion Survey Oral Health of the US Population. Chicago, IL: American Dental Association, 2004.
2. Donovan T, Heymann H. Perspectives. Tincture of time: a vital ingredient for dental success. J Esthet Restorative Dent 2011;23:133–135.
3. Gladwell M. The Outliers: Study of success. London: Penguin Books, 2009.
4. Hildebolt CF, Couture R, Garcia NM, Dixon D, Shannon WD, Langenwalter E, Civitelli R. Alveolar bone measurement precision for phosphor-plate images. Oral Surg Oral Med Oral Pathol Oral Radiol Endod 2009;108(3):e96–107.

5. Hopkins T. Selling. New York, NY: Hungry Minds Press, 2001.
6. Kavale K, Forness S. Auditory and visual perception processes and reading ability: a quantitative reanalysis and historical reinterpretation. Learning Disability Quarterly 2000;23.
7. Naisbitt J. High Tech. High Touch. New York, NY: Broadway Books, 1999.
8. Parks ET, Williamson GF. Digital radiography: an overview. J Contemp Dent Pract 2002;3(4):23–39.
9. Rout J, Brown J. Ionizing Radiation Regulations and the Dental Practitioner: 1. The Nature of Ionizing Radiation and Its Use in Dentistry. Dental Update 2012;39(3):191–203.
10. Toraman Alkurt M, Peker I, Sanal Ö. Assessment of repeatability and reproducibility of mental and panoramic mandibular indices on digital panoramic images. Int Dent J 2007;57:433–438.
11. Vlaar ST, van der Zel JM. Accuracy of dental digitizers. Int Dent J 2006;56:301–309.

Further reading

Faculty of General Dental Practitioners. Selection Criteria for Dental Radiography: a publication for the Faculty of General Dental Practitioners. 2nd edition. London: FGDP(UK), 2004.

Appendix 15-1

Checklist for intraoral camera views

Intraoral camera views can be set up as templates on the software so that they file and save directly into these formats. Views that should be recorded are detailed below.

Initial consultation

1. Patient's extraoral smile anterior view and both lateral views.
2. Mouth open, showing the entire mandibular arch.
3. Maxillary arch.
4. Maxillary right quadrant.
5. Maxillary left quadrant.
6. Mandibular left quadrant.
7. Mandibular right quadrant.
8. Mandibular lingual incisors.
9. Maxillary palatal incisors.
10. Incisal view of maxillary and mandibular anteriors looking at wear, bruxism, and eccentric anterior excursions.
11. Views of each individual posterior tooth from different sides; occlusal is essential.
12. Views of each existing restoration in the mouth. Multiple views of old amalgam restorations looking at restoration integrity and existing leakage, secondary caries, fractures, and chipping. Views of existing resin composite restorations looking for air bubbles, marginal integrity, contact points, and surface areas.
13. Areas of concern such a fractures, recession, carious lesions, fistulas, tooth wear from acid erosion, attrition, open crown margins, and porcelain wear or damage.
14. Soft tissue areas such as white lesions.
15. Lesions on the tongue, white or red.
16. Periodontal problems.

During treatment

1. Restoration replacement.
2. Prior to commencing restorative treatment: treatment to be done on that appointment.
3. Record the restoration to be replaced.
4. Once the restoration has been removed to show what is underneath.
5. Once all carious lesions have been removed to check that all caries removed as well as all existing amalgam.
6. Any existing cracks underneath the old restoration, exposure or other problems.
7. Once new restoration has been placed.
8. Before and after records can be saved on one file.

What's next?

1. What treatment will be needed at the next appointment, giving the patient a reason to return to complete the rest of the treatment.

2. Hygiene treatment: periodontal swelling, bleeding, inflammation, and stains on the teeth.

After treatment

Patient is shown pictures of how teeth looked before treatment and then after treatment so they can justify their investment and see how beautiful the teeth look with a natural tooth color restoration. This makes the restoration become invisible and return to good health.

Appendix 15-2

Checklist for intraoral digital radiographs

1. Radiology safety: machine testing, services, log and quality assurance, registration.
2. Beam aiming devices and accuracy, quality of the result.
3. Staff training.
4. Radiological prescription for exposure.
5. Filing of radiographs in the computerized system.
6. Templates and libraries created for storing radiographs within each patient's computerized record.
7. Interpretation with patients detailed knowledge.

16 Continuing Education

Cathy Jameson and Linda Greenwall

> *The fact is that your current level of knowledge and skill is becoming obsolete at a faster rate today than ever before. Your earning ability can be an appreciating or a depreciating asset, depending upon whether or not you are upgrading it or simply allowing it to become obsolete. This is a choice you are making, or failing to make every day.*
> *Brian Tracy (2010)*

There is no such thing as status quo. You are either choosing to go up or you are choosing to go down. If you become complacent, thinking that things are going just fine and that you do not need to do anything to improve, you are incorrect. While you are standing still, the rest of the world is passing you by. The world and everything in it, including you and your business, are constantly moving.

Since all things are in a constant state of movement and since you have the ability to make choices, why not make a choice to move forward, upward, and ahead. The choice is yours. Dr William James (1975) of Harvard University said that "The greatest evolution of my generation is the discovery that individuals, by changing their inner attitudes of mind, can change the outer aspects of their lives."

Yes, you have the ability to choose and to develop your life in a manner desired. The choice begins in your own mind. Your actions will immediately go to work to bring the major thought processes of your mind into a state of reality.

You have made a choice to build the aesthetic aspect of your dental practice. You want to make a difference in people's lives by enhancing their appearance and self image. You have talent and the education to support your goal. You have made the excellent decision to elevate yourself and your dental practice to the next level. There are places to go, heights to climb, areas of expertise to develop. The vehicle for your development is continuous education.

"It takes a great deal of study to be really good at aesthetics. A doctor [dentist] must be willing to spend the money and invest the time to take courses. He/she must always be a student seeking new skills in order to provide the very best care and achieve outstanding results for patients. Equally important is that the doctor [dentist] must be willing to invest money and time to provide appropriate skill development for team members in order to maintain their interest and knowledge. You can never learn too much!"

Dr Ken Hamlett (interview)

The path of continuous learning and continuous improvement can be not only enriching but also fun. W Edward Deming said, "Improve constantly and forever every process for planning, production and service" (Deming, 1994). Deming's operative words are "constantly and forever." No matter how much you may know or how well you are doing at the present time, learning should be "constant and forever."

When you make a choice to learn a new skill, whether a clinical, communicative, management, technological, or marketing skill, you may feel apprehensive or even afraid. You will be placing yourself in a mode of change. Change is not easy. It is, however, through the process of effective change that progress is made. Effective change takes place when all members of the team "buy into" the change and the reason behind it. The team that learns together grows together.

Peter Senge uses the term "team learning" to describe the process of continuous learning and development for both the individuals within an organization and for the organization itself. Senge says, "When teams are truly learning, not only are they producing extraordinary results, but the individual members are growing more rapidly than could have occurred otherwise" (Senge, 2006) (Fig 16-1).

Learning new and better ways makes good sense both personally and professionally. So why is change sabotaged in organizations? There are many reasons. Some of the reasons for resistance to change may be as follows:

- People may have tried something in the past without success, so they may think that the way things are being done at the present time is the best and only way.
- The leaders have not prepared the team members for the upcoming change and because team members have not been involved in the decision making process, they may resist.
- Team members may have become so engulfed in the "way things have always been here" that they become unwilling to step out of their comfort zone and try anything that is different. They may think that the status quo is "good enough." People may have drifted into complacency.
- A negative image or a lack of confidence may cause team members to question whether or not they can do something new and do it well. They

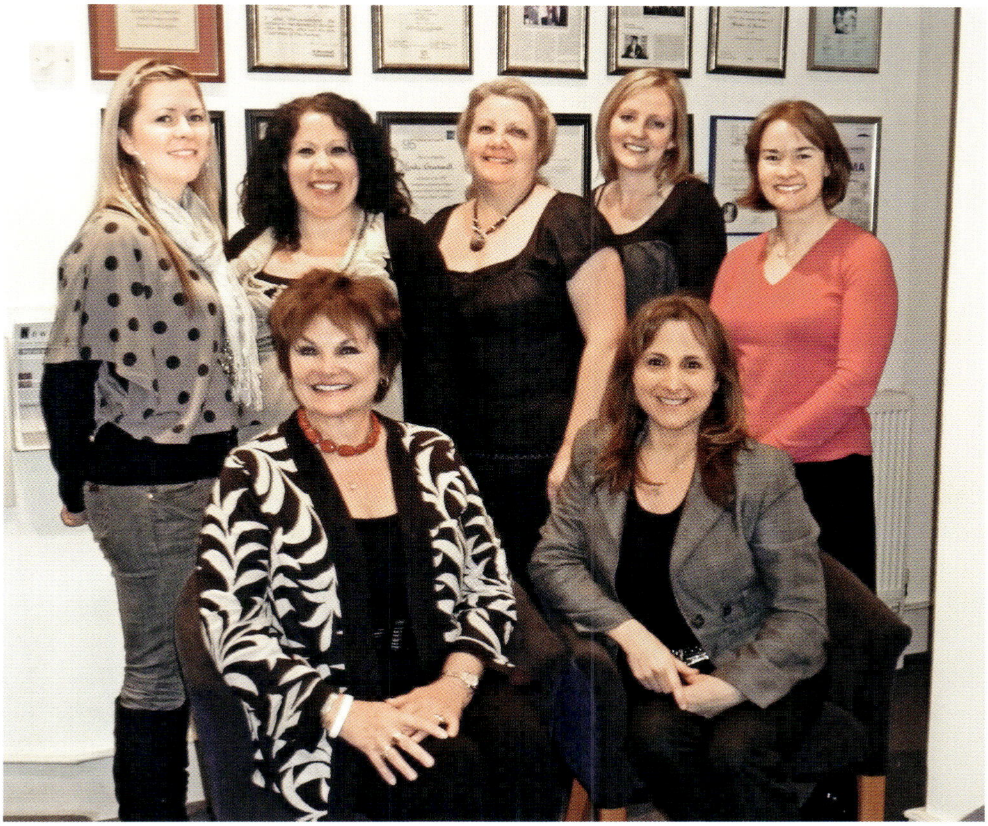

Fig 16-1 Dr Cathy Jameson teaching Dr Linda Greenwall's team.

may fear possible reprimand if they make a mistake. Leaders must be careful to support team members during any phase of change. While there may be mistakes, learning from mistakes can lead to improvement on the other side.

- Team members may "sabotage" progress by challenging a new idea before it has had a chance to incubate. They may negate the idea rather than take any responsibility for the risk that goes along with any new idea, skill or process.
- People may resist trying new ideas because they think it will take more work and effort on their part and they do not want to add anything to their job.

Integrate the following principles of change management:

- Be diligent in explaining why the new idea or system is desirable and how each person's role is imperative.
- Have a carefully constructed plan of action outlining what will be done, how it will be done, who will do what, and why (see Chapter 2).
- Always present new ideas in terms of how the change will benefit team members, the dental practice, and patients. Remember, behavior is driven by "what's in this for me" (LeBoeuf, 1985).
- Ask permission before you place additional responsibilities on someone's plate. Consider taking something off of their plate that is less productive.

- Gain support through a carefully developed coalition of team members working together toward the common goal (Jameson, 2010).

The basic principles of adult learning

In order for you and your team members to learn and to become competent in the new skills required for an aesthetic practice, incorporate the principles of adult learning into your continuing education program. Whether continuing education takes place in or out of the office, by following the basic principles of adult learning, your educational goals will become reachable. By making diligent efforts to incorporate new information and skills, you will find that you make steady progress.

Here are the steps of adult learning. These steps are applicable to any learning situation you encounter and embrace.

- Teach the system exactly as you wish it to be administered. Don't assume that anyone knows anything about the system. Take the time to go through each system intricately. You could do this at team meetings or, in some instances, one-on-one training by an instructor or coach may be best.
- Demonstrate how to perform the skills. Let others see or hear you performing the tasks. Do this both with and without patients.
- Have the trainee recap for the trainer what she thinks needs to be done, including how and why each step within the system is important and how it impacts other systems. Then have her perform the task with the trainer present but without patients.
- Have the trainer or mentor "shadow" the trainee as she is performing the task with patients.
- Evaluate the performance and give appropriate feedback in terms of what is working well and what needs adjustment or improvement. People want and need feedback. Feedback is motivational whether it addresses needed improvement or acknowledges progress.
- As systems change and evolve, make sure that these changes are reviewed with the entire team. Cross train any time there is a change in any system or procedure.

Dr Charles Puntillo believes in ongoing development and knows that he and his team, as well as his dental practice will never be perfect. His team constantly strives for excellence in all that they do. They believe that being on a continuous path of improvement is a good and productive path.

▶ *"I have an ongoing relationship with Jameson Management, Inc. They put us on the right track as we went through all of the systems to get them into ideal order. We have found that having a coach keeps us moving forward and gives new team members the guidance and preparation necessary for them to become productive quickly. We try to train them, but have found it more effective to have someone from outside the practice do the coaching."*

"In addition, we wanted to increase productivity and revenue every year and we do. The coaches see the little things that can add up to make a big difference. We get engulfed in the day to day activity and sometimes don't

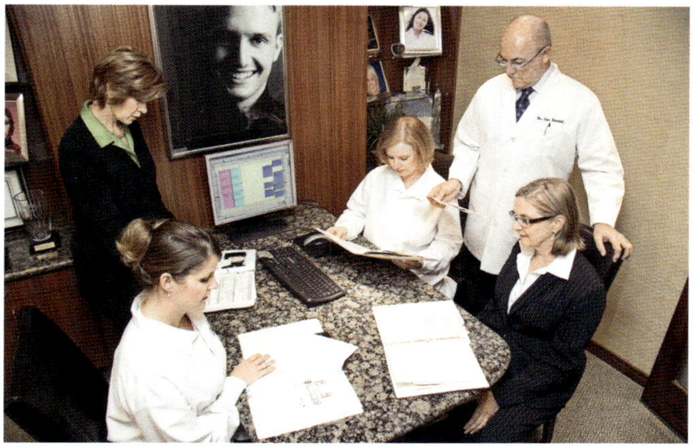

Fig 16-2a Dr Ken Hamlett's team cross-training.

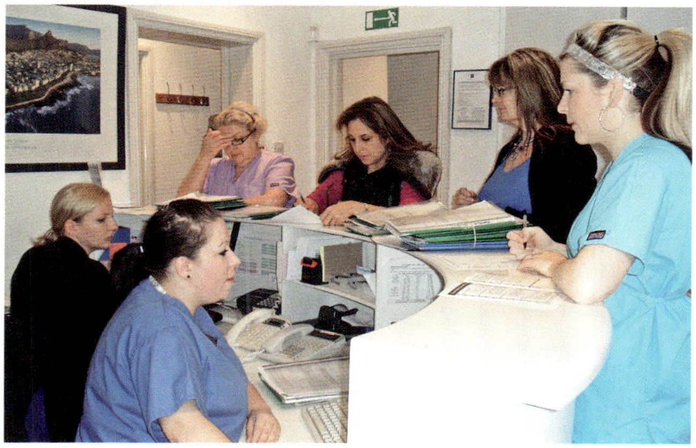

Fig 16-2b Dr Linda Greenwall's team cross-training.

see those fine aspects of the practice that they see. They make appropriate adjustments and the numbers go up proportionately. We continue to increase the production of the practice year after year. Continuing education through seminars, hands-on training and support of my coaches make that possible."

Dr Charles Puntillo (interview)

Dr John Jameson believes that the level and quality of dentistry goes up a notch each time a dentist takes an intense "hands-on" course. While lecture courses provide great insight and much can be learned in that situation, hands-on courses build confidence and capability.

Dr Jameson encourages doctors to have a program of continuing education in their dental practice. He incorporated the concept of a corporate university into his own dental practice. He recommends inviting representatives from supply companies, laboratories, technology companies, computer trainers, consultants, etc. to provide in-office skill development.

▶ *"Don't bother buying a piece of equipment, for example, if you do not intend to take full advantage of training and development. And don't think that one training session is enough. As the skill of your team advances, let the trainers help you go to the next level. Most practices use their technology, their computers, and many products to a minor degree. If you buy something, make a decision to invest in an ongoing development program. The time and money invested will be miniscule compared to the related increased productivity. You enhance your ability to diagnose, treatment plan, and educate with technology, photography, and systems that provide support."*

Dr John Jameson (interview)

Cross-training

An essential type of continuous education in your dental practice is constant cross-training (Fig 16-2). Everyone and everything in your organization needs to be duplicated. In that manner, your dental practice cannot be at risk if someone is unavailable. You do not want to stop progress because no one can carry out the necessary tasks that keep you on course. Plus, there is drastic danger if only one person knows the "ins and outs" of a system. What would you do if someone became unavailable or ill but no one else on the team knew what they did, how they did it, and where things were located? This includes your computer system.

It is important and efficient to have a specific person on the team "ultimately responsible" for each system. However, everyone on the team needs to understand how each system is set up, how it works, and how to administer that system. In addition, having intricately detailed descriptions of each system in your operation manual is mandatory. If you do not have an operations manual that details each system, including the expected end results, then this would be an excellent goal to set for yourself. In addition, this manual becomes an effective part of your new employee training manual. How can someone perform well if they are not clear about what to do, how to do it, and the expectations of their performance?

> *"We have written very specific job descriptions and expect each team member to become an expert in her responsibilities. We insist on continuing education and goal setting. Working well as a team takes a long time and a lot of hard work so we don't want a staff member leaving because they don't feel appreciated or feel they are in a dead end job. We want them to feel invested in the practice and respected for the professionals they are."*
>
> *Cindy Butler (interview), Business Administrator and Treatment Coordinator for Dr Charles Puntillo*

Identify who will be the immediate "back-up" should the need occur. For example: You may have a specific person who is "ultimately responsible" for making financial arrangements and for collecting fees. However, you need to make sure that another person can carry out those tasks. If you have one financial coordinator and she is out for some reason, the last thing you want is for the other team members to say to a patient, "Oh, Sherry is out today. I will just have her send you a statement when she gets back." That could lead to accounts receivable nightmares. Plan for the difficult situations to limit damage control.

As you are planning for your "damage control," outline carefully how the dental practice needs to respond if there is an absence of one of the providers—the dentist or hygienist. Having such a plan of action in place will provide a guideline for people to follow, as well as stress relief to everyone. Even if you have more than one dentist or hygienist, a plan of action regarding patient care, maintenance of the required level of productivity, and how to access temporary caregivers is a valuable part of your cross-training, your business plan, and your security.

Think of cross-training as business insurance. Everyone buys insurance but always hopes that it isn't needed. That doesn't stop us from making the

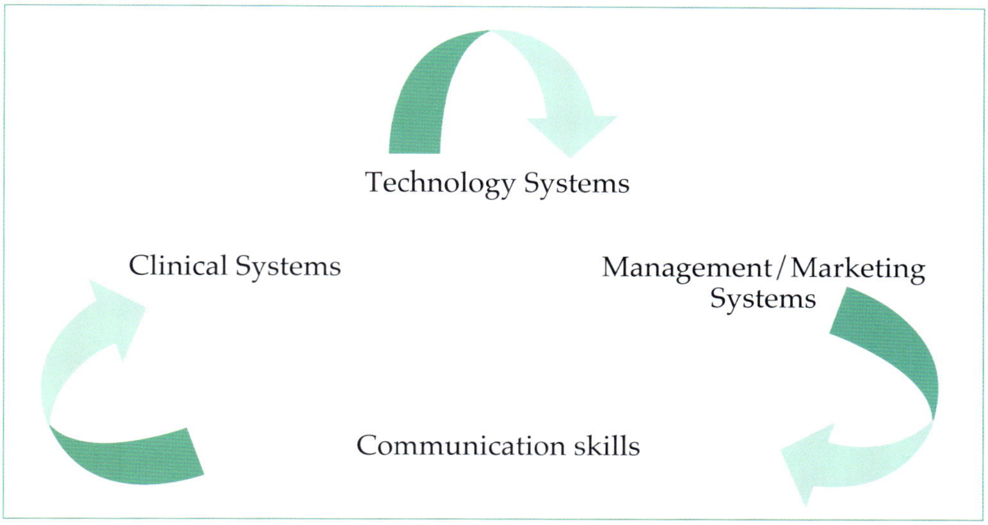

Fig 16-3 The circle of dental practice life.

wise investment in various types of insurance. Do the same thing with your dental practice. Invest time and effort into insuring the safety of your dental practice should someone be unavailable for any reason.

Options in continuing education

There are numerous ways in which learning can be accessed. As you develop your own plan for a corporate university, make sure to determine your goals, write out your strategic plan including how much money you are going to budget for continuing education. Make sure that the plan of continuing education includes a range of education that supports all members of the team. Even when the dentist goes to a clinical course, take the team members as well. The team members will be better able to support new clinical approaches if they are familiar with the method and technique, as well as the expected results of the new procedure. Balance your educational experiences to include clinical, technological, marketing and management, and communication. The circle of life in your dental practice includes all of these elements (Fig 16-3).

There are numerous options for continuing education that are available to you. These range from the traditional to the non-traditional. Here are a few modalities for continuing education:

- Seminars, lectures, workshops. These are available at dental conferences and conventions or can be offered by corporations, laboratories, or other supportive organizations and companies, such as manufacturers and suppliers, and by individuals. When you decide to go to a conference or convention where multiple courses are offered, study the program prior to going to the event. Decide who is going to attend which courses. For some courses, you will want the entire team in attendance. For other courses, you may wish to split up. Either way, schedule a team meeting soon after the conference and have different people on the team give a report of the course or courses they attended. Select activities from the courses that you wish to implement. Even if you gain one idea, that single concept can provide measurable improvement. Using the goal accomplishment worksheet

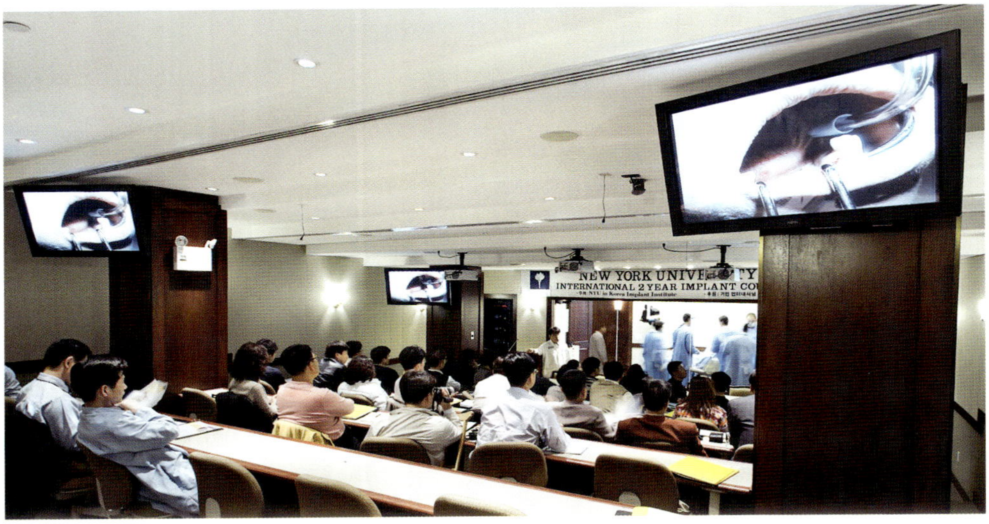

Fig 16-4 Dr Larry Rosenthal teaches at New York University College of Dentistry, New York.
Dr Rosenthal is the founder of Aesthetic Advantage, a hands-on course in aesthetics.

(Fig 2-5), outline a course of action by which you can integrate any new ideas into the dental practice. Then, evaluate your progress to make sure that you don't just attend another course only to do nothing with the information.

- Study clubs. These can either offer a variety of courses throughout a year or may offer a series of courses that focus on one specific topic, such as aesthetics.
- Courses offered by dental schools. The continuing education departments of many dental schools are extensive, cutting edge, and certified (Fig 16-4). These courses range from lectures and workshops to elaborate hands-on courses. Many of these are transmitted in real time to countries throughout the world.
- Webinars (eg, http://jamesonmanagement.com/webinars/).
- Home study. The materials for certain courses are offered through companies, organizations, and universities. Oftentimes testing is provided that goes along with such courses and continuing education credit is offered. Many of these courses can be found on the internet. Go to the websites of companies, organizations, or universities that promote the kind of information and study you desire. Courses may be available.
- Postgraduate institutes are available in most countries where advanced training through lecture, seminar, workshop, and hands-on training can be accessed (Fig 16-5). These institutes often host some of the most outstanding individuals in a particular field: aesthetics, implants, management, marketing, etc.
- On-line training is available now through various organizations. Learning and education will become more and more digital over time.
- Lunch and learn sessions given by the dentist or various team members. Share your own knowledge with your team. When a person presents material, they learn it even more powerfully. These presentations also build the confidence of team members and this translates to greater confidence with patients.
- In-office coaching: clinical, technological, marketing, and management.

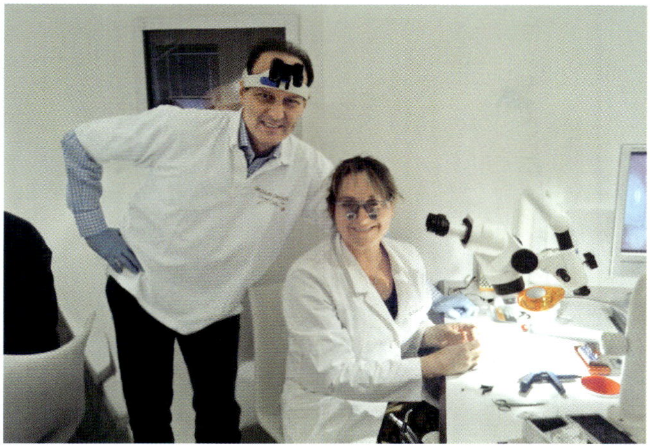

Fig 16-5 Dr Greenwall attending a hands-on workshop by Dr Didier Dietschi, Geneva.

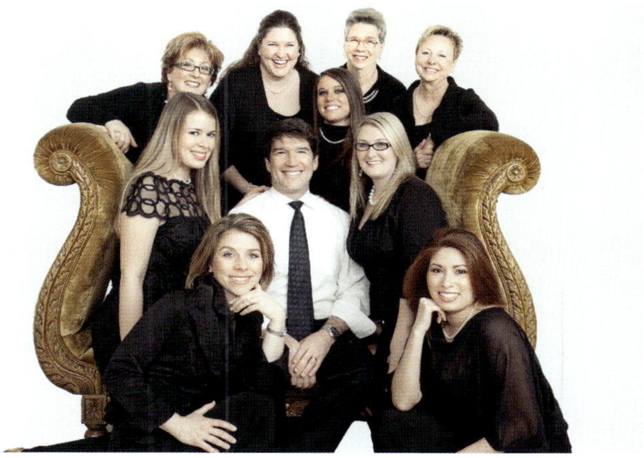

Fig 16-6 Dr Mark Hyman's team constantly pursues continuing education.

Dr Mark Hyman is a committed student himself but teaches thousands of dental professionals every year as a speaker in the dental industry.

▶ *"Continuing education is a given with any highly successful doctor and team. Our team sets a goal of 100 hours of continuing education a year for continuous improvement. We read books, have monthly 'lunch and learns', attend state and national meetings and have in-office coaching by Jameson Management, Inc. We love to learn and have fun doing it. If we are truly going to grow each year, continuing education must be a part of that growth."*

Dr Mark Hyman (interview) (Fig 16-6)

Continuing education in aesthetic dentistry

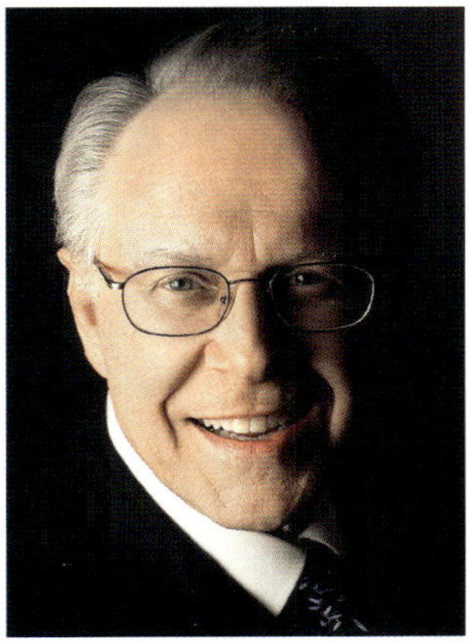

Dr Ron Goldstein

Stage 1

- Decide what interests you the most in dentistry.
- Focus on those areas. Continue learning in this field.
- Develop a passion for excellence.
- Takes everyone's course. Read all the surrounding literature.
- Determine who knows more and learn from them.
- Learn what you don't know.
- You continue learning until you become an authority in aesthetic dentistry and know more than most of your colleagues.
- Teach others.

Stage 2

- Find or develop the expertise in the aesthetic area and develop clinical expertise.

- Gain clinical experience though hands-on courses and within the dental practice.
- Practice these techniques again and again to get more experienced.

Stage 3

- Get a good intraoral camera and use it every day on every patient.
- Document every case success and failures. You learn more from failures.
- Continue learning throughout your dental career.

In summary

Be a lifelong learner. There is such excitement and renewed energy when knowledge becomes a welcomed part of your dental practice. Make the choice to commit to a life of continuous learning and education. Obviously, you have chosen to make a commitment to on-going development. Thus, you are reading this book and will be integrating the many strategies recommended into your dental practice.

From our own experience as dental educators, we see the confidence that evolves as dentists and teams expand their competencies in aesthetic dentistry. Continuing education is a vehicle for people to stretch, to grow, and to tap into their reserve of potential. Your decision to develop the aesthetic aspect of your dental practice is a good decision. Continuing education will be an ongoing part of your development. Who knows? One day you may be teaching others about your success in aesthetic dentistry.

Action steps

1. Review the goals you want to accomplish by building the aesthetic aspect of your dental practice, including your plan of action as to how you will accomplish those goals.
2. Create a strategic plan for continuing education that supports the goals and the plan of action that you have written.
3. Establish a budget that will be invested in continuing education for you and your team.
4. Explore the various kinds of continuing education and determine which type or types of continuing education would work best for you. Then, investigate who provides courses that are suited to your goals.
5. Designate a person on the team to gather information related to the various educational entities. Look for curriculum, costs, locations, time allotments, and expected end results.
6. Outline the entire year (or longer) and reserve dates on your calendar for the courses you choose.
7. Then, make the decision. Go for it. Know that when you work diligently to do the things you are being taught that your investment in time and money will come back to you quickly and multifold.

References

1. Deming WE. Out of the Crisis. Cambridge, MA: MIT Press, 1986.
2. James W. The Works of William James. Cambridge, MA: Harvard University Press, 1975.
3. Jameson C. The Impact of Training in Transformational Leadership on the Productivity of a Dental Practice. Minneapolis, MN: Walden University, 2010.
4. LeBoeuf M. GMP: The Greatest Management Principle in the World. New York, NY: Penguin Group, 1985.
5. Senge P. The Fifth Discipline. New York, NY: Doubleday, 2006.
6. Tracy B. Goals: How to Get Everything You Want—Faster Than You Ever Thought Possible. San Francisco, CA: Berrett-Koehler Publishers Inc, 2010.

17 In Conclusion

Cathy Jameson and Linda Greenwall

> *Never underestimate the power of the mind to disempower. Another rule: Never underestimate the power of clever people to help others to see the possibilities, to help generate a feeling of faith, and to change behavior.*
>
> *Kotter and Cohen (2002)*

Why aesthetics?

There are, of course, many reasons why aesthetic dentistry is of interest to you, the provider. Here are a few of the reasons.

- You love the challenge of performing the advanced techniques that are mandatory with aesthetic dentistry. You have achieved a high level of competence and find that these highly intricate procedures and challenging cases continue to stimulate your interest.
- You find it fulfilling to enhance a person's life by improving their appearance and self esteem.
- You are an artist as well as a scientist and want to maximize your aesthetic talents.
- You like having patients who are joyful when they come to the office and who are happy to climb into your chair. With aesthetic dentistry complaints are not the norm, compliments are the norm.
- The aesthetic cases generate significant revenue and bring financial health to your dental practice, to you, and to your team members.

All of these are excellent and valid reasons to increase the aesthetic aspect of your dental practice, and, of course, there are other reasons that are unique to you.

As you get ready to lead your team toward a prosperous, aesthetically oriented dental practice, lay the groundwork for the changes and development that must take place. Prepare your team for change by communicating your commitment to your vision in action and attitude. The focused energy of your team will be the fuel that drives each and every one of your projects. Thus, the end of this book reflects the beginning of this book. Clarify your vision and lead your team to incorporate success strategies that will bring that vision into a state of reality.

Success strategies in aesthetic dentistry

Dr Jill Wade, private practitioner, Frisco, Texas

Dr Jill Wade outlines the following factors that she considers essential for her success in her aesthetically focused dental practice.

- Setting and working toward the achievement of goals
- An excellent team
- A high level of technology
- Zest for continuing education
- Epitomizing "the business bounce factor": going above and beyond what is expected during each patient experience
- Being willing to change quickly when the environment or the economics of the times require
- Always practice dentistry, run the business, and live life with integrity.

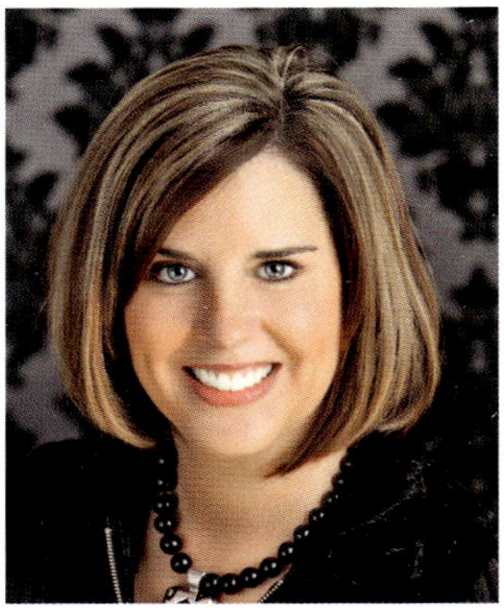

Practitioners, just like you, have made a conscientious decision to build the aesthetic aspect of their dental practice, have worked with commitment to make that happen, and are reaping the rewards of work well done. They find joy and fulfillment in their work and look forward to going to the dental practice. There is no reason not to have the dental practice of your dreams. This book has been all about defining and creating your "ideal" dental practice. From the beginning and throughout each chapter you have been given the step-by-step processes that have been incorporated by successful dental practices. You can do the same thing. You have been introduced to dental practices from different countries and different states in the USA. These practices thrive in both metropolitan and in rural areas. Thriving is not dependent on where you are. Thriving depends on your own mind set and on your own commitment.

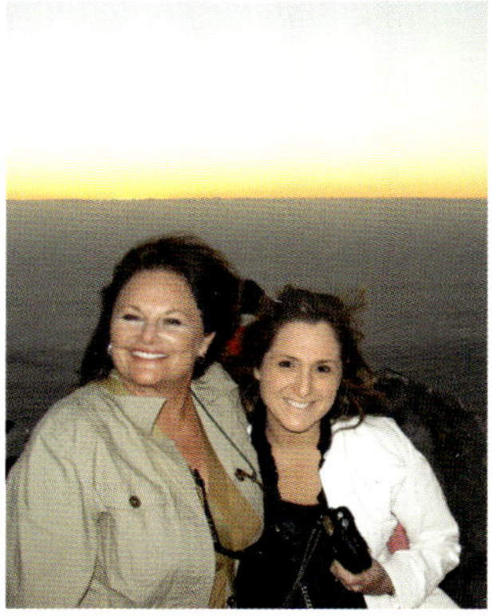

Fig 17-1 Drs Cathy Jameson and Linda Greenwall in Cape Town, South Africa.

Get your mind set. Confidence will lead you on.

Reference

1. Kotter J, Cohen D. The Heart of Change. Boston, MA: Harvard School Press, 2002.

Index

Q

R